# Atlas of
# HISTOPATHOLOGY

# Atlas of
# HISTOPATHOLOGY

**Ivan Damjanov** MD, PhD

Professor of Pathology
Department of Pathology and Laboratory Medicine
The University of Kansas School of Medicine
Kansas City, Kansas, USA

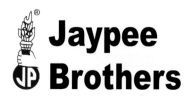

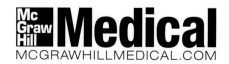

© 2012, Jaypee Brothers Medical Publishers

First published in India in 2011 by

 **Jaypee Brothers Medical Publishers (P) Ltd.**

*Corporate Office*
4838/24 Ansari Road, Daryaganj, **New Delhi** - 110002, India, +91-11-43574357
*Registered Office*
B-3 EMCA House, 23/23B Ansari Road, Daryaganj, **New Delhi** 110 002, India
Phones: +91-11-23272143, +91-11-23272703, +91-11-23282021,
+91-11-23245672, Rel: +91-11-32558559 Fax: +91-11-23276490, +91-11-23245683
e-mail: jaypee@jaypeebrothers.com, Website: www.jaypeebrothers.com

First published in USA by The McGraw-Hill Companies, 2 Penn Plaza, New York, NY 10121.
Exclusively worldwide distributor except South Asia (India, Nepal, Sri Lanka, Bhutan, Pakistan, Bangladesh,
Malaysia).

ISBN-13: 978-0-07-179712-2

ISBN-10: 0-07-179712-2

*Printed at* Replika Press Pvt. Ltd.

*This Atlas is dedicated to*
*our students and residents*

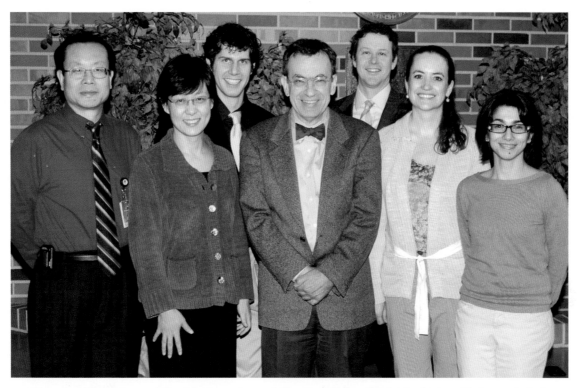

*The Authors from The University of Kansas School of Medicine (left to right):*
**Da Zhang, Fang Fan, Paul St. Romain, Ivan Damjanov,**
**Garth Fraga, Maura O'Neil, and Rashna Madan**

# Contributors

**Ivan Damjanov** MD, PhD
Professor of Pathology
The University of Kansas School of Medicine
Kansas City, Kansas, USA

**Katie L Dennis** MD
Assistant Professor of Pathology
The University of Kansas School of Medicine
Kansas City, Kansas, USA

**Fang Fan** MD, PhD
Associate Professor of Pathology
The University of Kansas School of Medicine
Kansas City, Kansas, USA

**Garth Fraga** MD
Assistant Professor of Pathology
The University of Kansas School of Medicine
Kansas City, Kansas, USA

**Rashna Madan** MD
Assistant Professor of Pathology
The University of Kansas School of Medicine
Kansas City, Kansas, USA

**Maura O'Neil** MD
Assistant Professor of Pathology
The University of Kansas School of Medicine
Kansas City, Kansas, USA

**Paul St. Romain** BA
Post-Sophomore Fellow in Pathology
The University of Kansas School of Medicine
Kansas City, Kansas, USA

**Da Zhang** MD
Associate Professor of Pathology
The University of Kansas School of Medicine
Kansas City, Kansas, USA

# *Preface*

Pathology as a medical discipline has been one of the cornerstones of medical education since the beginnings of the modern era of scientific medicine in the 19th century. The teaching of pathology has nevertheless changed considerably during that time and the emphasis has recently shifted from descriptive anatomic pathology to more dynamic aspects of this science such as pathophysiology. New vistas have been opened, like those made possible by molecular biology. These new trends have irrevocably altered our perspective not only of pathology but of medicine in general. The need to keep pace with the newest developments on the research front has also changed our approach to teaching of new generations of doctors as well.

Due to the constraints of time imposed by a hectic schedule of lectures, seminars, laboratory sessions and interim examinations, modern medical students spend less time at the autopsy table and medical museum and more time at the computer and interactive teaching sessions designed for the most efficient didactic impact. Histopathology, traditionally taught during the preclinical years with the use of optical microscopes, has been one of the "casualties" of modern medical school restructured curricula. The teaching of histopathology has been dramatically reduced in most US medical schools and consequently in many other parts of the world. Ironically, this de-emphasis imposed on histopathology happened just as clinical microscopy remerged as one of the most widely used and most critical diagnostic approaches. The number of microscopic examinations is constantly rising worldwide reflecting the wider use of biopsies and innovative techniques for obtaining tissue samples for diagnostic evaluation. The numbers of tissue samples removed for diagnostic purposes by surgical biopsy, endoscopy or fine needle aspiration biopsy has reached multiple millions per year in the US alone. The need for physicians who are qualified to interpret these samples has been greater than ever, and many countries report a shortage of diagnostic pathologists. This exigency combined with the fact that pathologists still teach histopathology to medical students and many junior physicians in training

highlights the need for additional investment into the didactic aspects of histopathology. It is also one of the reasons that we undertook the writing of this Atlas; the other reason being our firm belief that histopathology remains one of the key medical disciplines essential for the understanding of basic concepts, mechanisms of diseases, their causes and complications. For us ,it remains inconceivable that any medical doctor could graduate from his or her medical school without a strong foundation in basic microscopy of normal and pathologically altered human tissues.

As it logically follows from the above paragraph, histopathology can be perceived as a didactic discipline on one hand side and a diagnostic discipline on the other. A comprehensive Histopathology Atlas should cover both aspects of histopathology. With this notion in mind, we have prepared this Atlas with two goals in mind. The first one was to provide additional illustrations of basic pathologic processes and thus expand the horizons of *medical students* studying pathology during their preclinical years. The second goal was to provide a pictorial guide to *advanced students and clinical trainees* revisiting the arena of histopathology while preparing for specialty examinations in the clinical specialty of their choice. Many residents in internal medicine and its subspecialties, such as gastroenterology, nephrology, pulmonology, oncology and hematology are required to spend a month or two in pathology during their years of clinical training. Likewise, many residents in surgery and surgical subspecialties spend time in pathology, and are expected to become proficient in interpreting basic histopathologic findings. The same holds true for residents in many other clinical specialties such as neurology, dermatology or gynecology. We felt that all these residents might appreciate this *Atlas of Histopathology*, which was designed to enrich their clinical training and prepare them for a lifelong interaction with diagnostic pathologists. Last but not least, we hope that our own *pathology residents* will use this Atlas to master the basics of diagnostic microscopy. We wish them all a lot of luck and hope that this book will help them become better physicians.

**Ivan Damjanov**

# *Acknowledgments*

The Editor and all the Contributors to this Histopathology Atlas would like to express their thanks to Mr Jitendar P Vij (Chairman and Managing Director) of Jaypee Brothers Medical Publishers, New Delhi, India, for making possible the publication of this book. We also thank his staff whose technical support was absolutely critical for completing this project. We would also like to acknowledge the expert assistance of Mr Dennis Friesen, our departmental photographer at the University of Kansas, who helped us prepare the illustrations.

# Contents

1. **The Cardiovascular System** .................................................................... 1

Ivan Damjanov

Normal Histology   1
   Atherosclerosis   2
   Coronary Heart Disease   2
   Hypertension   3
   Rheumatic Heart Disease   3
   Infections of the Heart   4
   Cardiomyopathy   5
   Tumors of the Heart   5
   Vasculitis   5
Tumors of Blood Vessels   6

2. **The Respiratory System** .................................................................... 27

Paul St. Romain, Rashna Madan, Ivan Damjanov

Upper Respiratory System   27
   Sinonasal Inflammations   27
   Nasopharyngeal Tumors   27
Lungs   28
   Alveolar Disorders Impeding Respiration   28
   Bronchopulmonary Infections   29
   Immunologic Lung Diseases   31
   Interstitial Lung Diseases   31
   Pneumoconioses   32
   Chronic Obstructive Pulmonary Disease   33
   Pulmonary Neoplasms   33

3. **Hematopoietic and Lymphoid System** .................................................................... 57

Da Zhang

Normal Hematopoietic and Lymphoid System   57
   Anemia   57
   Microcytic Hypochromic Anemia   58
   Macrocytic Anemia   58
   Anemia Caused by Intrinsic Red Blood Cell Abnormalities   58
   Anemia Caused by Bone Marrow Failure   59
   Hemolytic Anemia   59
Leukemia   59
   Acute Myeloid Leukemia   60
   Acute Lymphoblastic Leukemia/Lymphoma   60
   Chronic Myeloid Leukemia   60
   Chronic Lymphocytic Leukemia   60
Lymphoma   61
   Hodgkin Lymphoma   61

4. **Digestive System** .................................................................... 83

Rashna Madan

Esophagus   83
   Developmental Anomalies   83
   Inflammatory and Infectious Conditions   83
   Preneoplastic Conditions and Neoplasms   84

*Stomach 85*
  *Developmental Anomalies 86*
  *Inflammatory and Infectious Conditions (Gastritis) and Gastropathies 86*
  *Polyps and Neoplasms 88*
*Small Intestine 90*
  *Developmental Anomalies 90*
  *Inflammatory and Infectious Conditions 90*
  *Polyps and Neoplasms 91*
*Colon 91*
  *Developmental Anomalies 92*
  *Inflammatory and Infectious Conditions 92*
  *Polyps and Neoplasms 94*
*Appendix 95*
  *Inflammatory and Infectious Conditions 96*
  *Neoplasms 96*

**5. Hepatobiliary System** ............................................................ **137**
*Maura O' Neil*
*Liver 137*
  *Inflammatory Diseases 137*
  *Metabolic Disorders 139*
  *Cirrhosis 139*
  *Neoplasms 139*
*Gallbladder 140*
  *Inflammation 140*
  *Neoplasms 141*

**6. Pancreas** .................................................................................... **159**
*Rashna Madan, Ivan Damjanov*
*Congenital and Inherited Conditions 159*
*Inflammatory Diseases 159*
*Neoplasms 160*
  *Tumors of the Exocrine Pancreas 160*
  *Tumors of the Endocrine Pancreas 161*

**7. The Urinary System** .............................................................. **177**
*Da Zhang, Ivan Damjanov*
*Normal Histology 177*
*Overview of Pathology 177*
  *Developmental Disorders 177*
  *Glomerular Diseases 178*
  *Vascular Kidney Diseases 180*
  *Infectious Diseases 180*
  *Neoplasms 180*

**8. The Male Genital System** ...................................................... **199**
*Ivan Damjanov*
*Testis 199*
  *Developmental Disorders 199*
  *Infections 199*
  *Neoplasms 200*
*Prostate 201*
  *Benign Prostatic Hyperplasia 201*
  *Neoplasms 201*
*Penis 201*
  *Neoplasms 202*

9. **Female Reproductive System** ............................................ **215**

*Fang Fan*

*Vulva, Vagina and Cervix   215*
   *Non-Neoplastic Epithelial Vulvar Disorders   215*
   *Non-Neoplastic Lesions of Cervix   216*
   *Human Papillomavirus Related Squamous Intraepithelial Lesions   216*
   *Invasive Squamous Cell Carcinoma   217*
   *Cervical Adenocarcinoma   217*
   *Vulvar Paget Disease   217*
*Uterine Corpus   217*
   *Endometritis   218*
   *Endometrial Hyperplasia   218*
   *Endometrial Epithelial Tumors   218*
   *Endometrial Stromal Tumors   219*
   *Smooth Muscle Tumors   219*
   *Carcinosarcoma   220*
*Fallopian Tube   220*
   *Acute and Chronic Salpingitis   220*
   *Tubal Pregnancy   221*
   *Carcinoma   221*
*Ovary   221*
   *Non-Neoplastic Cysts   221*
   *Endometriosis   221*
   *Surface Epithelial-Stromal Tumors   221*
   *Germ Cell Tumors   222*
   *Sex Cord-Stromal Tumors   222*
   *Metastatic Tumors   223*
*Pregnancy Related Changes   223*
   *Blighted Ovum   223*
   *Hydatidiform Mole   223*
   *Choriocarcinoma   224*

10. **Breast** ............................................................................ **253**

*Fang Fan*

*Normal Breast   253*
*Reactive and Inflammatory Lesions   254*
*Nonproliferative Fibrocystic Change   254*
*Adenosis   254*
*Intraductal Proliferative Lesions   254*
*Lobular Neoplasia   255*
*Fibroepithelial Lesions   256*
*Papillary Lesions   256*
*Invasive Breast Carcinoma   256*
*Male Breast Lesions   257*

11. **The Endocrine System** ................................................... **273**

*Paul St. Romain, Ivan Damjanov*

*Pituitary   273*
   *Neoplasms   273*
*Thyroid   274*
   *Goiter   274*
   *Thyroiditis   274*
   *Neoplasms   275*

*Parathyroid 276*
  *Hyperplasia 276*
  *Adenoma 276*
*Adrenal 277*
  *Acute Adrenal Insufficiency 277*
  *Chronic Adrenal Insufficiency 277*
  *Adrenal Cortical Hyperplasia 277*
  *Adrenal Cortical Adenoma 278*
  *Adrenal Cortical Carcinoma 278*
  *Pheochromocytoma 278*
  *Neuroblastoma 278*

**12. The Skin** ................................................................ **297**
*Garth Fraga*
*Genodermatoses 297*
*Inflammatory Dermatoses 297*
  *Spongiotic Dermatitis 297*
  *Psoriasiform Dermatitis 298*
  *Interface Dermatitis 298*
  *Disorders of the Hair Follicle 298*
  *Perivascular Dermatitis 299*
  *Granulomatous Dermatitis 299*
  *Vesiculobullous/Blistering Dermatitis 299*
*Infections and Infestations 300*
  *Bacterial Infections 300*
  *Viral Infections 300*
  *Fungal Infections 300*
  *Arthropods 300*
*Neoplasms 301*
  *Epidermal Neoplasms 301*
  *Melanocytic Neoplasms 301*
  *Mesenchymal Neoplasms 302*
  *Hematolymphoid Neoplasms 303*

**13. Bones, Joints and Soft Tissues** ........................................ **331**
*Katie L Dennis, Fang Fan*
*Bones 331*
  *Developmental Disorders 331*
  *Metabolic Disorders 332*
  *Inflammation 333*
  *Neoplasms and Related Lesions 333*
*Joints 334*
  *Osteoarthritis 335*
  *Rheumatoid Arthritis 335*
  *Gout 335*
  *Pigmented Villonodular Synovitis 335*
*Soft Tissue Tumors 335*
  *Tumors of Adipose Tissue 336*
  *Tumors of Fibrous Tissue 336*
  *Tumors of Skeletal Muscle 336*
  *Tumor of Uncertain Histogenesis 336*

**14. Skeletal Muscles** .................................................................... **355**

*Ivan Damjanov*

*Neurogenic Muscle Diseases   355*

*Genetic Muscle Diseases   356*

*Rhabdomyolysis   357*

**15 Central Nervous System** .......................................................... **367**

*Paul St. Romain, Ivan Damjanov*

*Normal Central Nervous System   367*

*Cellular Reactions to Injury   367*

   *Neuronal Injury   367*

   *Glial Reaction to Injury   368*

*Cerebrovascular Disease   368*

   *Cerebral Ischemia   368*

*Infections of the Central Nervous System   369*

   *Meningitis   369*

   *Encephalitis   369*

   *Subacute Sclerosing Panencephalitis   369*

   *AIDS Encephalopathy   369*

   *Spongiform Encephalopathies   370*

*Demyelinating Diseases   370*

   *Multiple Sclerosis   370*

*Neurodegenerative Diseases   370*

   *Alzheimer Disease   370*

   *Parkinson Disease   370*

   *Amyotrophic Lateral Sclerosis   371*

   *Subacute Combined Degeneration of the Spinal Cord   371*

*Neoplasms   371*

   *Astrocytic Tumors   371*

   *Oligodendroglioma   371*

   *Ependymoma   372*

   *Medulloblastoma   372*

   *Meningioma   372*

   *Schwannoma   372*

   *Hemangioblastoma   372*

   *Metastatic Tumors   372*

*Index* .................................................................................. *395*

# 1 The Cardiovascular System

*Ivan Damjanov*

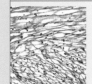

## Introduction

*The cardiovascular system consists of the heart and the blood vessels. The primary function of the heart is to pump the blood through the blood vessels and thus maintain the circulation. Through the arterial blood the tissues receive oxygen and the major nutrients, and through the venous blood they dispose of carbon dioxide and the metabolic degradation products.*

*The most important diseases of the cardiovascular system that cause distinctive histopathologic changes are as follows:*

- *Atherosclerosis*
- *Vascular changes induced by hypertension*
- *Coronary heart disease*
- *Rheumatic heart disease*
- *Infections of the heart*
- *Cardiomyopathy*
- *Tumors of the heart*
- *Vasculitis*
- *Tumors of blood vessels.*

## Normal Histology

*The heart* is a contractile organ that has three layers: (1) endocardium; (2) myocardium and (3) epicardium. The endocardium consists of an endocardial cell layer, continuous with the endothelium of blood vessels and a thin strand of connective tissue. The mural endocardium covers the inner surface of the cardiac chambers, and the valvular endocardium covers the valvular leaflets. The myocardium is composed of striated cardiac muscle cells arranged in a syncytium **(Fig. 1.1)**. The external surface of the heart is covered by a mesothelial layer separated from the myocardium by subepicardial fibrofatty tissue. The epicardium is in continuity with the inner mesothelial layer of pericardium.

*The blood vessels* can be divided into three groups: (1) arteries; (2) capillaries and (3) veins **(Figs 1.2A to D)**. All arteries have three layers (tunicae) including tunica intima, media and adventitia. The large arteries including the aorta are classified as *elastic arteries* because their tunica media consists predominantly of fenestrated elastic sheaths, admixed to collagen fibers and scattered smooth muscles. Smaller *muscular arteries* also have three distinctive layers but their tunica media is predominantly composed of smooth muscle cells. An internal and external elastic lamina are found on the internal or external side of the intima media. The muscular arteries extend into *arterioles*, which are composed of an endothelial layer and a smooth muscle cell layer. The arterioles extend into *capillaries*, which are continuous with *venules*. Capillaries have a thin wall made out endothelial cells lying on a basement membrane. The venules collect the deoxygenated blood from capillaries and deliver it into larger *veins*, through which the blood returns to the heart. The veins have a thinner wall than the arteries and their wall is not separated into distinct layers.

### Atherosclerosis

*Atherosclerosis* is a multifactorial disease affecting the aorta and major arteries such as the coronary, carotid or iliac arteries. The development of atherosclerosis occurs in several phases but it almost always begins with the insudation of lipids into the intima and media, and the appearance of lipid laden foamy macrophages in the inner layers of the artery **(Figs 1.3A to D)**. These changes lead to the formation of grossly visible *fatty streaks* which stimulate the proliferation of smooth muscle cells and fibroblasts, and an additional influx of macrophages. These cells accumulate lipids and release growth factors stimulating further for the deposition of collagen and the formation of *fibrofatty plaques*. With time many of the fat-laden cells die releasing lipids into the interstitial space and thus leading to formation of an *atheroma*, the characteristic lesion of full-blown atherosclerosis. Atheromas are complicated by secondary changes, such a *calcification, ulceration of the endothelium and thrombosis*, and weakening of the arterial wall leading to the formation of *aneurysms*.

### Coronary Heart Disease

*Coronary heart disease* is a major complication of generalized atherosclerosis, but often it may occur as the only aspect of atherosclerosis or it may be disproportionally more pronounced than the atherosclerosis of other arteries. Coronary atherosclerosis leads to a narrowing of the lumen of coronary arteries, thus reducing the blood supply to the myocardium. Slowly progressive narrowing of coronary arteries causes angina pectoris or chronic congestive heart failure. Sudden occlusion of the lumen of coronary arteries due to the formation of a thrombus over a ruptured atheroma may cause a myocardial infarct.

*Coronary atheromas* are traditionally subdivided into two groups: (1) *soft atheromas* and (2) *hard atheromas* **(Figs 1.4A to D)**. Predominantly soft atheromas have a central core composed of cholesterol rich lipidized amorphous detritus, which is separated from the lumen of the artery by a thin fibrous cap. This fibrous cap may rupture, whereupon the content of atheroma enters the lumen of the artery causing thrombosis. Such thrombi may occlude the coronary partially, causing angina pectoris, or completely, causing an infarction. Hard atheromas are composed of fibrous connective tissue which tends to calcify. Progressive fibrosis and calcification may cause marked narrowing presenting clinically as angina pectoris or congestive heart failure.

*Myocardial infarct* is a localized area of ischemic necrosis of myocardium caused in most instances by a thrombotic occlusion of a coronary artery or its major branches. Ischemia will produce predictable biochemical and ultrastructural changes in cardiac myocytes within several minutes. If the blood flow is restored within 20 minutes, some of the reversibly injured myocytes can be rescued. The irreversibly damaged cardiac myocytes will show signs of *contraction band necrosis* **(Fig. 1.5)**, the hallmark of myocardial reperfusion injury.

The cardiac myocytes irreversibly damaged by hypoxia and anoxia, and the entire area of infarction undergo typical microscopic changes which are progressive and time dependent. The first signs of infarction include *necrosis* of cardiac myocytes which become eosinophilic. Myocardial cell death is sequentially followed by signs of *acute inflammation, chronic inflammation, granulation tissue formation and fibrosis.*

Microscopic examination of the infarcted heart may be used to date the onset of the infarction **(Figs 1.6A to D)**. During the later hours of the first postinfarction day, the cytoplasm of ischemic damaged myocytes becomes eosinophilic, and the cardiac myocytes begin loosing their nuclei. During the second postinfarction day, the infarcted areas are invaded by neutrophils which start removing the damaged cardiac myocytes. Neutrophils infiltrating the infarction start dying 1–2 days thereafter, and accordingly a typical 3 day infarction will consist of necrotic eosinophilic myofibers and pyknotic or fragmented white blood cell nuclei. Toward the end of the first week, the infarct becomes gradually invaded by macrophages and a vascularized granulation tissue starts forming. Over the next few weeks, the granulation tissue is gradually replaced by avascular fibrous tissue forming a collagenous scar 5–8 weeks after the onset of ischemia.

## Hypertension

*Cardiac hypertrophy* is one of the most common complications of hypertension. It predominantly affects the left ventricle and is associated with widespread hypertrophy of cardiac myocytes **(Figs 1.7A and B)**. The hypertrophic cardiac myocytes contain more abundant cytoplasm and contractile elements. Their nuclei are enlarged and appear hyperchromatic due to an increased amount of their constituent DNA. In longitudinal sections the nuclei appear wider and longer than normal, whereas on cross sections they have irregular outlines due to invaginations of the nuclear membrane. The increased surface of the nuclear membrane allows more efficient exchange between the large nucleus and the more abundant cytoplasm of hypertrophic cells.

*Arterial changes* caused by hypertension are seen in the aorta, elastic and muscular arteries as well as arterioles. In the aorta and elastic arteries hypertension is one of the major adverse influences accelerating the development of atherosclerosis. In muscular arteries, like the interlobar or intralobar arteries of the kidney, hypertension leads to *intimal* and *medial fibrosis* and narrowing of the arterial lumen **(Figs 1.8A and B)**.

*Arteriolar changes* are the most prominent histopathologic sign of hypertension and are most prominent in the kidneys **(Fig. 1.9A)**. In longstanding slowly evolving (benign) hypertension there is prominent *hyalinization of renal arterioles.* It is associated with eosinophilic homogenization of the wall of the arterioles and narrowing of their lumen. Most prominent hyalinization of renal arterioles is seen in diabetes mellitus, indicating that the metabolic changes can produce similar changes as hypertension. It is worth of a notice that arteriolar hyalinization can occur even without hypertension or diabetes, as typically seen in the spleen of the elderly patients **(Fig. 1.9B)**. Involution of postmenopausal ovaries is also accompanied by hyalinization of arterioles and small arteries.

*Rapidly progressive (malignant) hypertension* may cause *proliferative arteriolitis*, with concentric "onion-skin-like" proliferation of smooth muscle cells **(Fig. 1.10A)**. These changes, which markedly narrow the lumen of the arterioles, presumably protect glomeruli from excessive blood influx. Uncontrolled rapid onset of malignant hypertension may cause *fibrinoid necrosis* of renal arterioles **(Fig. 1.10B)**. In extreme cases fibrinoid necrosis may involve even glomerular capillaries and thus cause rapidly progressive renal failure.

*Aortic dissection*, previously known as dissecting aneurysm of the aorta, is a frequently lethal complication of hypertension **(Figs 1.11A to D)**. It most often occurs in persons who have aortic atherosclerosis, but it may also affect younger persons with constitutively weak aorta and those suffering from genetic connective tissue diseases such as Marfan syndrome. In all these cases the aortic wall shows nonspecific changes such as fragmentation and loss of elastic fibers, accumulation of acid mucopolysaccharides in the form of myxoid amorphous material, generalized loss of normal architecture. All these changes lead to a separation of one layer of the aortic wall from another. The blood stream dissects the vessel wall by penetrating between the layers of the aorta. This may lead to the formation of a second lumen, which often ruptures causing a massive fatal hemorrhage.

## Rheumatic Heart Disease

Rheumatic carditis is a clinical-pathologic feature of rheumatic fever, an immunologically mediated systemic disease complicating streptococcal throat infection. It may present as acute nonbacterial endocarditis, myocarditis, pericarditis or pancarditis involving all parts of the heart.

*Rheumatic endocarditis* presents in acute stages of the disease as endocarditis usually involving the cusps of the mitral or the aortic valves. Initially valvulitis presents as a deposition of fibrin and the formation of fibrin-rich nodules or excrescences, known as "vegetations" **(Fig. 1.12A)**. These changes are not diagnostic and can resemble any other form of nonbacterial thrombotic endocarditis. On the mural endocardium the inflammation will more likely present with diagnostic changes which include the formation of *Aschoff bodies* **(Fig. 1.12B)**. Aschoff bodies consist of macrophages, occasional multinucleated giant cells and scattered lymphocytes which accumulate around a central area composed of amorphous fibrinoid material. Valvular vegetations elicit the formation of granulation tissue in the valves. The proliferating vessels within the granulation tissue will ultimately organize the vegetations and at the same time produce deformities of the valves (Fig. 1.12C). Like in other forms of wound healing the granulation tissue transforms into a fibrous scar, which usually undergoes calcification (Fig. 1.12D). Such deformed valves cannot function properly and are also prone to bacterial superinfection.

*Rheumatic myocarditis* presents with the formation of Aschoff bodies, which are the microscopic hallmarks of rheumatic fever (Figs 1.13A and B). Over time the macrophages are replaced by fibroblasts which form a spindle shaped fibrous scar, usually in the vicinity of myocardial blood vessels.

*Rheumatic pericarditis* is associated with nondiagnostic histopathologic changes which usually include nonspecific chronic inflammation and an extensive fibrin rich exudate (Figs 1.14A and B). The exudate covers the epicardial surface of the heart and the parietal mesothelial surfaces of pericardial sac. After a few days the granulation will grow into the fibrin exudate and organize it over a period of a few weeks. The granulation tissue will then transform into a fibrous scar covering the heart and obliterating the pericardial cavity, clinically presenting as constrictive pericarditis.

### Infections of the Heart

Infections of the heart can be caused by viruses and bacteria, and less often by fungi or protozoa. These infections may present pathologically and clinically as: (a) endocarditis; (b) myocarditis; or (c) pericarditis.

*Endocarditis* is most often caused by bacteria, such as *Streptococcus* or *Staphylococcus*, which account together for more than 75% of all infections. Endocarditis caused by other bacteria is less common. Fungal infections are seen in immunosuppressed or chronically emaciated persons.

Infectious endocarditis presents most often with formation of fibrin-rich vegetations on the surface of valvular endocardium (Figs 1.15A to D). Inside the aggregates of fibrin one may identify bacteria or fungi with special stains. The vegetations are invaded by the granulation tissue which forms inside the valves, contributing to the vascularity of these almost avascular structures. Granulation will grow into the fibrinous base of vegetations, sealing them firmly to the valve. The surface portions of the vegetations are more friable and can detach forming septic emboli, which are carried by blood to distal parts of the arterial circulation. Endocarditis has a high mortality but it may also progress into a chronic form, resulting in scarring and valvular deformities. In chronic stages of endocarditis the valves become partially hyalinized and may calcify, but in most instances they also retain a hypervascular central core, which is also in part infiltrated with chronic inflammatory cells.

*Myocarditis* is most often caused by viruses, but it may be found also in patients who have bacterial sepsis, and some disseminated fungal and parasitic diseases. Immunologically mediated myocarditis may be seen in autoimmune diseases in persons with drug hypersensitivity reactions. Granulomatous myocarditis is a feature of sarcoidosis. Giant cell myocarditis is a rare form of chronic inflammation of unknown etiology.

*Viral myocarditis* is characterized by single cell necrosis of cardiac myocytes surrounded by infiltrates composed predominantly of lymphocytes (Fig. 1.16A). *Hypersensitivity myocarditis* usually represents an adverse reaction to drugs including infiltrates of eosinophils (Fig. 1.16B). *Bacterial myocarditis*, usually seen in sepsis and immunosuppressed patients such as those with AIDS, usually presents with microscopic abscesses or foci of myocardial necrosis surrounded by neutrophils (Fig. 1.16C). *Chagas disease*, a systemic disease common in South America may present with myocarditis; cysts of *Trypanosoma cruzi* may be seen in cardiac myocytes (Fig. 1.16D).

*Pericarditis* is most often caused by viruses presenting as a serous inflammation. This inflammation usually heals spontaneously and therefore it is rarely seen in pathology practice. Bacterial infections of the pericardium presents usually in the form of a purulent or fibrinopurulent exudate (Fig. 1.17). The fibrin-rich exudate is organized by an ingrowth of granulation tissue, which ultimately leads to fibrotic scarring and obliteration of the pericardial cavity. Fibrotic pericarditis may clinically present as constrictive pericarditis.

## Cardiomyopathy

*Cardiomyopathy* is a name given to a group of primary myocardial diseases for which the exact cause cannot be always identified. Under this term it is customary to include genetic myocardial diseases, myocardial diseases in some systemic diseases, drug and toxin induced or vitamin deficiency conditions, and diseases of unknown etiology.

On the basis of macroscopic finding cardiomyopathies are usually divided into three groups: (a) dilated; (b) hypertrophic and (c) restrictive cardiomyopathies. In most instances the microscopic changes in the myocardium are nonspecific and include fibrosis or hypertrophy of the cardiac myocytes **(Figs 1.18A and B)**.

*Amyloidosis* is one of the rare forms of cardiomyopathy that presents with pathognomonic histopathologic changes. The disease can be diagnosed by heart biopsy which typically shows accumulation of amyloid fibrils in the interstitial spaces **(Figs 1.19A and B)**. Amyloid may be seen in the blood vessels and the cardiac valves as well. Amyloid deposits typically cause a restrictive cardiomyopathy preventing the heart from dilating during diastole. Amyloid may also interfere with the blood supply and thus ultimately cause atrophy and loss of cardiac myocytes.

*Glycogenoses*, such as glycogen storage disease type II (Pompe disease), may present with cardiomyopathy due to the accumulation of glycogen in cardiac myocytes **(Fig. 1.20)**. Deposits of glycogen in the myocardial cells, which appear vacuolated on light microscopy, can be demonstrated by electron microscopy or by special stains such as the periodic acid Schiff (PAS) reaction.

## Tumors of the Heart

Primary tumors of the heart are rare, and even metastases from other sites are found only exceptionally.

*Atrial myxoma* is the most common benign tumor of the heart. It usually develops from the interatrial septum or the valvular endocardium. It presents as a pedunculated polypoid mass composed microscopically of loose myxoid connective tissue **(Figs 1.21A and B)**.

## Vasculitis

*Vasculitis* is a term used for inflammatory diseases of the blood vessels. Although in some cases, vasculitis may be caused by bacteria or other infectious pathogens. In most instances it is caused by immunological mechanisms.

Vasculitis may be subdivided into several groups depending on the size and type of blood vessels involved. Here we shall illustrate the most common forms of vasculitis.

*Giant cell aortitis or Takayasu disease* is a granulomatous inflammation involving the aorta of young or middle aged women **(Figs 1.22A and B)**. The inflammation may weaken the aorta and lead to formation of aneurysms, or it may cause narrowing of aorta and its major branches, especially on the arch of aorta.

*Temporal arteritis* is the most common form of arteritis. It involves the temporal artery and its major branches, and affects typically older persons. It presents as a transmural granulomatous inflammation disrupting the internal elastic lamina and causing a narrowing of the arterial lumen **(Figs 1.23A to C)**. Histologically the inflammatory infiltrates contain numerous lymphocytes, macrophages and giant cells, thus resembling giant cell aortitis.

*Polyarteritis nodosa* is an immune complex mediated type III hypersensitivity reaction involving medium sized and small arteries **(Figs 1.24A and B)**. The deposition of immune complexes are associated with fibrinoid necrosis of the vessel wall and transmural inflammation. Thrombotic occlusion of the arteries and the formation of microaneurysms through the weakened or partially disrupted vessel wall are common complications.

THE CARDIOVASCULAR SYSTEM

*Hypersensitivity vasculitis* involves small blood vessels, such as dermal arterioles, venules and capillaries **(Figs 1.25A and B)**. It may present as acute leukocytoclastic vasculitis or chronic perivasculitis. Leukocytoclastic vasculitis is characterized by infiltration of small dermal vessels and adjacent connective tissue with neurotrophils. In chronic immunologically mediated vasculitis the infiltrates consist of lymphocytes and plasma cells. Most reactions of this type represent an adverse hypersensitivity reaction to drugs or foreign antigens. Any tissue could be involved but the disease is most often diagnosed in skin biopsies.

*Tumors of Blood Vessels*

Tumors of blood vessels are very common and most of them are benign. Malignant vascular tumors are rare.

*Hemangioma* is the most common benign tumor composed of small blood vessels **(Fig. 1.26)**. It occurs in the skin and many internal organs.

*Angiofibroma* is a benign vascular tumor of the nasal passages of young men **(Fig. 1.27)**. It is composed of irregularly shaped (staghorn-like) and dilated thin walled vessels surrounded by fibrous tissue. Due to their vascularity these friable tumors tend to bleed profusely.

*Angiosarcoma* is a rare malignant soft tissue tumor composed of neoplastic endothelial cells **(Figs 1.28A and B)**. Tumor cells form irregularly shaped vascular spaces and solid strands invading adjacent tissue.

*Kaposi sarcoma* is a malignant endothelial cell tumor related to infection with human herpes virus 8 and occurs most often in persons suffering from the acquired immunodeficiency syndrome (AIDS) **(Figs 1.29A and B)**. The tumor may present in the form of hemorrhagic patches and nodules on the skin, but it may involve lymph nodes and other internal organs as well.

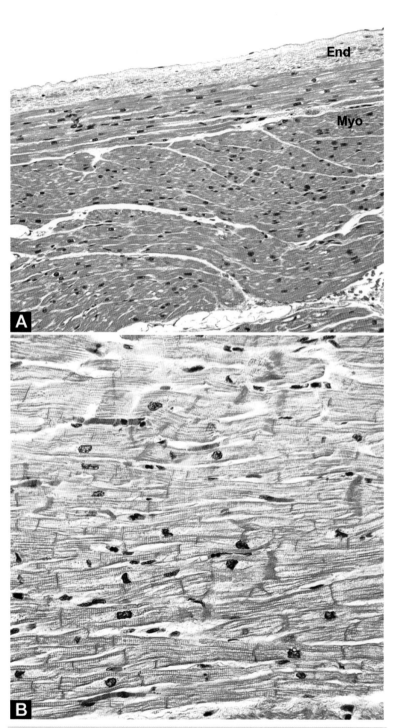

**Figs 1.1A and B:** Normal myocardium
**A.** The thin inner layer of heart, endocardium (End), is composed of loose connective tissue covered with an endothelial layer. The myocardium (Myo) is composed of striated muscle cells. **B.** Myocardium is composed of cardiac myocytes arranged in a syncytium.

THE CARDIOVASCULAR SYSTEM

CHAPTER

**1**

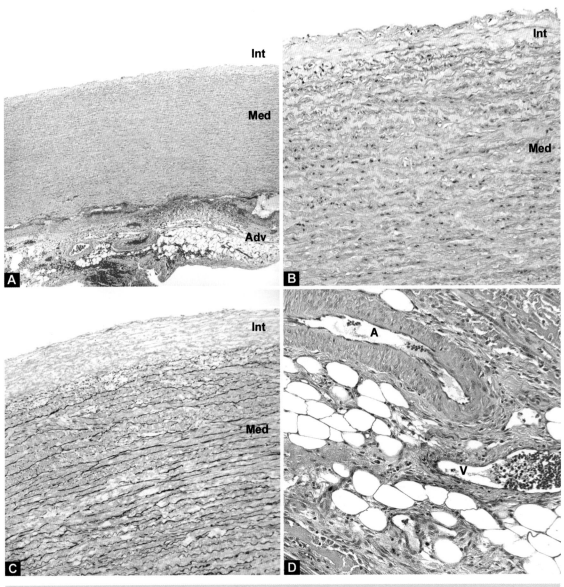

**Figs 1.2A to D:** Normal blood vessels

**A.** Aorta is an elastic artery which has three layers: tunica intima (Int); tunica media (Med) and tunica adventitia (Adv). **B.** High magnification shows loosely structured tunica intima (Int) and media (Med) composed of extracellular matrix and smooth muscle cells. **C.** Elastica Van Gieson special stain outlines the elastic lamellae black illustrating the abundance of elastic tissue in the media of the aorta. **D.** Smaller muscular artery (A) has a thick wall mostly composed of smooth muscle cells; a vein (V) has a thinner wall.

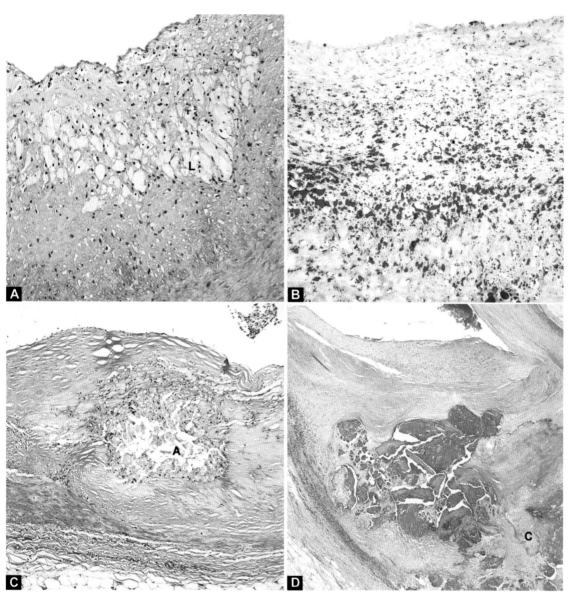

**Figs 1.3A to D:** Atherosclerosis of the aorta

**A.** In early stages of atherosclerosis there is accumulation of lipids (L) in the inner layers of the aorta, which give the aorta a vacuolated appearance in routine H&E section. **B.** Special stain (Oil red O), stains the lipids red, proving that the aortal wall contains an increased amount of lipids. **C.** Progression of atherosclerosis is accompanied by the formation of atheroma (A), which in microscopic slides appears as a cavity filled with lipid and amorphous loosely structured cell detritus. Most of the lipid has been extracted from the tissue during the preparation of slides, and therefore parts of atheroma appear like empty spaces. **D.** Hardening of the atheroma which has been replaced with hyalinized collagen (red) and deposits of insoluble bluish calcium salts (C).

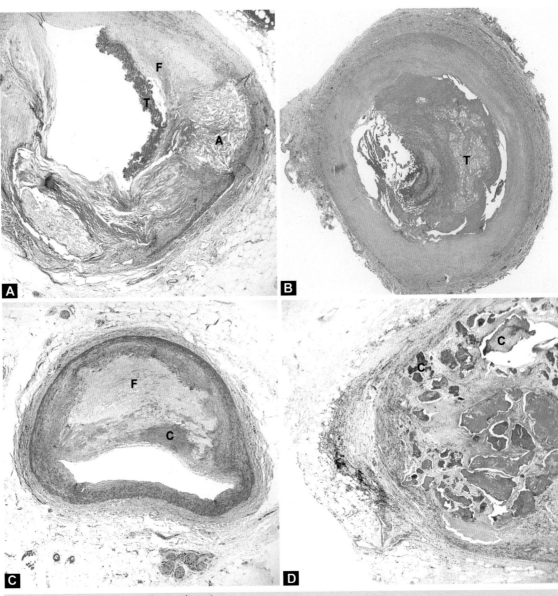

**Figs 1.4A to D:** Coronary atherosclerosis

**A.** Soft atheroma (A) consists of cholesterol rich amorphous material covered with a fibrous cap (F). Cholesterol crystals have been washed out during the processing of the tissue leaving behind cleft-like "empty" spaces. The lumen of the artery contains a fibrin rich thrombus (T) attached to the fibrous cap (F) of the atheroma. One may assume that the leaks in the fibrous cap have initiated the formation of the thrombus. **B.** This coronary artery contains a large thrombus (T). This section was taken distally from the complete occlusion of the coronary artery by a thrombus overlying a ruptured soft atheroma. **C.** Hard atheroma is composed of fibrous tissue (F) which has replaced the lipid core. Note the thick hyalinized fibrous cap (C) overlying the lighter staining loosely structured fibrous core. **D.** Massive calcification occludes almost completely the lumen of the coronary artery. Calcified artery must be decalcified prior to sectioning and most of the calcium has been removed leaving behind eosinophilic hyalinized collagen and only a few bluish specks of calcium salts (C). The cracks in the calcified material are also artificially induced during the processing of the tissue.

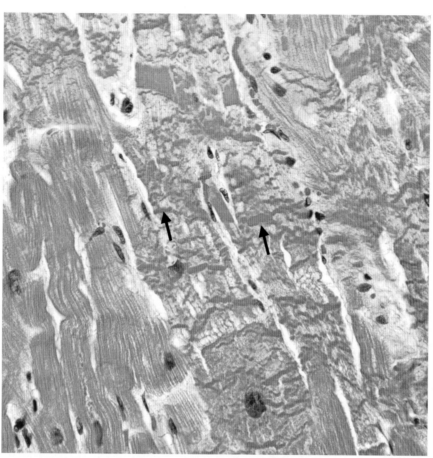

**Fig. 1.5:** Reperfusion of myocardial infarction

Early reperfusion of an infarction will save some cardiac myocytes, but some other cells will undergo contraction band necrosis (arrows).

ATLAS OF HISTOPATHOLOGY

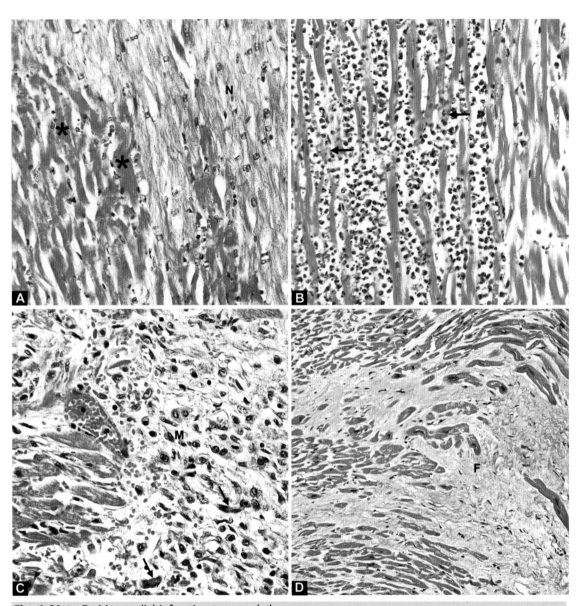

**Figs 1.6A to D:** Myocardial infarction-temporal changes

**A.** Around 20 hours after occlusion of the coronary artery, the infarcted cardiac myocytes lack nuclei and have eosinophilic cytoplasm (asterisks), in contrast to the normal cardiac myocytes on the right side of the figure (N). **B.** 3-day-old infarction is infiltrated with numerous neutrophils phagocytizing the dead cardiac myocytes (arrows). **C.** A week old infarction is characterized by infiltrates of macrophages (M) and new blood vessel formation (arrows). **D.** 3 months after the onset of the coronary occlusion, the infarcted cardiac myocytes have been replaced by fibrous tissue (F).

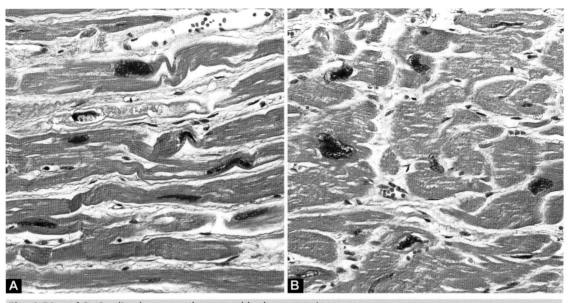

**Figs 1.7A and B:** Cardiac hypertrophy caused by hypertension

**A.** Longitudinally sectioned cardiac myocytes have enlarged hyperchromatic (dark blue) nuclei and abundant cytoplasm. **B.** On cross section the nuclei appear irregularly shaped.

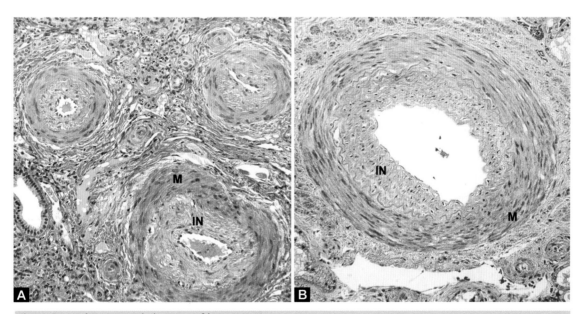

**Figs 1.8A and B:** Arterial changes of hypertension

**A.** Small renal arteries show thickening of their intima (IN) and media (M). **B.** Medium sized branch of the renal artery shows intimal fibrosis (IN) and an increased number of smooth muscle cells in the media (M).

THE CARDIOVASCULAR SYSTEM

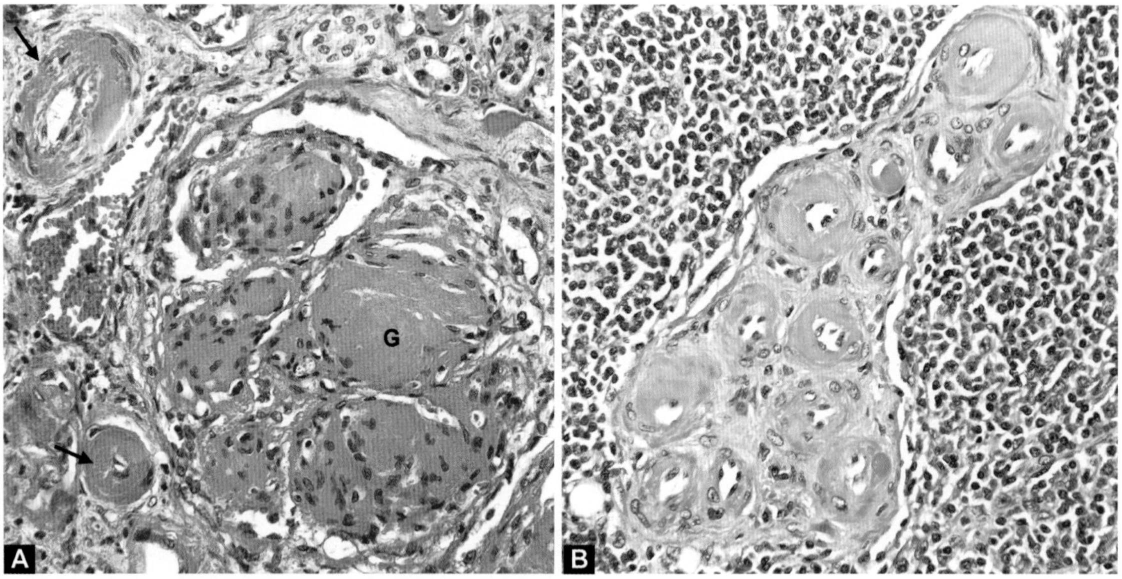

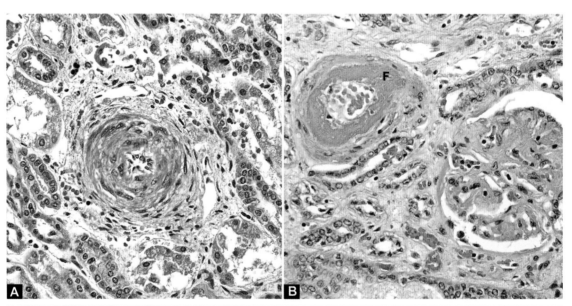

**Figs 1.9A and B:** Hyalinization of arterioles

**A.** Next to the partially hyalinized glomerulus (G) affected by diabetes mellitus, there are two hyalinized renal arterioles (arrows). Hyalinized arterioles have thick homogeneously eosinophilic walls. Hyalinized parts of the glomerulus have the same appearance like the arterioles. **B.** Hyalinized arterioles in the spleen of this elderly person resemble those induced by diabetes and hypertension in the kidney, even though they are not necessarily related to these two diseases.

**Figs 1.10A and B:** Malignant hypertension

**A.** Concentric proliferative arteriolitis characterized by an increased number of concentrically layered smooth muscle cells gives the arterioles an "onion skin" appearance. **B.** Fibrinoid necrosis (F), presenting as bright red homogenization of the wall of this small renal artery is another complication of uncontrollable malignant hypertension of rapid onset.

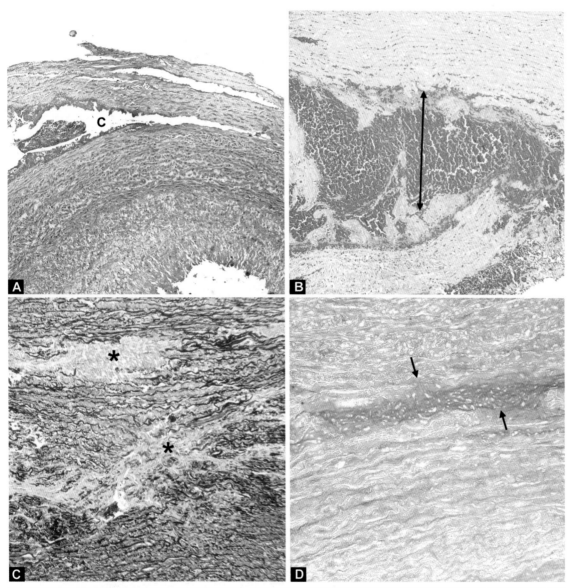

**Figs 1.11A to D:** Aortic dissection

**A.** Separation of layers of the aortic wall causes longitudinal clefts (C). **B.** The blood fills the space in the dissected aortic wall (arrow). **C.** Elastic stain shows fragmentation and disruption of elastic fibers (black) and formation of clefts that contain afibrillar amorphous material (asterisks). **D.** Alcian blue stains blue the acid mucopolysaccharides accumulating in the tissue clefts devoid of elastic fibrils (arrows).

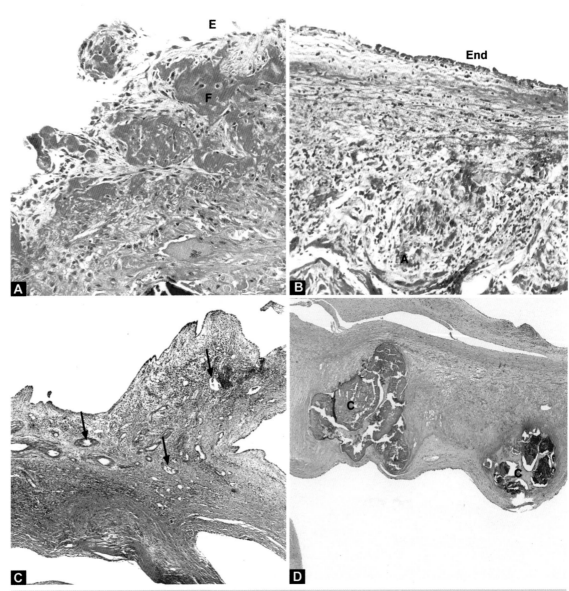

**Figs 1.12A to D:** Rheumatic endocarditis

**A.** Endocarditis initially presents with deposits of fibrin (F) partially covered on its luminal surface by proliferating reactive endocardial cells (E). **B.** Subendocardial inflammation of this ventricle is associated with chronic inflammation and formation of typical Aschoff bodies (A). The luminal surface of the endocardium (End) is covered with prominent endothelial cells, but appears intact. **C.** In later stages of rheumatic endocarditis the valve is deformed by proliferating granulation tissue that contains numerous blood vessels (arrows). **D.** End stage chronic endocarditis is characterized by irregular fibrosis and nodular calcification (C).

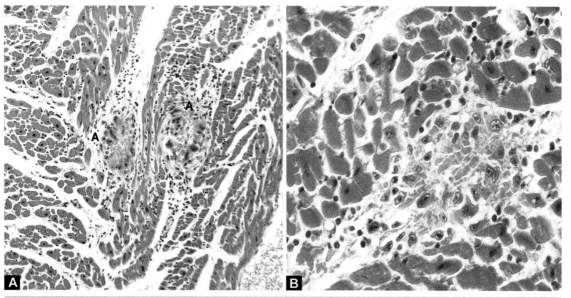

**Figs 1.13A and B:** Rheumatic myocarditis

**A.** Aschoff bodies (A) in the myocardium appear as aggregates of macrophages and lymphocytes surrounding amorphous centrally located material. **B.** Higher magnification view of another Aschoff body shows macrophages with vesicular nuclei and rope-like or granular chromatin.

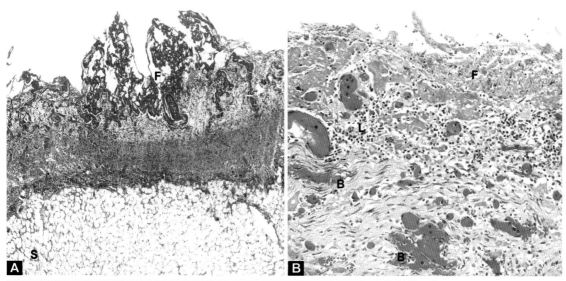

**Figs 1.14A and B:** Rheumatic pericarditis

**A.** The inflammation is characterized by chronic inflammation of the epicardium and exudation of fibrin (F) on the external surface of the heart. The subepicardial (S) fat tissue is not inflamed. **B.** Another case of fibrinous pericarditis illustrating the surface layer of fibrin (F), lymphocytic infiltrates (L) and granulation tissue containing numerous newly formed vessels filled with blood (B).

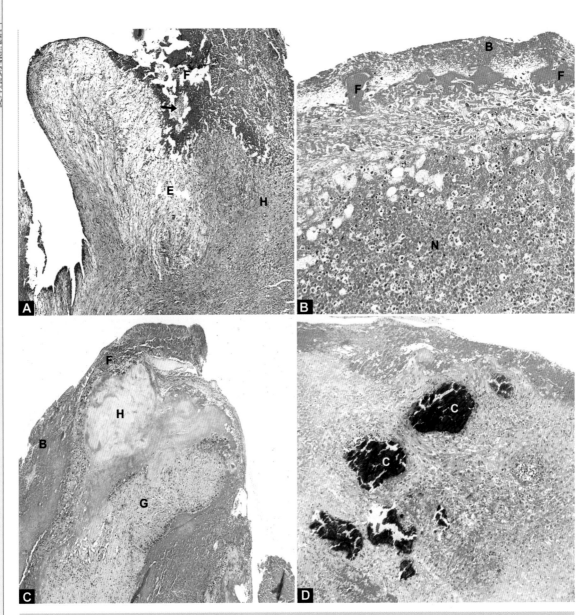

**Figs 1.15A to D.** Infectious endocarditis

**A.** In subacute bacterial endocarditis the surface of this deformed valve is covered with fibrin (F) admixed to groups of neutrophils (arrow). The matrix of the valve appears edematous (E) in some areas and fibrotic and hypercellular (H) in others. The slit spaces corresponding to newly formed small blood vessels, in sharp contrast to normal valves which are almost avascular (not shown here). **B.** Surface of the valvular vegetation caused by bacterial infection consists of several layers: the lowermost bluish layer composed of lysed neutrophils (N) is covered with a layer of fibrin (F) and a surface layer of coagulated blood (B). **C.** Chronic bacterial endocarditis has caused hyalinization of a portion of the valve (H), whereas the other portion consists of fibrotic vascular granulation tissue (G). The surface is focally covered with fibrin (F) and clotted blood (B). **D.** Chronic fungal endocarditis is characterized by an infiltrate of macrophages and lymphocytes on the valve (not included in the figure). There are also several foci of dystrophic calcification (C). Fungi are not seen without a special stain.

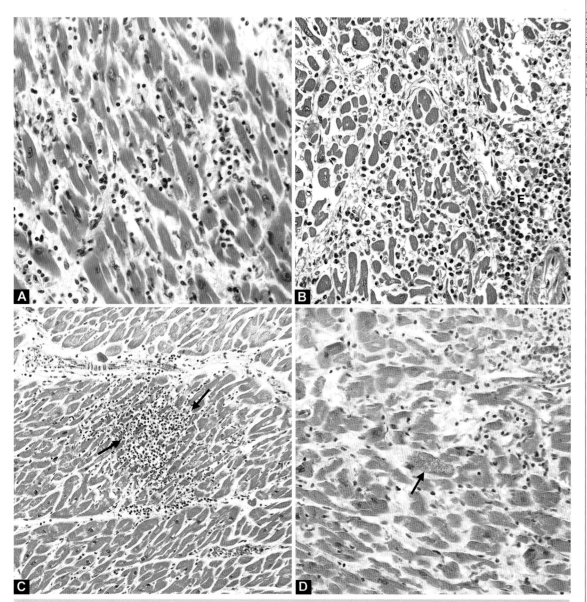

**Figs 1.16A to D:** Myocarditis

**A.** This viral myocarditis is characterized by abundant lymphocytic infiltrates, which can be seen between the cardiac myocytes. **B.** Hypersensitivity myocarditis which developed as an adverse drug reaction is in this case characterized by infiltrates dominated by eosinophils (E). **C.** Bacterial infection of the myocardium is characterized by foci of neutrophils forming a microscopic abscess (between two arrows). **D.** Myocarditis of Chagas disease is caused by *Trypanosoma cruzi* forming cysts, one of which is shown here in a cardiac myocyte (arrow). Note also chronic inflammatory cells in the right upper corner.

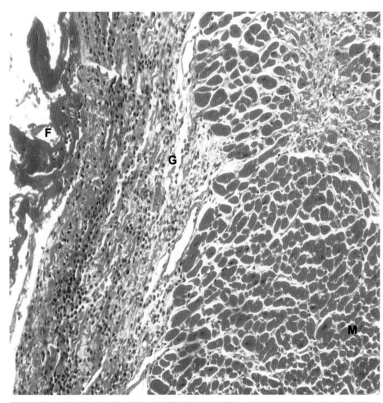

**Fig. 1.17:** Pericarditis

The inflammation of the epicardium is characterized by a surface exudate of fibrin (F) covering macrophage rich granulation tissue (G). The inflammation extends to the myocardium in the upper part of the figure. Most of the myocardium (M) is however not affected.

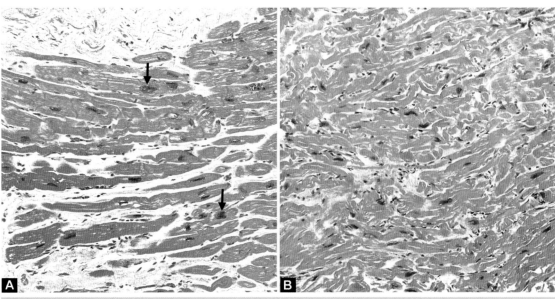

**Figs 1.18A and B:** Cardiomyopathy

**A.** Dilated cardiomyopathy is in this characterized by fibrosis and hypertrophy of the remaining cardiac myocytes (arrows). **B.** In hypertrophic congenital cardiomyopathy there is an apparent disarray of hypertrophic cardiac myocytes which are not arranged in the usual manner parallel to one another.

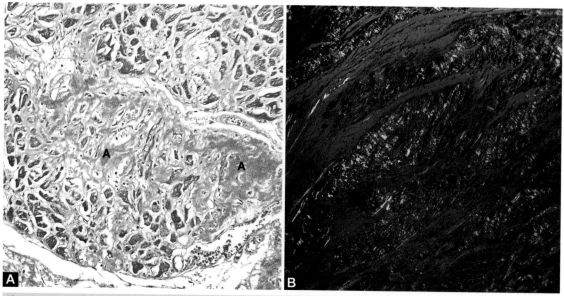

**Figs 1.19A and B:** Cardiac amyloidosis

**A.** Amyloidosis presents with accumulation of amorphous eosinophilic material (A), partially replacing cardiac myocytes or constricting those that remain. **B.** When stained with Congo red and examined under polarized light, the red stained amyloid appears apple green.

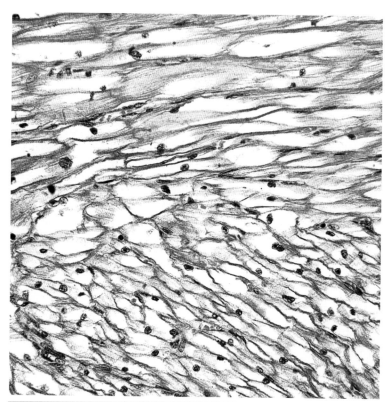

**Fig. 1.20:** Cardiac glycogenosis

Glycogenosis type II (Pompe disease), presents with accumulation of glycogen in the cardiac myocytes which have clear (empty) cytoplasm.

THE CARDIOVASCULAR SYSTEM

CHAPTER

**1**

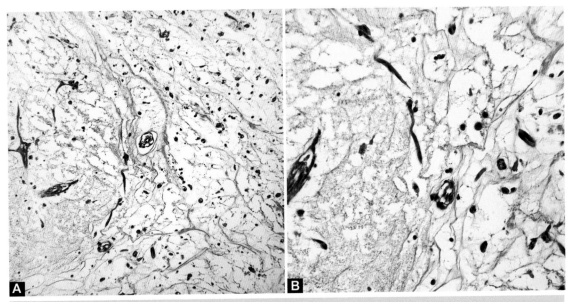

**Figs 1.21A and B:** Atrial myxoma

**A.** This benign tumor is composed of spindle cells and thin walled blood vessels embedded in eosinophilic myxoid material. **B.** Higher power view of spindle-shaped cells in the myxoid stroma.

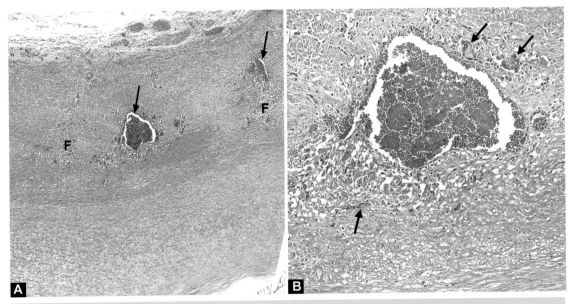

**Figs 1.22A and B:** Giant cell aortitis

**A.** The inflammation in the wall of the aorta is associated with fraying of the connective tissue (F) and formation of blood filled spaces (arrows). **B.** Higher magnification shows that inflammatory infiltrate contains multinucleated giant cells (arrows).

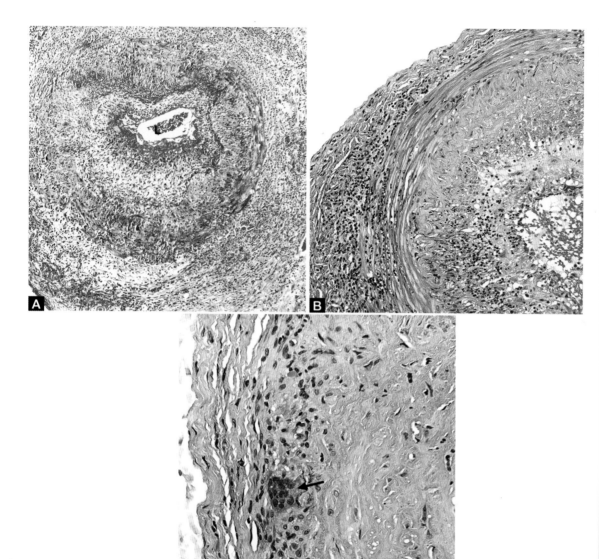

**Figs 1.23A to C:** Temporal arteritis

**A.** This granulomatous transmural inflammation causes narrowing of the arterial lumen. Trichrome stain shows fibrin (red) on the inside of the lumen and disrupted smooth muscle cell layer (red), as well as bluish fibrous tissue. **B.** The inflammatory infiltrates consists of lymphocytes and macrophages permeating all three layers of the temporal artery. **C.** Scatted multinucleated giant cells are also found (arrow).

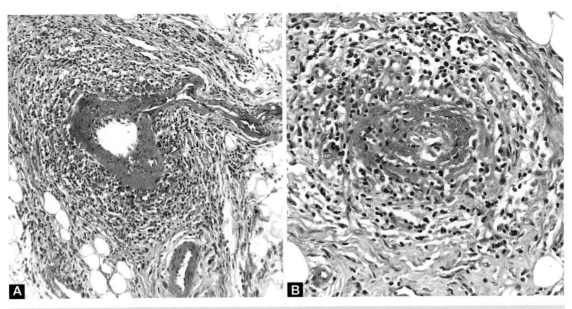

**Figs 1.24A and B:** Polyarteritis nodosa

**A.** This inflammation of a medium sized artery is characterized by a fibrinoid necrosis (pink) of its intima and transmural inflammation. **B.** Fibrinoid material has occluded this small artery which also shows transmural inflammation.

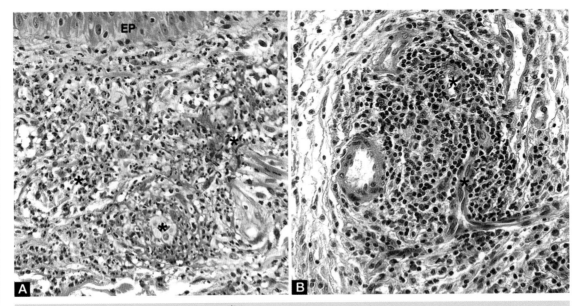

**Figs 1.25A and B:** Hypersensitivity vasculitis

**A.** Leukocytoclastic vasculitis involving the small dermal vessels (asterisks) which are surrounded and partially permeated with acute inflammatory cells. Epidermis (EP) is not involved. **B.** Small dermal blood vessels (asterisks) are surrounded by chronic inflammatory cells, mostly lymphocytes and scattered plasma cells.

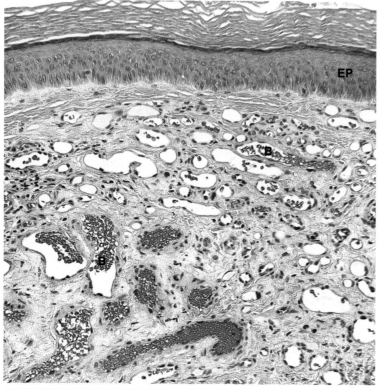

**Fig. 1.26:** Hemangioma

This dermal tumor is composed of dilated capillaries, partially filled with blood (B). The neoplastic capillaries are lined by cells that do not differ from normal endothelial cells. The surface epidermis (EP) is intact.

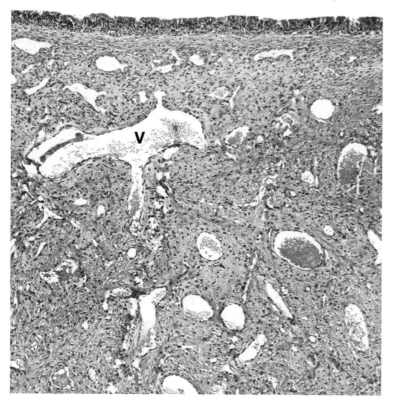

**Fig. 1.27:** Angiofibroma

This nasal tumor is composed of dilated, staghorn-shaped thin-walled blood vessels (V) surrounded by fibrous tissue.

THE CARDIOVASCULAR SYSTEM

CHAPTER

**1**

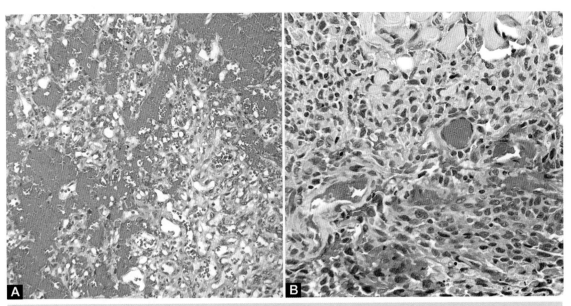

**Figs 1.28A and B:** Angiosarcoma

**A.** This malignant soft tissue tumor is composed of highly atypical endothelial cells lining irregular spaces, some of which contain blood. **B.** Higher magnification shows atypical nuclei forming sheets between abortively formed vessels filled with blood.

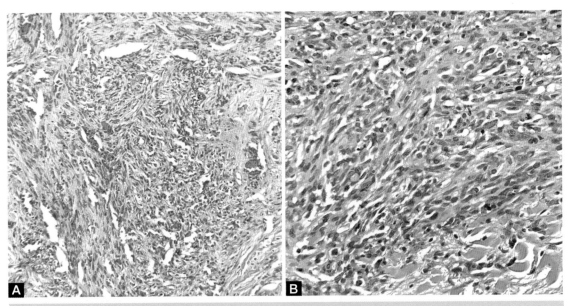

**Figs 1.29A and B:** Kaposi sarcoma

**A.** This tumor of subcutaneous tissue is composed of spindle-shaped cells and extravasated blood in the intercellular spaces. **B.** Higher magnification view of tumor cells with spindle-shaped nuclei and slit-like spaces filled with blood.

# 2 The Respiratory System

*Paul St. Romain, Rashna Madan, Ivan Damjanov*

## Introduction

*The respiratory system may be divided anatomically and functionally into two parts: (a) an upper conducting portion that does not directly participate in gas exchange and (b) a lower respiratory portion that directly involves in gas exchange. In this chapter we will describe some of the salient changes of the upper respiratory system but will mostly deal with the pathologic changes involving the lower respiratory system, i.e. the bronchi and lungs.*

## Upper Respiratory System

The mucosa of the nasal cavity, nasal sinuses, nasopharynx and trachea is lined by pseudostratified ciliated columnar epithelium, also known as respiratory epithelium **(Figs 2.1A and B)**. The only notable exception is the vocal cords of the larynx, which are lined by stratified squamous epithelium. The walls of the trachea and bronchi contain mucous-secreting goblet cells, submucosal glands and bundles of smooth muscles reinforced by an external layer of cartilage.

The most important diseases of the upper respiratory system are:
- Inflammations
- Neoplasms.

### Sinonasal Inflammations

Inflammations of the nasal mucosa and nasal sinuses represent some of the most common human diseases. They may be caused by: (a) infections or (b) allergies to exogenous antigens **(Figs 2.2A and B)**.

*Infectious rhinitis* is most often caused by viruses. Microscopically it presents as edema of the nasal mucosa accompanied by infiltrates of lymphocytes. Bacterial superinfections are common, and inflammation may become mucopurulent or chronic, spreading to the nasal sinuses. As in other sites, these bacterial infections present microscopically with infiltrates of neutrophils dominating in the acute stages of the disease, and infiltrates of lymphocytes, plasma cells and macrophages in the chronic stages of infection. In *chronic mucopurulent sinusitis* the sinuses contain mucus permeated with neutrophils and chronic inflammatory cells.

*Allergic rhinitis* is also characterized by edema and infiltrates of inflammatory cells. In addition to lymphocytes and plasma cells, the inflammatory infiltrate includes eosinophils and mast cells. Long-standing allergic rhinitis may produce *nasal polyps*. These polyps represent redundant folds of the edematous and inflamed respiratory mucosa. Nasal polyps may be sessile or elongated (hanging on a stalk and protruding into the nasal cavity or the sinuses). Microscopically they consist of edematous mucosa infiltrated with chronic inflammatory cells.

### Nasopharyngeal Tumors

Nasopharyngeal tumors may be classified as benign or malignant. The most important benign tumors are sinonasal papillomas, and the most important malignant tumors are squamous cell carcinomas.

*Sinonasal papillomas* are benign tumors arising from the respiratory epithelium of the nose or nasal sinuses. They may be classified as: (a) exophytic or (b) inverted **(Figs 2.3A and B)**. *Exophytic papillomas* are composed of papillae, which have a central vascular core lined by benign squamous epithelium. Parts of the papillae may be covered with ciliated respiratory epithelium. *Inverted papillomas* are composed of similar benign epithelial cells which form nests and sheets invaginating and extending into the underlying stroma. Inverted papillomas are locally invasive tumors that may recur if not removed completely during surgery.

*Nasopharyngeal carcinomas* present microscopically as squamous cell carcinomas which can be classified as: (a) keratinizing carcinomas; (b) nonkeratinizing carcinomas or (c) undifferentiated carcinomas **(Figs 2.4A and B)**. *Keratinizing and nonkeratinizing squamous cell carcinomas* resemble squamous cell carcinomas of the skin or oral cavity and are typically composed of groups of nests and cords of squamous cells, with or without apparent keratinization. *Undifferentiated nasopharyngeal squamous cell carcinomas* are composed of large nonkeratinizing epithelial cells with vesicular nuclei. These tumor cells do not have sharply outlined cell membranes and form syncytium-like sheets. Tumor cells are intermingled with lymphocytes, which accounts for the tumors erroneously being called *lymphoepitheliomas*. Epstein-Barr virus can be identified in most undifferentiated squamous nasopharyngeal tumors, and it is thought to play a role in their pathogenesis.

## Lungs

The lungs consist of bronchi, bronchioli, alveolar ducts and alveoli **(Fig. 2.5)**. The bronchi are lined by ciliated respiratory epithelium, which also contains goblet cells and scattered neuroendocrine cells. They have a wall composed of smooth muscle cells, cartilage and mucus glands. The bronchioli have a thinner wall and are lined by cuboidal epithelium. Bronchioles lack cartilage but are wrapped in a layer of smooth muscle that determines airway diameter. The alveoli are lined by simple squamous epithelium (type I pneumocytes), which shares a basement membrane with underlying capillaries to facilitate gas exchange. The alveoli and their associated capillaries are often referred to together as the "alveolar-capillary unit" in order to emphasize the functional interdependence of alveoli and capillaries. Type II pneumocytes in the alveoli are cuboidal cells that make up less than 10% of alveolar lining, but hold the important task of producing pulmonary surfactant. Alveolar macrophages (dust cells) are found in some alveoli, where they phagocytose any particulate matter not removed by the trachea-bronchial mucociliary apparatus. The lungs are encased in pleura, which is a fibroepithelial tissue derived from mesothelium on the surface of the developing lungs.

The most important diseases of the lung are:
• Alveolar disorders impeding respiration
• Bronchopulmonary infections
• Immunological lung diseases
• Interstitial (restrictive) lung diseases
• Pneumoconioses
• Chronic obstructive pulmonary disease
• Pulmonary neoplasms.

### Alveolar Disorders Impeding Respiration

Respiration involves inhalation and exchange of gases through the alveolar wall into the alveolar capillaries. Respiration may be impeded by any obstruction of the airways; however, here we will discuss only pathologic conditions that impede gas exchange at the level of the alveolar-capillary unit, such as: (a) atelectasis; (b) neonatal respiratory distress syndrome; (c) pulmonary edema and congestion; (d) acute respiratory distress syndrome in adults and (e) pulmonary alveolar proteinosis.

*Atelectasis* denotes a collapse of alveoli resulting in airless lungs **(Fig. 2.6)**. Atelectasis may have many causes. Irrespective of the cause, the alveolar spaces always appear collapsed and their diameter is reduced or almost inapparent. *Compression atelectasis* results from compression of lungs by pleural effusion or air (pneumothorax). In *resorption atelectasis*, airway obstruction leads to absorption of the oxygen in the alveoli with eventual development of negative pressure distal to the obstruction and alveolar collapse on the affected side. *Patchy atelectasis* occurs multifocally in the lungs due to collapse of a group of alveoli. It is related to local deficiency of pulmonary surfactant or a lack of elastic recoil that normally keeps the alveoli open. *Contraction atelectasis* occurs typically underneath the pleura and is usually related to pulmonary fibrosis or lesions of the pleura. Atelectasis is reversible in most instances.

*Neonatal respiratory distress* in prematurely born infants is a consequence of atelectasis. This form of atelectasis related to incomplete expansion of the lungs results from underproduction of functionally active (adult-type) pulmonary surfactant. Due to the collapse of the alveoli, gas exchange may take place only in the alveolar ducts. Since these ducts are not lined by pneumocytes, the inhaled oxygen damages their cell lining. The dead cells leave a denuded surface which is covered with fibrin exudates, known as *hyaline membranes*. Microscopically, the lungs appear atelectatic, whereas the open alveolar ducts and even respiratory bronchioli are lined by fibrin-rich hyaline membranes **(Figs 2.7A and B)**. There is usually no inflammation, but the alveolar capillaries appear dilated and congested. Neonatal respiratory distress syndrome previously had a high mortality, but this has been dramatically reduced with modern treatment.

*Pulmonary edema* is characterized by accumulation of fluid in the alveolar spaces in the form of a transudate or exudate. Transudate most often develops due to increased pressure in the pulmonary veins. Most often it is found in heart failure, when it is typically associated with venous and capillary pulmonary congestion and focal intra-alveolar hemorrhages **(Figs 2.8A and B)**. The fluid in the alveoli has a low concentration of proteins and contains no white blood cells. It thus differs from exudate, which contains more proteins and also inflammatory cells. Protein-rich exudate is usually found in early stages of pneumonia or diffuse alveolar damage (DAD) which is discussed below.

*Acute respiratory distress syndrome (ARDS)* is a clinical term used for a number of conditions characterized pathologically by DAD **(Figs 2.9A and B)**. The ARDS may have numerous causes, which among others include various forms of shock, sepsis, pneumonia, trauma and inhalation of hot fumes or chemical irritants. The common denominator of these conditions is injury to the *alveolar-capillary unit*, followed by disruption of the alveolar lining and capillaries, and inflammation at the site of injury. Elaboration of proinflammatory cytokines results in neutrophil margination and diapedesis into the interstitium, and activation of the coagulation cascade with formation of capillary microthrombi. The alveolar damage is "patched up" by fibrin-rich exudate forming alveolar *hyaline membranes*. The microscopic findings in DAD include accumulation of edema fluid in the alveoli, formation of hyaline membranes, congestion and focal necrosis of alveolar type I pneumocytes. If the patient recovers from the initial injury, type II pneumocytes proliferate to give rise to new type I pneumocytes that will line the alveoli. In later stages of repair granulation tissue may grow into the alveoli organizing the fibrin. Granulation tissue that persists within the alveoli will with time transform into intra-alveolar fibrous scars obliterating the airspaces. The ARDS still has a very high mortality, and most patients who survive have residual chronic respiratory problems.

*Pulmonary alveolar proteinosis* is a rare disease that may impede gas exchange in the alveoli. It may be congenital or acquired secondary to other underlying disorders. Most cases are of the acquired type and occur in adulthood. The formation of antibodies to granulocyte macrophage-colony stimulating factor (GM-CSF) in these individuals leads to impaired function of alveolar macrophages and the accumulation of gelatinous surfactant in the alveoli. This fluid filling the alveolar spaces appears pink, finely granular or amorphous in H&E stained slides **(Fig. 2.10)**. The alveoli themselves are normal and there are no microscopic signs of inflammation.

## Bronchopulmonary Infections

The respiratory tract is vulnerable to airborne pathogens, aspiration of saprophytic or potentially pathogenic oral and nasopharyngeal bacteria, and hematogenous spread of microbes from other sites. Individuals with a dysfunctional mucociliary apparatus (e.g. Kartagener syndrome with ciliary immotility) and those with suppressed cough reflex (e.g. unconscious persons due to stroke, drug addicts or chronic alcoholics) are especially vulnerable. Infection that involves the lung is called *pneumonia*, which is pathogenetically classified as: (a) *community-acquired* and (b) *hospital-acquired*. Pneumonias can be further subclassified etiologically into several groups such as: (a) *bacterial (alveolar) pneumonia*; (b) *viral (interstitial) pneumonia*; (c) *fungal pneumonia* and (d) *pulmonary tuberculosis*.

*Bacterial pneumonia* occurring in the community is most often caused by *Streptococcus pneumoniae*. *Staphylococcus aureus* is an important cause of secondary bacterial pneumonia superimposed on viral infections. *Klebsiella pneumoniae* is the most common cause of gram negative bacterial pneumonia. Gram negative bacteria and *S. aureus* are the most common causes of hospital-acquired bacterial pneumonia. Two histological patterns may be recognized and the disease is thus classified as: (a) bronchopneumonia or (b) lobar pneumonia. *Bronchopneumonia*, which is also known as *lobular pneumonia*, is typically patchy and focal, limited to branches of the bronchial tree and adjacent alveoli (**Figs 2.11A and B**). *Lobar pneumonia* is more serious, involving the entire lobe or more than one lobe of the lungs. It may develop from bronchopneumonia in debilitated patients. It is characterized by four stages of inflammation (**Figs 2.12A and B**). In the first phase, called the phase of *congestion*, numerous bacteria are present and vasculature is engorged. In the next phase, called *red hepatization*, a massive inflammatory exudate fills the alveoli, spreading through the pores of Kohn. It is accompanied by extensive hyperemia of capillaries, imparting a red color to the lung parenchyma when examined macroscopically. In the third phase, called *gray hepatization*, the alveoli are filled with inflammatory cells and fibrin, which expand the alveoli compressing the capillaries. In the final phase, called the phase of *resolution*, the exudate is completely resorbed by macrophages with a variable degree of residual fibrosis.

*Viral pneumonia* is most commonly caused by various strains of influenza virus type A. Cytomegalovirus is an important cause in immunosuppressed patients, patients with AIDS and chemotherapy-treated cancer patients. In contrast to alveolar exudates of bacterial pneumonia, the infiltrates of viral pneumonia are primarily localized to the interstitium (**Figs 2.13A and B**). Radiologically they present with reticular opacities diagnosed as *interstitial pneumonia*. The inflammation typically involves both lungs. Microscopic features include widening of the alveolar septae and infiltration of the alveolar septae by mononuclear cells. Alveolar damage is typically associated with protein-rich pulmonary edema and fibrin-rich hyaline membranes. Virus-induced multinuclear cells are seen in pneumonia caused by measles virus. Cytomegalovirus may cause enlargement of cells containing basophilic intranuclear and cytoplasmic inclusions.

*Fungal pneumonia* occurs most often in immunocompromised persons, but some fungal pathogens may affect healthy individuals as well. Fungal pathogens are readily demonstrable in tissue sections impregnated with silver. *Candida albicans* and *Aspergillus fumigatus* affect debilitated and immunosuppressed persons. They usually provoke a mixed inflammatory response affecting the bronchi and alveoli. *Aspergillus* also characteristically invades blood vessels, and septated hyphae with acute-angle branching can be visualized crossing into blood vessel lumens (**Figs 2.14A and B**). *Pneumocystis jiroveci* almost exclusively affects immunocompromised persons. It produces a frothy or bubbly proteinaceous alveolar exudate that contains the fungi (**Figs 2.15A and B**). Dimorphic fungi, such as *Histoplasma capsulatum*, *Blastomyces dermatitidis* and *Coccidioides immitis*, are known to occasionally cause symptomatic infection in normal hosts. Infections usually result in the formation of granulomas with central necrosis containing the causative organisms (**Figs 2.16A and B**).

*Pulmonary tuberculosis* is the most common manifestation of infection with *Mycobacterium tuberculosis*. In most instances the infection results in the formation of granulomas (**Figs 2.17A and B**). In individuals with active cell-mediated immunity, the *primary tuberculosis* infection is walled off into a granuloma (Ghon focus), which has a central caseous necrosis due to the presence of bacterial mycolic acid. A pulmonary granuloma accompanied by a granuloma in a mediastinal lymph node is termed a Ghon complex. Over time, these granulomas may calcify, but still contain bacteria which may serve as centers for reactivation of infection. Reactivation causes the typical lesions of *secondary* *tuberculosis*, which may be found in the lungs or extrapulmonary locations. Hematogenous spread in the lungs results in the formation of numerous small granulomas, typical of miliary tuberculosis. Systemic hematogenous spread may cause lesions in the kidney, bones, brain and many other organs. Secondary spread may also occur through the expectorated sputum, which may affect the larynx. Swallowed infected sputum may cause gastrointestinal tuberculosis, which most often presents with lesions of the ileocecal region.

## Immunologic Lung Diseases

The lungs may be the primary organs affected in autoimmune disease, but they are additionally often caught in the crossfire of systemic diseases. The most important immunological diseases involving the lung are: (a) asthma; (b) hypersensitivity pneumonitis; (c) sarcoidosis and (d) Wegener granulomatosis.

*Asthma* is a disease of large airways characterized by chronic inflammation combined with episodic, reversible bronchospasm. Episodes are most commonly related to an IgE mediated, Gel and Coombs type I hypersensitivity reaction (*atopic asthma*). In other cases the asthmatic attacks are precipitated by industrial or environmental air pollutants, smoking, drugs (such as aspirin) or exercise (*non-atopic asthma*). Over time, repeated airway inflammation leads to characteristic microscopic changes of all layers of the airway, including mucous cell and submucosal gland hyperplasia, thickening of the basement membrane and bronchial smooth muscle, and chronic inflammation with an increase in vascularity in the lamina propria **(Figs 2.18A and B)**. Occasionally aggregates of an eosinophil-derived protein called galectin-10 may form so-called Charcot-Leyden crystals.

*Hypersensitivity pneumonitis* is a spectrum of diseases in which an inappropriate immune response is mounted to an inhaled antigen, resulting in damage to small airways. Examples related to commonly recognized antigens include farmer's lung, pigeon breeder's lung and humidifier/air-conditioner lung. Unlike asthma, large airways are not generally affected, and the hypersensitivity reaction is probably a mixed Gel and Coombs type III/IV (humoral and cell mediated immunity). Microscopic features include chronic interstitial inflammation, fibrosis and noncaseating granulomas (in two-thirds of patients) **(Figs 2.19A and B)**.

*Sarcoidosis* is a systemic autoimmune disease of unknown etiology. The disease has a striking predilection for African Americans. Affected individuals may have characteristic abnormalities of cell-mediated immunity; however, the defining feature of the disease is multi-organ involvement by noncaseating granulomas, especially in the lungs and hilar lymph nodes. The lung lesions are usually small and are generally located near bronchi, lymphatic channels or blood vessels. Stellate inclusions within the giant cells (asteroid bodies) and calcified aggregates of proteins (Schaumann bodies) may be present but are not pathognomonic for sarcoidosis **(Fig. 2.20)**.

*Wegener granulomatosis* classically affects the upper respiratory tract (chronic sinusitis), lower respiratory tract (pneumonitis and cavitary lung lesions) and kidneys (crescentic glomerulonephritis). Antibodies to proteinase-3, an antigen found in the cytoplasm and on the surface of neutrophils, are probably involved in the pathogenesis of the disease by causing neutrophil degranulation and lesions in small blood vessels. These antibodies are readily detected in serum of affected patients and thus are also diagnostically useful. Pulmonary lesions include vasculitis involving small and medium sized vessels, and confluent granulomas with central necrosis **(Figs 2.21A and B)**. Areas of necrosis are arranged in a "geographic pattern" (i.e. irregularly shaped, like outlines of countries in a geographic atlas), and tend to be confluent, which leads to formation of cavitary lesions. Healing lesions may show primarily fibrosis and scarring, and recanalization of the thrombi occluding the damaged blood vessels.

## Interstitial Lung Diseases

This group of diseases is characterized by inflammation of the alveolar interstitium, resulting in fibrosis that is referred to as "honeycomb lung" in its severe end-stage form. Clinically, they present with a restrictive pattern of pulmonary function tests, and so are often referred to as restrictive lung diseases. The etiology of the interstitial lung diseases is poorly understood. The most important interstitial lung diseases are: (a) idiopathic pulmonary fibrosis; (b) desquamative interstitial pneumonia and (c) cryptogenic organizing pneumonia.

*Idiopathic pulmonary fibrosis* is a progressive disease of unknown etiology that carries a poor prognosis. The disease is a diagnosis of exclusion and depends on presence of certain clinical, radiologic and pathologic features. The pathologic findings are termed usual interstitial pneumonia (UIP), which is characterized by a mixture of areas of normal-appearing lung combined with cellular areas of mild fibrosis (early lesions) and areas of dense collagenous fibrosis **(Figs 2.22A to D)**. The areas of dense fibrosis destroy the normal architecture of the lung to form cystic spaces (honeycomb fibrosis). A varying degree of chronic inflammation may be present in the bronchi or in the fibrous tissue.

*Desquamative interstitial pneumonia* is a smoking-associated interstitial lung disease. The precise etiologic mechanism is unknown, but complete recovery can be made with smoking cessation and immunosuppressive therapy. Microscopically, macrophages with brown cytoplasmic pigment fill the alveolar spaces. These macrophages were originally thought to be desquamated pneumocytes, hence the misnomer for this disease. Alveolar walls are thickened, fibrotic and infiltrated with chronic inflammatory cells **(Figs 2.23A and B)**.

*Cryptogenic organizing pneumonia* (also known as *bronchiolitis obliterans organizing pneumonia* or BOOP) is a disease of unknown etiology characterized by obliteration of the alveolar lumina. The hallmark of this disease is fibroblastic granulation tissue forming balls or spindles (*Masson bodies*) in the alveoli, alveolar ducts and even bronchioli **(Figs 2.24A and B)**. All Masson bodies in a lung appear to be at the same stage of organization. Interstitial fibrosis is relatively mild or absent. It is worth noting that similar intra-alveolar plugs composed of granulation tissue may be seen in healing stages of bacterial pneumonia or various forms of ARDS, but in such cases the organizing granulation tissue is usually in various stages of organization, and residual inflammatory exudate or hyaline membranes are readily recognized.

## Pneumoconioses

Despite the best efforts of the mucociliary apparatus, inhaled fine particulate matter can settle into the alveoli. Alveolar macrophages provide some degree of protection by phagocytosing these particles, but chronic inhalation can overwhelm the ability of the alveolar macrophages to clear debris. Hence, this category of lung diseases is called pneumoconioses (dusty lung diseases). Although most individuals will show mild or no symptoms, in a minority the particles will cause enough local damage and fibrosis to cause a restrictive (interstitial) lung disease.

*Coal miner pneumoconiosis* is a professional disease that has historically affected workers employed in mining and processing of coal. Inhalation of carbon dust results in accumulation of black pigment in alveolar macrophages and pulmonary lymphatics known as *anthracosis* **(Figs 2.25A and B)**. Some degree of anthracosis may be detected in the lungs of smokers or city dwellers and generally is clinically inconsequential. However, in coal miners exposed to dust that contains not only carbon particles but also other more fibrogenic minerals, progressive massive fibrosis of the lungs can develop over a period of years. Inhalation of silica results in the formation of fibrotic nodules and areas of confluent pulmonary fibrosis known as *anthracosilicosis*.

*Asbestosis* is a fibrotic lung disease caused by chronic inhalation of asbestos particles. Asbestos is an industrial silicate that forms fibers, which can penetrate deeply into the lung and even reach the pleura. Here, these fibers cause oxidative damage and may even bind other inhaled toxins such as those found in cigarette smoke. Hence, chronic asbestos exposure is a risk factor for lung carcinoma and malignant mesothelioma, and smoking synergistically increases risk for lung carcinoma. As is characteristic for the pneumoconioses, the lungs show diffuse interstitial fibrosis. Asbestos fibers can be seen on H&E as golden brown rods "ferruginous bodies" **(Figs 2.26A and**

**B).** The brown color likely comes from ferritin that is acquired when phagocytic cells attempt to remove the asbestos fiber.

### Chronic Obstructive Pulmonary Disease

Chronic obstructive pulmonary disease (COPD) is characterized by irreversible airway obstruction as measured by pulmonary function tests. Over 90% of cases can be attributed to cigarette smoking, although the majority of smokers never develop the disease. The two prototypical manifestations of COPD are: (a) chronic bronchitis and (b) emphysema; however, most patients have a mixture of features of both diseases.

*Chronic bronchitis* is the manifestation of COPD in large airways. It is a clinical diagnosis, defined as three months of productive cough of unknown origin in two consecutive years. Damage to large airways by cigarette smoke induces chronic inflammation, submucosal gland hyperplasia and protective goblet cell or squamous cell metaplasia **(Figs 2.27A and B)**. The result is mucous overproduction and productive cough, along with the possibility of progression to squamous dysplasia and carcinoma. Cigarette smoke also damages the mucociliary apparatus, predisposing the individual to infection. The severity of disease can be gauged microscopically by measurement of the ratio of thickness of the submucosal gland layer to the total mucosal thickness (Reid index). A normal Reid index is 0.4.

*Emphysema* is a form of COPD characterized by destruction of alveoli distal to the terminal bronchioles **(Figs 2.28A and B)**. It is thought to result from a relative increase in protease activity over antiprotease activity in the lung, resulting in damage to the elastic tissue of the lung. This elastic tissue normally pulls the small airways open, so the ensuing loss of radial traction by small airways on one another causes them to collapse during expiration, creating functional airway obstruction. The role of cigarette smoke in this process is mediated by reactive oxygen species that inactivate the antiprotease α1-antitrypsin and recruit damaging inflammatory cells (mainly neutrophils and macrophages) to the alveoli. Congenital deficiencies in α1-antitrypsin can result in emphysema even in the absence of cigarette smoking. Emphysema resulting from cigarette smoking is classically centriacinar (affects the respiratory bronchioles primarily, not the alveoli) and is most severe in the upper lobes. By contrast, α1-antitrypsin deficiency typically affects the lower lobes more severely in a panacinar pattern.

### Pulmonary Neoplasms

Primary lung cancer is the most common cancer diagnosis in the world (excluding skin cancers); in the United States it is the second most common non-skin cancer in men and in women, trailing only prostate and breast cancer, respectively. The vast majority of those affected are cigarette smokers, and there is substantial epidemiological and molecular evidence that the carcinogens (over 1,200 identified) in cigarette smoke cause the panel of genetic mutations that lead to malignant transformation.

The most important histologic types of lung cancer are: (a) squamous cell carcinoma; (b) adenocarcinoma; (c) bronchioloalveolar carcinoma; (d) large cell (undifferentiated) carcinoma; (e) small cell carcinoma; (f) carcinoid; (g) mesothelioma and (h) metastases. However, the most important distinction clinically is whether the cancer is small cell carcinoma or non-small cell carcinoma, due to differences in treatment between the groups of tumors. Overall, lung tumors have a poor prognosis and account for more cancer deaths in the United States than any other type of cancer.

*Squamous cell carcinoma* classically arises from central bronchi in the lung. Although there is normally not squamous epithelium in the bronchi, the chronic injury caused by cigarette smoke can lead to squamous metaplasia, followed by dysplasia, carcinoma in situ and invasive squamous cell carcinoma. Thus, these tumors are etiologically highly associated with smoking. They are notorious for producing parathyroid hormone-related peptide—resulting in hypercalcemia. Microscopically these tumors are indistinguishable from squamous cell carcinomas arising in other sites **(Figs 2.29A and B)**.

*Adenocarcinoma* is now the most common variant of lung cancer. For unknown reasons it more commonly occurs in women and in peripheral airways, where it is thought to arise from bronchial epithelium. This common origin of adenocarcinoma and squamous cell carcinoma is highlighted by occasional tumors that express both growth patterns. Adenocarcinoma of the lung may display acinar, papillary, bronchioloalveolar and solid variants. In general, it is histologically indistinguishable from adenocarcinoma originating from other sites. Immunohistochemical stains are used to distinguish metastatic from primary lung adenocarcinomas. Pulmonary adenocarcinomas typically react with antibodies to thyroid transcription factor 1 (TTF-1), and cytokeratin CK7, and do not react with the antibodies to CK20 (Figs 2.30A and B).

*Bronchioloalveolar carcinoma* is an important subtype of adenocarcinoma with a more favorable prognosis and indolent course than other types. It occurs at terminal bronchioles, where it is thought to originate from stem cells. The tumor cells may produce mucin, and do not invade surrounding structures. This unique growth pattern is often referred to as "lepidic" (scaly), and neoplastic cells may be described as butterflies sitting on top of a fence (Figs 2.31A and B).

*Large cell (undifferentiated) carcinoma* is a very poorly differentiated malignant tumor characterized by large, anaplastic cells with prominent nucleoli and frequent mitoses. These tumors may have foci that are architecturally and immunohistochemically suggestive of squamous, adenocarcinomatous or neuroendocrine differentiation (Figs 2.32A and B). Hence, it is thought that these tumors are probably very poorly differentiated variants of other histologic subtypes.

*Small cell carcinoma* is a highly malignant tumor of neuroendocrine origin with a strong relationship to smoking. The tumor is composed of sheets of small cells, which have hyperchromatic oval or round nuclei and scant cytoplasm; this accounts for molding of closely spaced nuclei. Frequent mitoses and necrosis betray this tumor's malignant potential. Necrosis may be so extensive as to cause cellular build-up on adjacent vascular walls, resulting in basophilic staining of vasculature (Azzopardi effect). Immunohistochemical stains to typical neuroendocrine markers are generally positive, and electron microscopy reveals neurosecretory granules in the cytoplasm of tumor cells (Figs 2.33A and B). Paraneoplastic syndromes related to hormonal secretion are common.

*Carcinoid tumors* are locally invasive neuroendocrine tumors of low malignancy. They generally occur in younger patients than do other types of lung cancer and are less strongly associated with smoking. Tumor cells appear benign and grow in nests and trabeculae (Figs 2.34A to D). Neurosecretory granules visible by electron microscopy are present in the cytoplasm. Immunohistochemically these cells typically react with the markers for neuroendocrine cells, such as chromogranin or synaptophysin. The release of serotonin from some tumors accounts for the associated clinical constellation of symptoms, such as facial flushing, bronchospasm and intestinal spasm with bouts of diarrhea, known as carcinoid syndrome.

*Mesothelioma* is a malignant tumor arising from the parietal or visceral pleura (mesothelium). As discussed previously, it is highly associated with asbestos exposure. Embryologically, the mesothelium may give rise to epithelial and stromal tissues. Hence, the tumor may show either one of these patterns or have a biphasic pattern, including both epithelial and stromal cells (Figs 2.35A to D). The tumor is highly malignant, and prognosis is poor.

*Metastases* to the lung most commonly arise hematogenously and present as multiple small nodules. The lung is the most common organ of distant metastasis in the body. The histologic pattern of the tumor mirrors that of the primary cancers, which are most often adenocarcinomas (Fig. 2.36). Metastatic adenocarcinomas may resemble primary pulmonary adenocarcinomas of the lung, and immunohistochemistry must be used to determine the nature of the tumor. Primary adenocarcinomas usually react with antibodies to TTF-1 and keratin CK7, whereas colonic adenocarcinoma are TTF-1 and CK7 negative, and keratin CK20 positive.

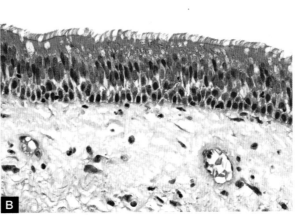

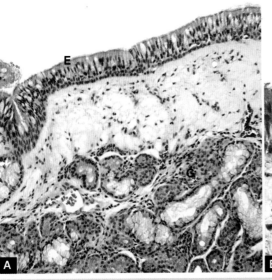

**Figs 2.1A and B:** Normal nasal respiratory mucosa

**A.** The surface is covered with ciliated pseudostratified epithelium (E) that also contains scattered goblet cells. In the lamina propria there are seromucous glands (G). **B.** Higher magnification illustrates the ciliated pseudostratified epithelium and the loosely structured upper portion of the lamina propria.

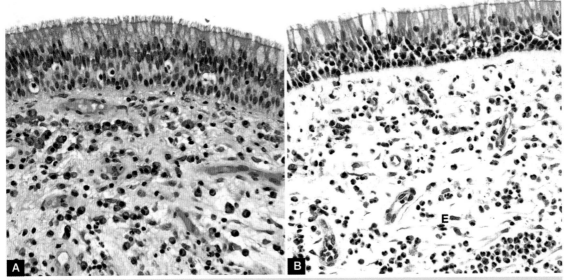

**Figs 2.2A and B:** Chronic nasal inflammation

**A.** Chronic infectious rhinitis presents with an infiltrate of lymphocytes, plasma cells and macrophages in the lamina propria. **B.** Allergic rhinitis is characterized by infiltrates of chronic inflammatory cells intermixed with prominent eosinophils (E) in the lamina propria. Basophils are also present but they cannot be easily recognized without special stains.

THE RESPIRATORY SYSTEM

CHAPTER

**2**

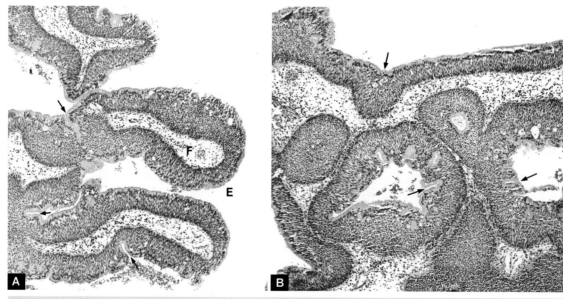

**Figs 2.3A and B:** Sinonasal papilloma

**A.** Exophytic papilloma is composed of papillae which have a central fibrovascular core (F) and non-keratinizing squamous epithelium (E). Foci of respiratory epithelium may be seen as well (arrows). **B.** Inverted papilloma resembles the exophytic papillomas and is on its surface covered with non-keratinizing squamous epithelium with foci of respiratory epithelium (top arrow). This epithelium invaginates into the underlying stroma forming solid or cystic nests which may contain foci of respiratory epithelium (bottom arrows).

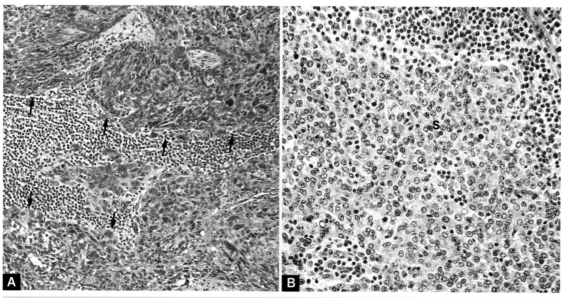

**Figs 2.4A and B:** Nasopharyngeal carcinoma

**A.** Nonkeratinizing squamous cell carcinoma is composed of squamous cells arranged into nests sharply demarcated from the lymphocyte rich stroma. Arrows indicate the outer border of epithelial tumor nests. **B.** Undifferentiated squamous cell carcinoma is composed of nonkeratinizing squamous cells (S). Tumor cells that have clear vesicular nuclei, indistinct cytoplasm and are intermixed with lymphocytes.

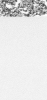

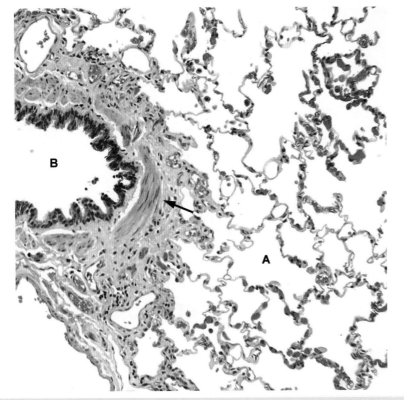

**Fig. 2.5:** Normal lung

The bronchiolus (B) lined by cuboidal epithelium surrounded by bundles of smooth muscle cells (arrow). The adjacent alveolar ducts and alveoli (A) have thin walls that contain capillaries.

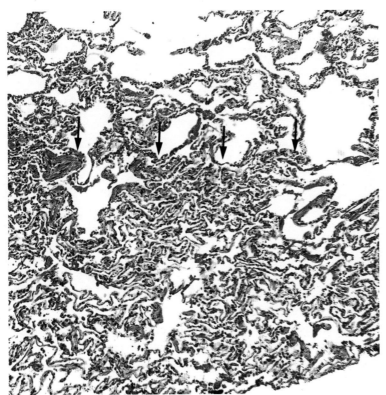

**Fig. 2.6:** Atelectasis

The border between the normally aerated alveoli in the upper part of the figure and the airless atelectatic alveoli in the lower part of the figure is marked with arrows.

THE RESPIRATORY SYSTEM

CHAPTER

**2**

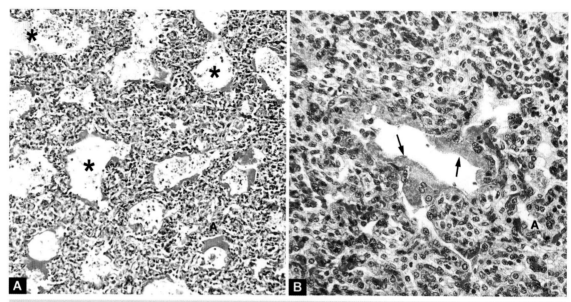

**Figs 2.7A and B:** Neonatal respiratory distress syndrome

**A.** An overview photograph of the lung shows dilated respiratory bronchioli and alveolar ducts (asterisks) lined by hyaline membranes, and atelectasis of alveoli (A) around them. **B.** Higher magnification figure illustrates the hyaline membranes (arrows) and atelectatic alveoli (A).

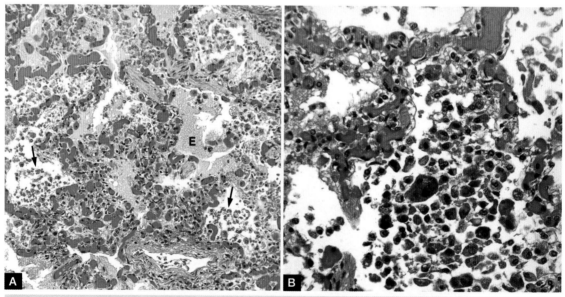

**Figs 2.8A and B:** Pulmonary edema and congestion

**A.** The alveolar capillaries are dilated and filled with blood, some of which has spilled into their lumens (arrows). Lumen of some alveoli also contains proteinaceous (eosinophilic) edema fluid (E). **B.** Chronic congestion showing hemosiderin-laden alveolar macrophages within an alveolar duct and alveoli.

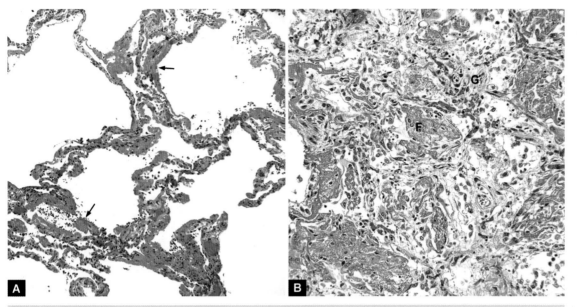

**Figs 2.9A and B:** Acute respiratory distress syndrome
**A.** The dilated alveoli and alveolar ducts are lined by fibrin rich hyaline membranes (arrows). The clear spaces in the alveoli were most likely filled with low protein-content edema fluid that was washed out during processing of the lung tissue for the preparation of microscopy slides. **B.** Hyaline membranes cannot be removed readily from the alveoli. If the patient survives ARDS, granulation tissue (G) fills the alveoli growing into the fibrin (F) in a manner similar to the organization of intravascular thrombi or wound healing.

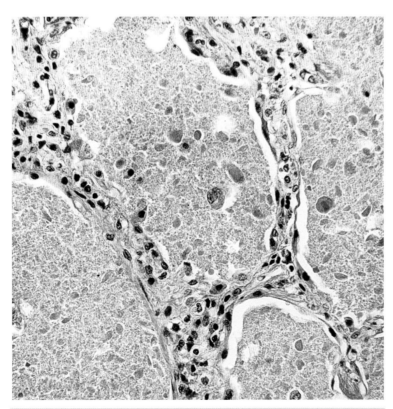

**Fig. 2.10:** Alveolar proteinosis
Almost all alveoli are filled with finely granular eosinophilic material.

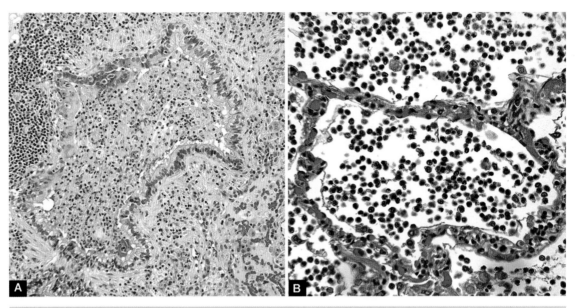

**Figs 2.11A and B:** Bronchopneumonia

**A.** The bronchus contains a protein rich acute inflammatory exudate, predominantly composed of neutrophils.
**B.** The adjacent alveoli have congested walls and contain acute inflammatory cells in their lumen.

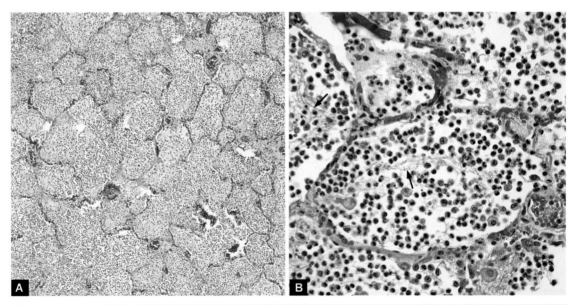

**Figs 2.12A and B:** Lobar pneumonia

**A.** All alveoli are filled with acute inflammatory cells. **B.** At higher magnification the intra-alveolar exudate appears composed of neutrophils, some of which have condensed (pyknotic) nuclei, and thin strands of fibrin (arrows).

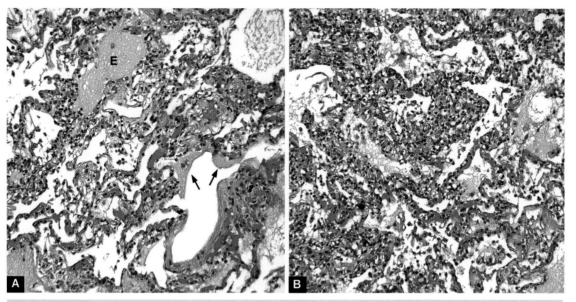

**Figs 2.13A and B:** Interstitial pneumonia caused by viruses

**A.** The alveoli are mostly open but some contain edema fluid (E) or hyaline membranes (arrows). The inflammatory cells in the wall of the alveoli contribute to their thickening and rigidity thus preventing them from collapsing. **B.** Another example of interstitial inflammation contributing to the thickening of the alveolar walls. The alveolar lumens appear mostly open, but some contain eosinophilic edema fluid.

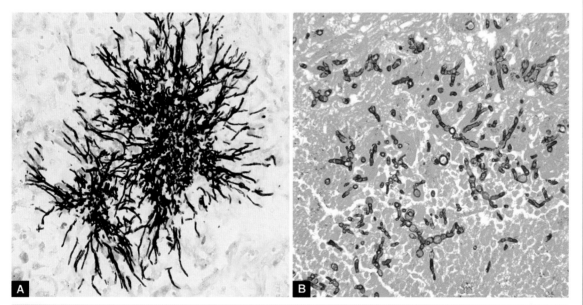

**Figs 2.14A and B:** Aspergillus pneumonia

**A.** Fungal hyphae (black) forming a cluster are demonstrated here with a special silver impregnation stain. **B.** Fungal hyphae and yeast forms (black) are seen in the staining necrotic material replacing parts of the lung parenchyma, which stains green in this figure (silver stain).

THE RESPIRATORY SYSTEM

CHAPTER

**2**

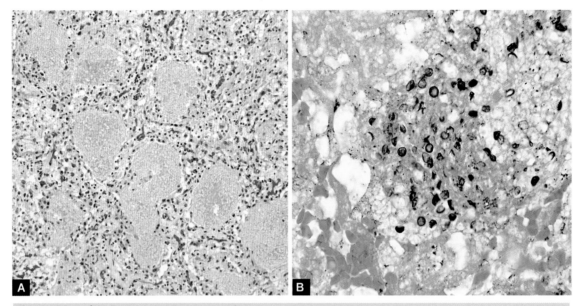

**Figs 2.15A and B:** Pneumocystis pneumonia

**A.** Alveoli are filled with bubbly proteinaceous alveolar exudate. **B.** *Pneumocystis jiroveci* can be demonstrated in the intra-alveolar exudate with the silver impregnation technique, which stains the fungal cysts black.

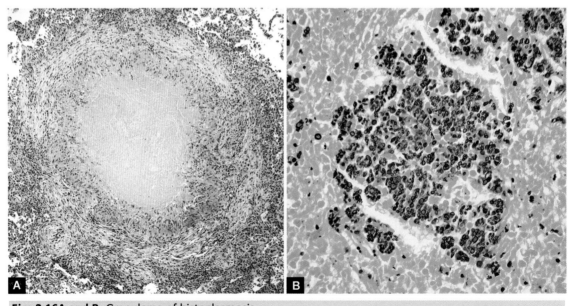

**Figs 2.16A and B:** Granuloma of histoplasmosis

**A.** The granuloma has a necrotic center surrounded by epithelioid macrophages and lymphocytes. Similar granulomas are found in tuberculosis. **B.** Histoplasma capsulatum can be demonstrated in the necrotic material with silver impregnation technique.

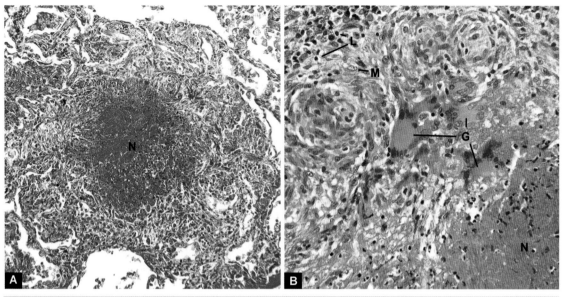

**Figs 2.17A and B:** Tuberculosis

**A.** Necrotizing granuloma of miliary tuberculosis has a necrotic center (N) ringed by epithelioid macrophages and lymphocytes. **B.** At higher magnification the necrotic center (N) is composed of amorphous granular eosinophilic material. Epithelioid macrophages (M) have clear vesicular nuclei, whereas the lymphocytes appear dark and round (L). There are also scattered multinucleated giant cells (G).

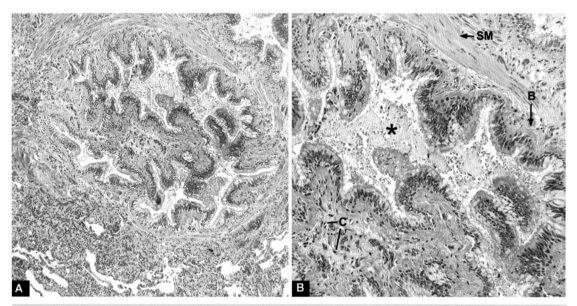

**Figs 2.18A and B:** Asthma

**A.** The bronchioli are dilated, irregularly shaped and surrounded by bundles of hypertrophic smooth muscle cells. **B.** At higher magnification one may see mucus in the lumen of the bronchiolus (asterisk), the thick epithelial basement membrane (B), bundles of smooth muscle cells (SM) and inflammatory cells (C).

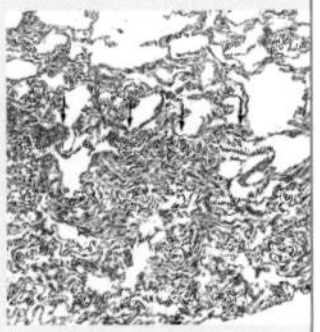

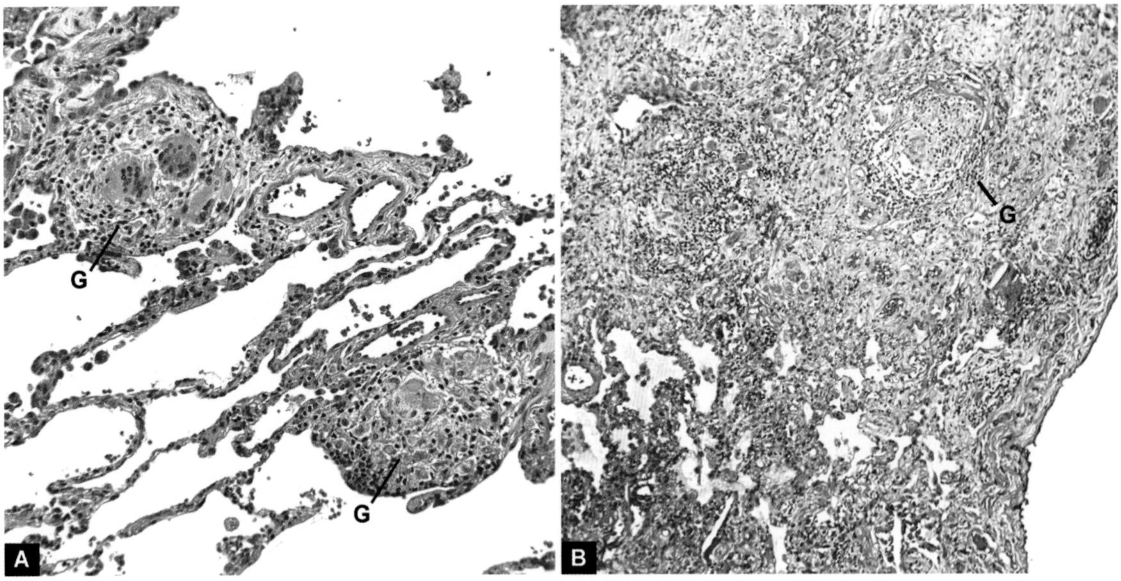

**Figs 2.19A and B:** Hypersensitivity pneumonitis

**A.** The alveolar walls contain loosely structured noncaseating granulomas (G). **B.** In advanced stages of the disease there is prominent fibrosis replacing alveoli, some of which are still preserved in the lower part of the figure. In the areas of fibrosis there are granulomas (G).

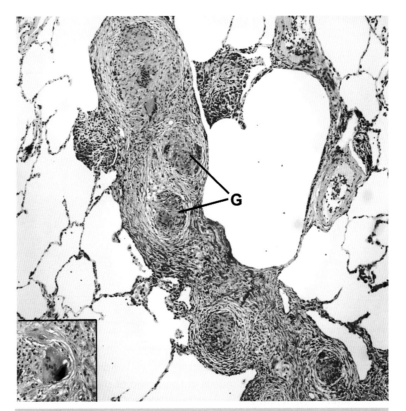

**Fig. 2.20:** Sarcoidosis

Multiple well-formed, noncaseating granulomas (G) are found in the alveolar walls. Surrounding alveoli appear normal. Inset shows calcification within a giant cell (Schaumann body).

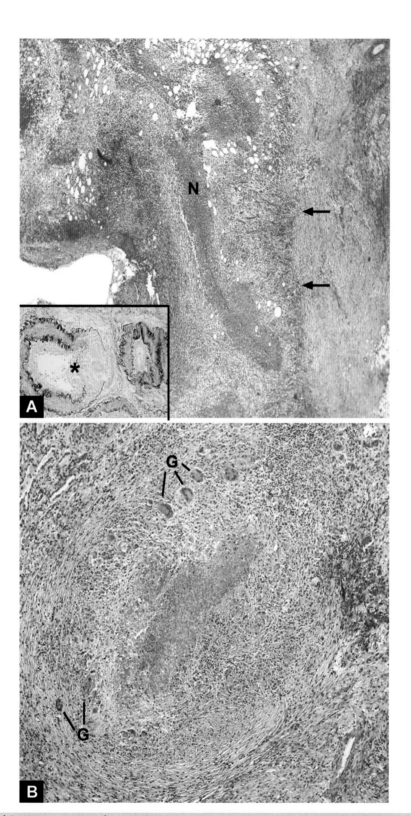

**Figs 2.21A and B:** Wegener granulomatosis

**A.** Irregular areas of necrosis (N), related to areas of inflammation (arrows). The inset shows a focally destroyed wall of an inflamed pulmonary artery (asterisk). The slide was stained with the elastica Van Gieson stain, which stains the elastic laminae black and demonstrates the lack of elastic tissue in part of the vessel wall. **B.** Higher magnification of another area shows that the area of irregular necrosis is surrounded by granulomatous inflammation containing giant cells (G).

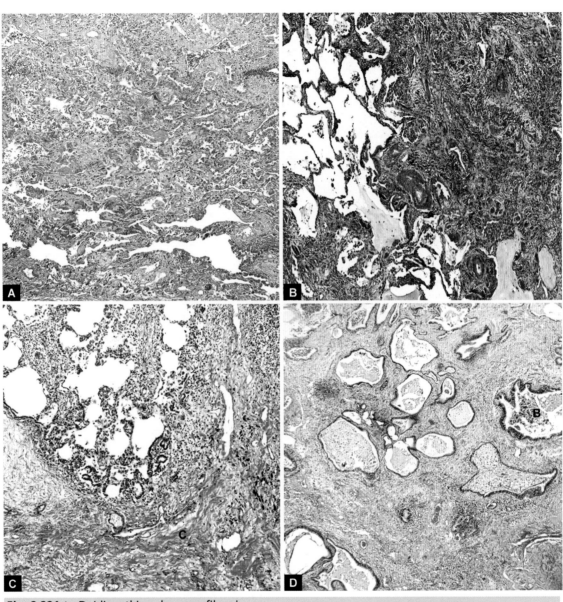

**Figs 2.22A to D:** Idiopathic pulmonary fibrosis

**A.** Normal alveoli have been destroyed and are replaced by fibrous tissue. **B.** Special stain (trichrome) used to stain the connective tissue blue shows that the alveoli are preserved only in the left part of the figure .On the right the alveoli have been replaced by fibrous tissue. **C.** Irregular airspaces surrounded by thick fibrous tissue infiltrated with chronic inflammatory cells. Parts of the lung are replaced with solid fibrous scars composed of hyalinized collagen (C), which stains red with eosin. **D.** Advanced pulmonary fibrosis replacing the alveoli and surrounding irregularly shaped terminal parts of the bronchial tree (B), commonly known as "honeycomb lung".

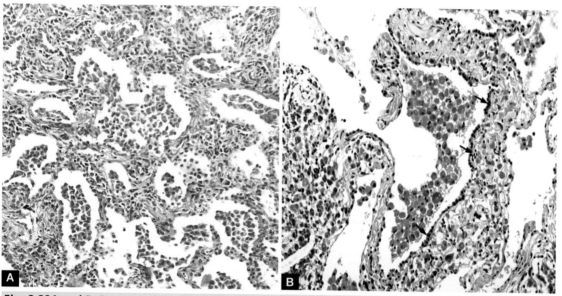

**Figs 2.23A and B:** Desquamative interstitial pneumonia

**A.** The alveoli are infiltrated with chronic inflammatory cells and appear thickened, whereas the alveolar lumen contains aggregates of macrophages. **B.** Higher power view of intra-alveolar macrophages showing that these cells have a brownish cytoplasm. Air spaces are lined by cuboidal cells (arrows).

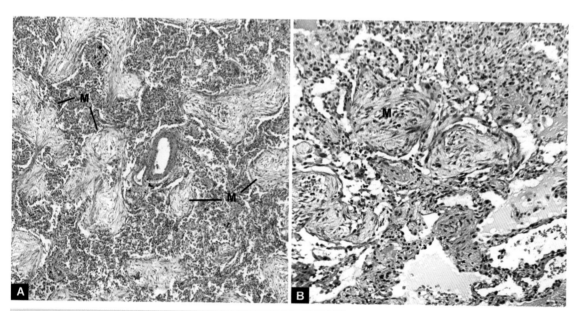

**Figs 2.24A and B:** Cryptogenic organizing pneumonia

**A.** The alveoli are filled with loosely structured fibroblastic Masson bodies (M). **B.** At higher magnification alveolar Masson bodies (M) appear composed of fibroblasts and thin walled capillaries.

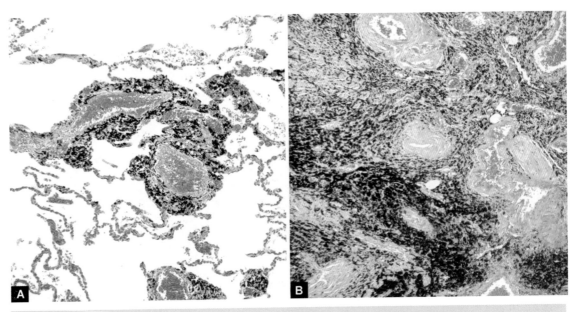

**Figs 2.25A and B:** Anthracosis

**A.** Carbon particles accumulate in the fibrotic alveolar walls. **B.** A fibrotic scar contains large amounts of anthracotic pigment.

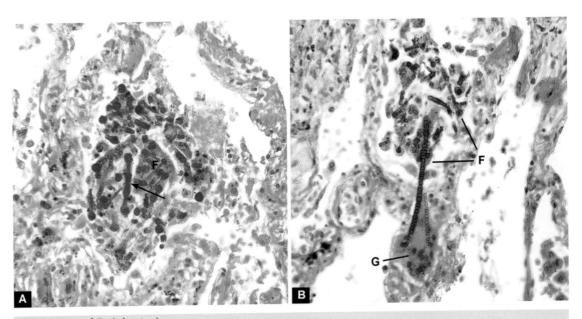

**Figs 2.26A and B:** Asbestosis

**A.** Ferruginous bodies (F) appear brown and form aggregates in fibrotic parts of the lung. Some of them are dumbbell-shaped (arrow). **B.** Some ferruginous bodies (F) may be very long and are engulfed in foreign body giant cells (G).

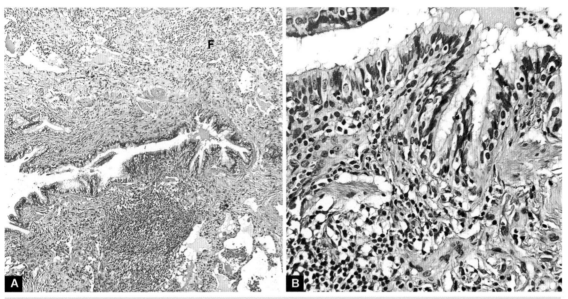

**Figs 2.27A and B:** Chronic bronchitis

**A.** Dilated irregularly shaped bronchiolus has a thickened wall infiltrated with inflammatory cells and is surrounded by fibrous tissue (F) replacing the alveoli. **B.** At higher magnification one may see the hyperplastic bronchial epithelium and chronic inflammatory cells in the wall of the bronchus.

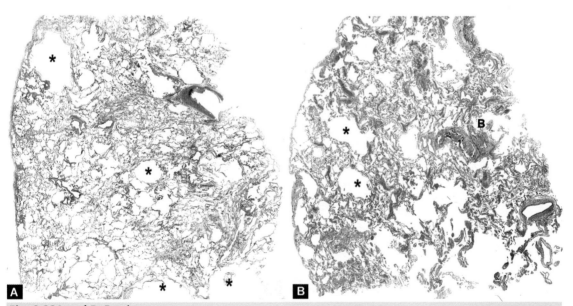

**Figs 2.28A and B:** Emphysema

**A.** A panoramic view of the emphysematous lungs shows irregularly dilated terminal airspaces (asterisks). **B.** Dilatation of the terminal airspaces (asterisks) is in this case associated with chronic inflammation of the bronchioli (B) and adjacent fibrotic alveoli.

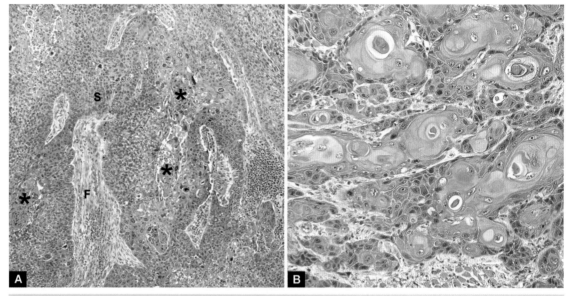

**Figs 2.29A and B:** Squamous cell carcinoma

**A.** The tumor is composed of nests and strands of keratinizing squamous epithelium (S) surrounded by fibrous stroma (F). Keratinized centers are marked with asterisks. **B.** Another squamous cell carcinoma shows prominent foci of concentric keratinization (keratin pearls).

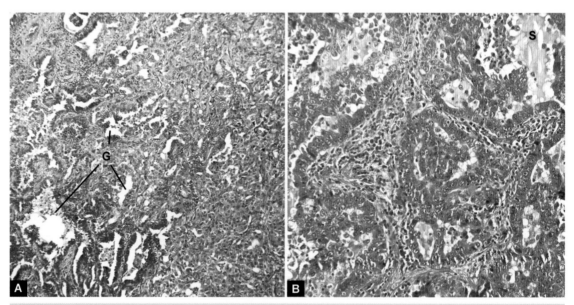

**Figs 2.30A and B:** Adenocarcinoma

**A.** Tumor forms duct-like or gland-like structures (G), which on the right side of the figure appear collapsed or consolidated. **B.** Tumor cells arranged into interconnected stands enclose lumina, imparting them a gland-like or duct-like appearance. Some ducts contain secretory material (S).

ATLAS OF HISTOPATHOLOGY

CHAPTER

**2**

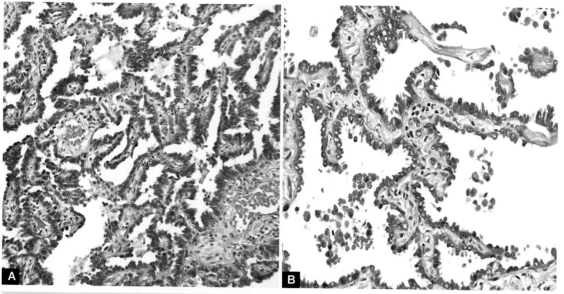

**Figs 2.31A and B:** Bronchioloalveolar carcinoma
**A.** Cuboidal tumor cells cover the inner side of fibrotic alveoli, which still appear "empty", i.e. filled with air.
**B.** Higher power view of the fibrotic alveoli lined by hyperchromatic cuboidal tumor cells. Note the widely open alveolar spaces, and lack of invasion of the tumor cells into the stroma.

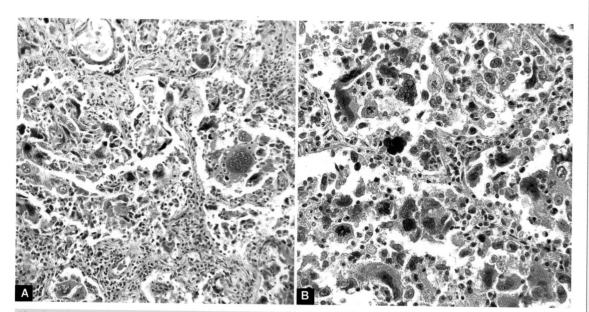

**Figs 2.32A and B:** Large cell undifferentiated carcinoma
**A.** The tumor is composed of cells that vary in size and shape, arranged without any distinct pattern. **B.** This tumor is composed of hyperchromatic cells, many of which have very large, irregularly shaped nuclei.

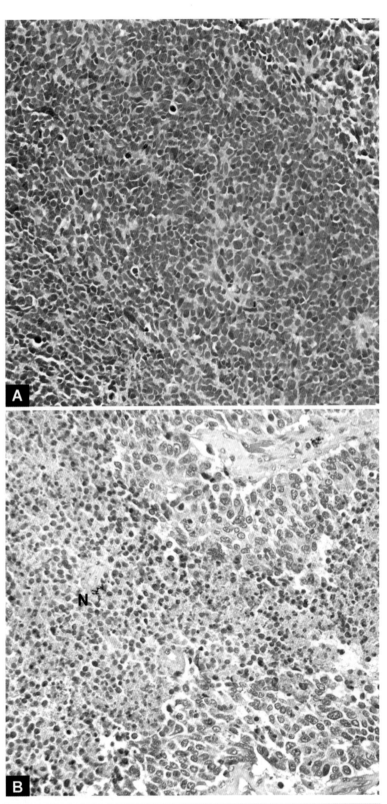

**Figs 2.33A and B:** Small cell carcinoma

**A.** The tumor is composed of densely compacted cells that have oval shaped dark blue nuclei and scant cytoplasm. **B.** Another view of the tumor showing areas central necrosis (N).

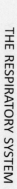

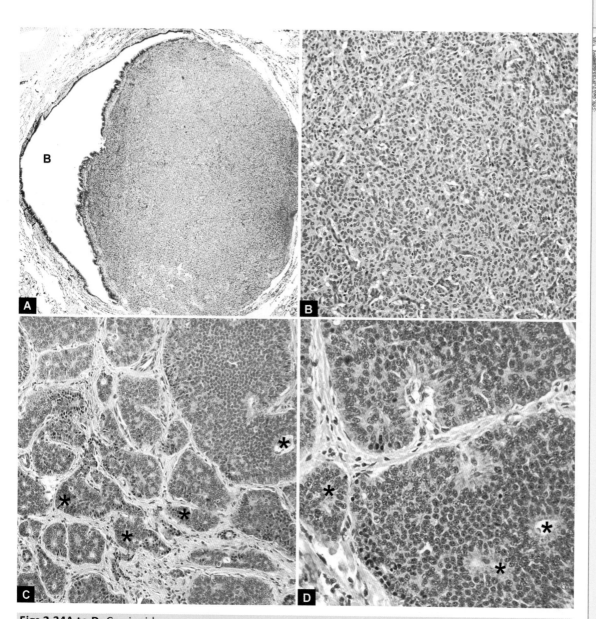

**Figs 2.34A to D:** Carcinoid

**A.** A round sharply demarcated submucosal tumor is deforming the lumen of this bronchiolus. **B.** The tumor is sheets of cells that have uniform round nuclei. **C.** Tumor cells form nests. Within nests there are blood vessels that appear like "empty spaces" (asterisks). **D.** The nests of tumor cells are sharply demarcated from the stroma. Small blood vessels are denoted with asterisks. The lumens of the vessels are surrounded by tumor cell cytoplasm while the nuclei are more peripherally located.

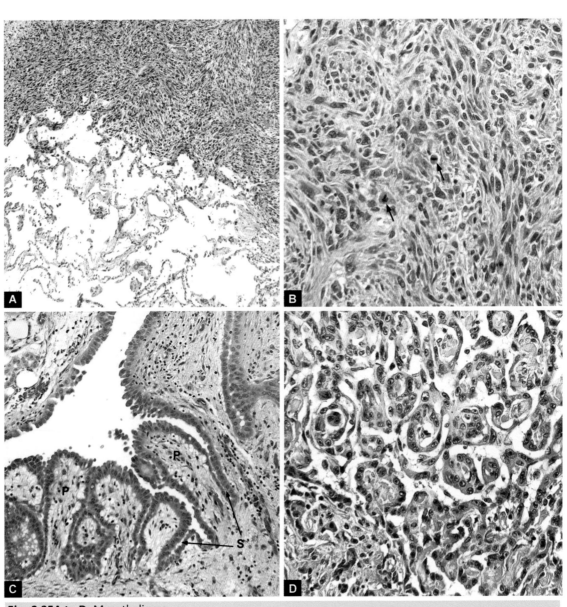

**Figs 2.35A to D:** Mesothelioma

**A.** The tumor is on the external side of the lung and does not invade into the alveoli. **B.** This sarcomatous mesothelioma is composed of cells with hyperchromatic spindle shaped nuclei resembling fibroblasts. Mitotic figures are indicated with arrows. **C.** Epithelial mesothelioma forms papillae (P), projecting with narrow slit-like spaces (S) between them. **D.** Epithelial mesothelioma composed of cuboidal cells forming interlacing cords, papillae, and lining slit-like spaces.

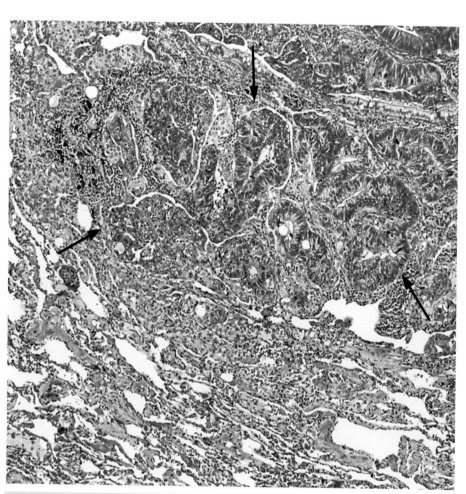

**Fig. 2.36:** Metastatic adenocarcinoma from a colonic primary
The tumor is composed of hyperchromatic cells forming irregular duct-like and gland-like structures (arrows).

# 3 Hematopoietic and Lymphoid System

*Da Zhang*

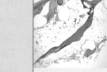

## Introduction

*The peripheral blood is composed of plasma and blood cells, including erythrocytes, or red blood cells (RBCs); leukocytes or white blood cells (WBCs); and thrombocytes or platelets. The most important diseases of the hematopoietic system include the following:*
* *Anemia*
* *Leukemia*
* *Lymphoma and related neoplastic diseases such as multiple myeloma.*

## Normal Hematopoietic and Lymphoid System

In a broader sense, the hematopoietic system includes not only the peripheral blood and the bone marrow (Figs 3.1A to C) but also the lymph nodes and organ-related lymphoid tissue, the spleen and the thymus. The lymph nodes and the organ-related lymphoid tissue play an important role in the defense of the body and participate in the immune response to adverse external as well as internal influences. The thymus plays a crucial role in the formation of the T-cell portion of the immune system. The spleen and the liver are the primary sites for the removal of aged blood cells.

## Anemia

Anemia is a reduction of the circulating red blood cell mass recognized as a reduced number of erythrocytes or decreased concentration of hemoglobin or both. This common disorder, affecting 25–30% of the population, is diagnosed by examining the RBCs in peripheral blood and measuring the concentration of hemoglobin. Additional tests that are sometimes needed include, among others: bone marrow biopsy, electrophoretic studies of hemoglobin and molecular biological studies of genes controlling heme and globin synthesis. On the basis of these studies anemias can be *classified pathogenetically* into three major groups: (a) anemia due to blood loss; (b) anemia due to abnormal RBC or hemoglobin production and (c) anemia due to increased RBC destruction (hemolysis).

Morphologic classification of anemias is based on microscopic examination of peripheral blood smears, which is nowadays supplemented by instrumental measurements of the size of RBC and their hemoglobin content. These measurements are used to calculate the mean corpuscular volume (MCV), mean corpuscular hemoglobin (MCH) and mean corpuscular hemoglobin concentration (MCHC).

Microscopically, anemias can be classified into several groups including: (a) *microcytic anemia*; (b) *macrocytic anemia*; (c) *spherocytosis*; (d) *sickle cell anemia*; (e) *acanthocytosis*. Further classification can be performed by using additional tests, used to identify intrinsic hemolytic anemias due to *genetic hemoglobin abnormalities,* such as *sickle cell anemia or thalassemia*. Presence of antibodies to red blood cell components is helpful in identifying *autoimmune hemolytic anemias*. Bone marrow biopsy is used to assess the capacity of the hematopoietic bone marrow to produce RBC, and is essential for diagnosing *aplastic* and *myelophthisic anemia*.

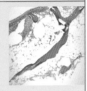

## Microcytic Hypochromic Anemia

*Microcytic hypochromic anemia* is most often a consequence of iron deficiency. Overall the RBCs vary in size and shape, i.e. show *anisocytosis* and *poikilocytosis* **(Fig. 3.2A)**. Many cells are small (microcytic) and have a large pale central areas reflecting their low hemoglobin content (*hypochromic*). Small pale elliptical "cigar-shaped" cells are known as *elliptocytes*. Crenated RBCs are called *acanthocytes*. The deficiency of iron can be readily corrected by providing iron orally when many cells increase their hemoglobin content and resemble *spherocytes*. Bone marrow is sometimes performed to exclude other forms of anemia and to confirm that the marrow contains normal erythroid cells and does not contain iron **(Figs 3.2B to D)**. Typically, the bone marrow contains no hemosiderin, and accordingly the bone marrow biopsy stained with the Prussian blue will not show any bluish pigment.

## Macrocytic Anemia

*Macrocytic anemia* is usually caused by vitamin $B_{12}$ or folate deficiency. The deficiency of these essential nutrients affects DNA synthesis and impedes the maturation of all hematopoietic cells. In the peripheral blood smears, the RBCs are enlarged and vary in size and shape technically described as macrocytosis, anisocytosis and poikilocytosis of erythrocytes **(Fig. 3.3A)**. Another common finding is the hypersegmentation of polymorphonuclear leukocytes. The bone marrow is hypercellular due to compensatory erythroid hyperplasia and contains numerous megaloblasts **(Fig. 3.3B)**, replacing normal erythroid precursors (normoblasts). Megaloblasts have large nuclei and very little cytoplasm because of asynchrony in the maturation of nuclei and the cytoplasm of erythroid precursors. The precursors of leukocytes are also enlarged, and the inhibition of thrombocytopoiesis results in hypersegmentation of megakaryocytes.

## Anemia Caused by Intrinsic Red Blood Cell Abnormalities

These chronic hemolytic anemias are typically caused by mutations of genes encoding skeletal and cell membrane proteins or hemoglobin. Defective proteins or hemoglobins cause RBC abnormalities which predispose RBC to accelerated hemolysis. Clinically these abnormalities present as *chronic intrinsic hemolytic anemia*.

*Hereditary spherocytosis* is the name for a group of hemolytic anemias caused by mutation of genes encoding one of the RBC structural proteins such as spectrin, ankyrin or other cell membrane, or cytoskeletal proteins. Instead of the normal biconcave shape of normal RBC, the spherocytes are round and more fragile, prone to hemolysis during their passage through the spleen. In the peripheral blood smears, spherocytes lack the central pale area and appear homogeneously red **(Fig. 3.4A)**. Spherocytosis is accompanied by splenomegaly resulting from the pooling of abnormal RBC in the splenic red pulp, where these blood cells undergo hemolysis **(Fig. 3.4B)**.

*Sickle cell anemia* results from a defect in the synthesis of beta globin that leads to the formation of S-hemoglobin. This abnormal hemoglobin polymerizes in deoxygenated blood, thus causing RBC deformities, or precipitation of abnormal hemoglobin in the center of RBC, giving them a targetoid appearance **(Fig. 3.5A)**. Sickling accompanied by thrombi formation tends to cause infarcts in many organs, including bones, kidney, brain or the spleen. The spleen undergoes fibrosis and shrinkage **(Fig. 3.5B)**. It may be reduced to a very small size or completely infarcted and reduced to a fibrotic scar (autosplenectomy).

*Thalassemia* is a name for a group of congenital microcytic hypochromic anemia caused by a defect of the globin alpha or beta gene. In addition to hypochromia, there is also poikilocytosis and anisocytosis or RBC **(Fig. 3.6A)**. Abnormal hemoglobin formed due to a defective alpha or beta chain accumulates in the cells in the form of central densities giving RBCs a targetoid appearance **(Fig. 3.6B)**. Abnormal RBCs are hemolyzed, causing an erythroid hyperplasia in the bone marrow. Nucleated RBCs may be released into the peripheral blood from such a hyperplastic bone marrow.

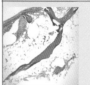

### Anemia Caused by Bone Marrow Failure

*Aplastic anemia* is characterized by a depletion of all hematopoietic cell precursors from the bone marrow. The term is used as a synonym for total bone marrow failure because it involves not only the precursors of RBCs but the WBCs and platelets as well. Clinically it presents with normocytic normochromic anemia, leukopenia and thrombocytopenia. The bone marrow is depleted of hematopoietic cells and contians only fat cells, a few fibroblasts or scattered lymphocytes **(Fig. 3.7)**.

*Myelofibrosis* is characterized by an overgrowth of the bone marrow with fibroblasts, replacing the normal hematopoietic cells **(Fig. 3.8A)**. *Primary myelofibrosis* is classified as a form of *myelodysplastic syndrome*, and is typically associated with the appearance of extramedullary hematopoiesis in the liver and spleen **(Figs 3.8B and C)**. Peripheral blood contains typical "tear drop-like erythrocytes". *Secondary myelofibrosis* may occur following radiation and chemotherapy.

*Myelophthisic anemia* is caused by tumors infiltrating the bone marrow and replacing the normal hematopoietic cells **(Fig. 3.9)**. Bone marrow may be infiltrated with hematopoietic and lymphoid neoplasms, metastatic carcinomas or macrophages accumulating there in the course of lipid storage diseases.

### Hemolytic Anemia

*Hemolytic anemia* is a name for a number of diseases characterized by accelerated destruction of RBC. The causes of hemolysis may be classified as *intrinsic* to RBC or *extrinsic*. The intrinsic factors include a variety of structural RBC abnormalities, which have been discussed above. The extrinsic factors include: (a) *antibodies*, which are typically found in chronic autoimmune hemolytic anemias; (b) *infections* affecting the RBC such as malaria and (c) *microangiopathic diseases*, such as thrombotic thrombocytopenic purpura (TTP) or disseminated intravascular coagulation (DIC), causing RBC destruction mechanically. The diagnosis of these diseases is based on clinical and laboratory findings, and the microscopic examination of the peripheral blood is used only to confirm the diagnosis. Suffice to say that all hemolytic anemias are associated with increased accumulation of hemosiderin in the macrophages of the spleen, liver and bone marrow, and hyperbilirubinemia clinically presenting as jaundice. In all autoimmune hemolytic anemias RBC in peripheral blood assume the shape of spherocytes, similar to those in hereditary spherocytosis. Bone marrow typically shows erythroid hyperplasia.

*Microangiopathic diseases*, such as DIC or TTP, are associated with acquired deformities of RBC best seen in peripheral blood smears. These deformities take many forms and are described by such names as crenated burr cells or helmet cells (schistocytes) **(Fig. 3.10)**. Similar changes are seen in patients who have anemia caused by the mechanical destruction of RBCs by heart valves.

## Leukemia

Leukemias are clonal disorders of myeloid and lymphoid progenitor cells presenting with proliferation of neoplastic cells in the bone marrow or lymphoid tissues respectively, and the appearance of their descendants in blood. Leukemias are classified as: (a) acute or (b) chronic. *Acute leukemias* comprise two main categories: (a) acute myeloid leukemia (AML) and (b) acute lymphoblastic leukemia. *Chronic leukemia* comprises two major groups: (a) chronic myelogenous leukemia and (b) chronic lymphocytic leukemia. According to 2008 WHO classification, each of these categories comprises several subtypes that are defined on the basis of their cell morphology and differentiation, cytogenetic and molecular studies. In the 2008 WHO classification they are listed under the categories of myeloproliferative neoplasm, mature B cell neoplasms and mature T and NK cell neoplasms which include several important diseases such as chronic myelogenous leukemia (CML), CLL, hairy cell leukemia and Sézary syndrome.

## Acute Myeloid Leukemia

*Acute myeloid leukemia (AML)* is a heterogeneous group of diseases, which are classified, according to WHO, into four groups: (a) AML with recurrent genetic abnormalities; (b) AML with myelodysplasia-related changes; (c) AML, therapy related and (d) AML, not otherwise specified. The WHO classification can be correlated with the French-American-British (FAB) classification which includes the following subcategories:

M0: AML minimally differentiated

M1: AML without maturation

M2: AML with myelocytic maturation

M3: AMLwith t(15;17) (q22;11-22)

M4: AML with myelomonocytic differentiation

M5: AML with myelomonocytic maturation

M6: AML with erythroid maturation

M7: AML with megakaryocytic maturation

In all forms of AML the bone marrow contains at least 20% myeloid blasts, which may also be found in the peripheral blood **(Figs 3.11A and B)**.

## Acute Lymphoblastic Leukemia/Lymphoma

*Acute lymphoblastic leukemia/lymphoma (ALL),* the most common malignancy of infancy and early childhood, can be classified into two groups: (a) *B-ALL* composed of immature B (pre-B), accounting for 85% of all cases and (b) *T-ALL* composed of immature T (pre-T), accounting for 15% of all cases. Both forms of ALL may present as leukemia with bone marrow infiltration or lymphoma involving the lymphoid tissue **(Figs 3.12A to D)**. Neoplastic cells are immunohistochemically positive for terminal deoxynucleotidyl transferase (TdT), which can be demonstrated by enzyme histochemistry in the nuclei of neoplastic cells or by flow cytometry analysis. Two forms of ALLs (mentioned above) show considerable overlap in clinical manifestations, although T-ALL more often involves the thymus, lymph nodes and the spleen.

## Chronic Myeloid Leukemia

*Chronic myeloid leukemia (CML)* is a myeloproliferative neoplasm. The hallmark of CML is the Philadelphia (Ph) chromosome comprising the translocation of t(9;22) chromosome and resulting in the formation of the BCR/ABL fusion gene. The peripheral blood smears show an increased number of granulocytes in excess of 50,000 per microliter in all stages of maturation **(Figs 3.13A and B)**. In addition to segmented neutrophils, the peripheral blood smears not only contain myeloblasts, promyelocytes, myelocytes, metamyelocytes and band forms but also basophils **(Figs 3.14A and B)**. The bone marrow is hypercellular bone (> 90%) and is infiltrated with neoplastic cells. Leukemic cells may infiltrate other tissues, most prominently the spleen and the liver, and form tumors of soft tissues called myeloid sarcoma (chloromas). In about two-thirds of cases, the disease ends in a blast crisis and death.

## Chronic Lymphocytic Leukemia

*Chronic lymphocytic leukemia (CLL)* is one of the mature B cell neoplasms. The CLL is characterized by an increased number of lymphocytes in the circulating blood and lymph nodes, spleen and liver. Neoplastic cells express either kappa, or lambda, chains of immunoglobulins reflecting their monoclonality. They resemble mature lymphocytes and express surface immunoglobulins such as normal B cells. The peripheral blood smears contain numerous lymphocytes **(Figs 3.15A to C)**. The smears also contain smudge cells, an artifact produced by preparation of the smears, probably reflecting the increased fragility of neoplastic cells. The CLL infiltrates lymph nodes and the white pulp of the spleen, but it may involve the bone marrow and the liver as well.

*Hairy cell leukemia* is another mature B cell neoplasm. This B-cell leukemia can be recognized morphologically and presents with a clinically distinct picture. The neoplastic cells contain round nuclei and well developed cytoplasm that has a ruffled surface extending into short villi (hairs) **(Figs 3.16A and B)**. Hairy cell leukemia typically infiltrates the spleen, diffusely obliterating its normal architecture.

*Chronic T-cell lymphoma/leukemia* may present in several forms. *Sézary syndrome* is a T-cell leukemia characterized by the appearance of relatively mature T cells in the circulating blood **(Fig. 3.17A)**. Mycosis fungoides is closely related to neoplastic condition in which neoplastic T-cells infiltrate the skin **(Fig. 3.17B)**. Such cells have deeply indented or lobulated nuclei and scant cytoplasm.

## Lymphoma

The term malignant lymphoma includes a variety of neoplastic disorders of lymphoid cells, which are subdivided into two groups: (a) *non-Hodgkin lymphoma* and (b) *Hodgkin lymphoma*. All these disorders represent clonal proliferation of T or B lymphocytes and their common or distinctly specific precursors. Non-Hodgkin lymphomas can be further classified as: (a) *precursor lymphoid neoplasm*; (b) *mature B cell neoplasms* and (c) *mature T and NK cell neoplasms*.

The most important lymphomas to be illustrated here are: (a) acute lymphoblastic lymphoma—a lymphomatous form of lymphoblastic leukemia **(Figs 3.18A and B)**; (b) follicular lymphoma **(Fig. 3.19)**; (c) CLL/small lymphocytic lymphoma (SLL) **(Figs 3.20A and B)**; (d) diffuse large B cell lymphoma **(Figs 3.21A and B)**; (e) Burkitt lymphoma **(Figs 3.22A and B)** and (f) multiple myeloma/solitary plasmacytoma **(Figs 3.23A and B)**.

### Hodgkin Lymphoma

Hodgkin lymphoma is a form of lymphoma that occurs in two histological types: (a) *classical Hodgkin lymphoma* and (b) *nodular lymphocyte predominant Hodgkin lymphoma*.

*Classical Hodgkin lymphoma* has four subtypes: (a) nodular sclerosis; (b) mixed cellularity; (c) lymphocytes rich and (d) lymphocytes depleted. *Nodular sclerosis Hodgkin lymphoma* is the most common subtype accounting for two-thirds of all cases. Microscopically it is characterized by the deposition of broad bands of collagen subdividing the lymph node into several smaller nodules **(Fig. 3.24A)**. Like other subtypes of Hodgkin lymphoma, it contains the diagnostic *Reed-Sternberg cells*, which are typically bilobed and have prominent nucleoli surrounded by a clear halo **(Fig. 3.24B)**.

*Nodular lymphocyte predominant* is an uncommon form of Hodgkin lymphoma accounting for 5% of all cases. The involved lymph nodes have a nodular appearance and are infiltrated with small lymphocytes and macrophages. Instead of the classical Reed-Sternberg cells, this variant contains so-called L&P variant or "popcorn" cells.

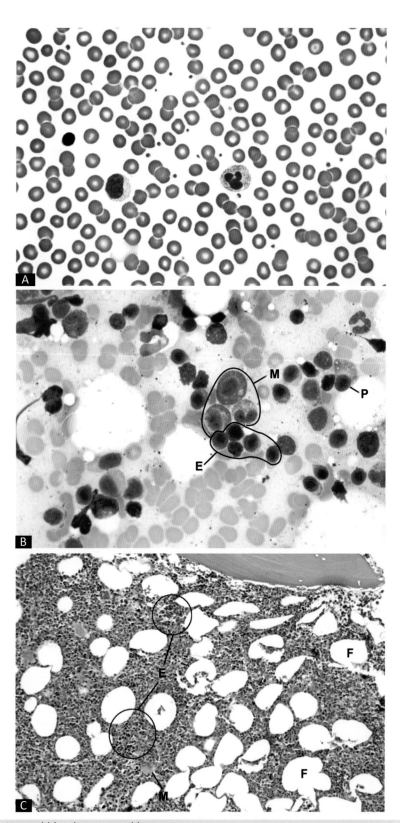

**Figs 3.1A to C:** Normal blood smear and bone marrow

**A.** The peripheral smear contains predominantly RBCs and a few scattered nucleated WBCs. From left to right one may see a lymphocyte, a monocyte and a neutrophil. **B.** Aspirate of bone marrow contains predominantly nucleated precursors of mature peripheral blood cells such as myeloid (M) and erythroid (E) cells. The bone marrow contains also plasma cells (P), macrophages and megakaryocytes (not shown). **C.** Bone marrow biopsy contains bone spicules (red) and hematopoietic cell admixed with fat cells (F). Myeloid precursors predominate. Erythroid precursors (E) form groups recognizable by their dark round nuclei.

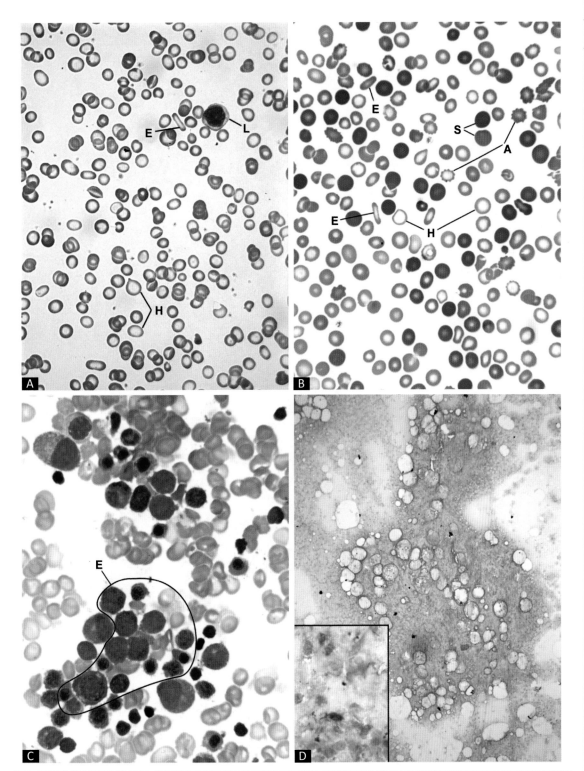

**Figs 3.2A to D:** Iron deficiency anemia

**A.** Peripheral blood smear shows variation in size and shape of erythrocytes, but most cells are small as compared with the normal lymphocyte (L). Some cells are hypochromic (H) and have a large central pale area. Elliptocytes (E) have an elongated shape. **B.** This smear taken after iron treatment shows fewer hypochromic (H) cells, whereas many others appear darker red, without a central halo, resembling spherocytes (S). There are also cigar-shaped elliptocytes (E) and crenated cells called acanthocytes (A). **C.** Bone marrow aspirate contains groups of nucleated erythrocyte precursors (E). **D.** Bone marrow aspirate stained with Prussian blue stain shows no hemosiderin, which is however normally present in the bone marrow (blue stained material in the inset).

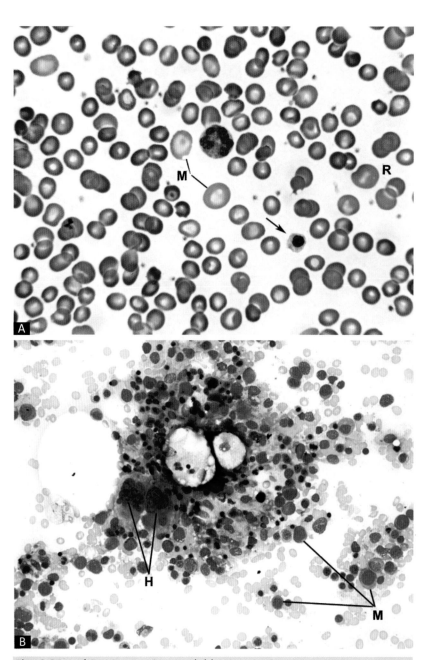

**Figs 3.3A and B:** Macrocytic megaloblastic anemia

**A.** Peripheral smear show marked variation in size and shape of RBC. Macrocytes (M) are enlarged and have a wider central pale area. There are also reticulocytes (R), immature RBC which have a bluish cytoplasm due to the presence of RNA, and nucleated red blood cell (arrow). The neutrophil shows hypersegmentation of the nucleus, which has six segments. **B.** Bone marrow aspirate is hypercellular and contains large RBC precursors called megaloblasts (M) and hypersegmented megakaryocytes (H).

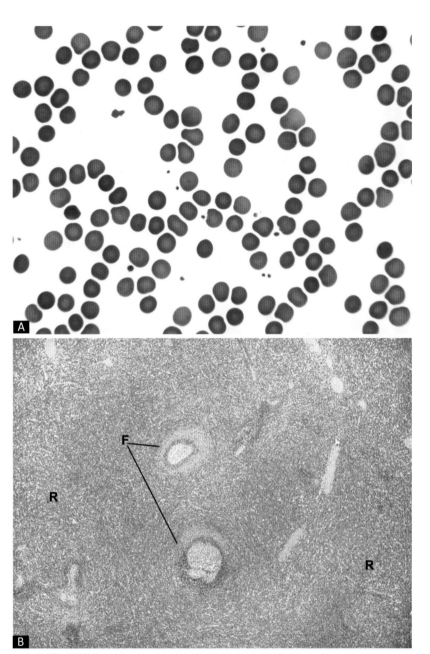

**Figs 3.4A and B:** Spherocytosis

**A.** Peripheral blood smear contains spherocytes, i.e. RBC which appear round, uniformly red lacking central pallor. **B.** Spherocytosis results in splenomegaly due to the pooling of abnormal RBC in the sinusoids of the red pulp (R) of the spleen. The splenic follicles (F) are normal.

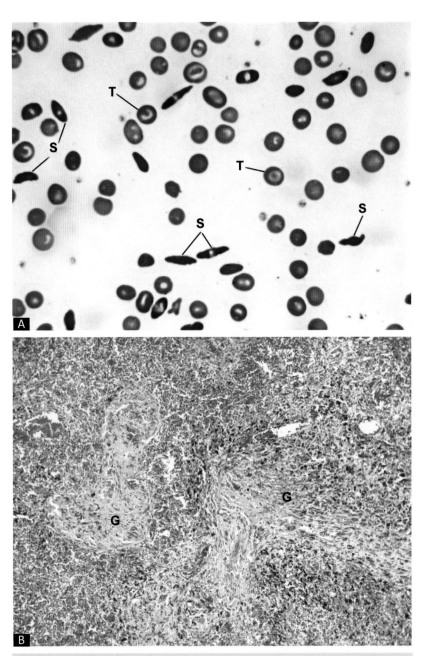

**Figs 3.5A and B:** Sickle cell anemia

**A.** Peripheral blood smear contains numerous sickle cells (S) and target cells (T). **B.** Infarction of the spleen results in the formation of fibrotic hemosiderin rich scars, called Gamna-Gandy bodies (G).

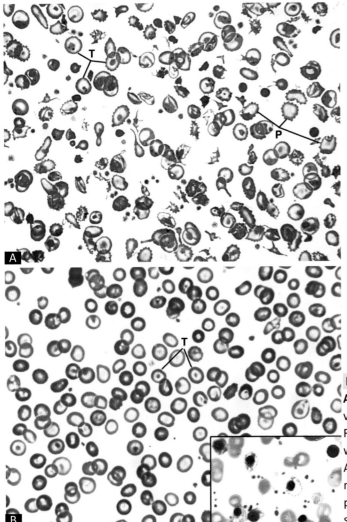

**Figs 3.6A and B:** Thalassemia

**A.** Peripheral blood smear shows marked variation in size and shape of RBC. Many RBCs have large central pale areas (P), whereas others appear targetoid (T). **B.** Another example of thalassemia showing numerous hypochromic cells with central pale areas and targetoid cells (T). The inset shows numerous nucleated RBCs.

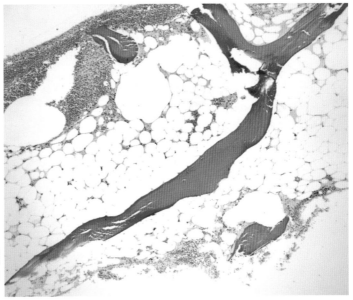

**Fig. 3.7:** Aplastic anemia

The hematopoietic bone marrow has been replaced by fat cells.

HEMATOPOIETIC AND LYMPHOID SYSTEM

CHAPTER

**3**

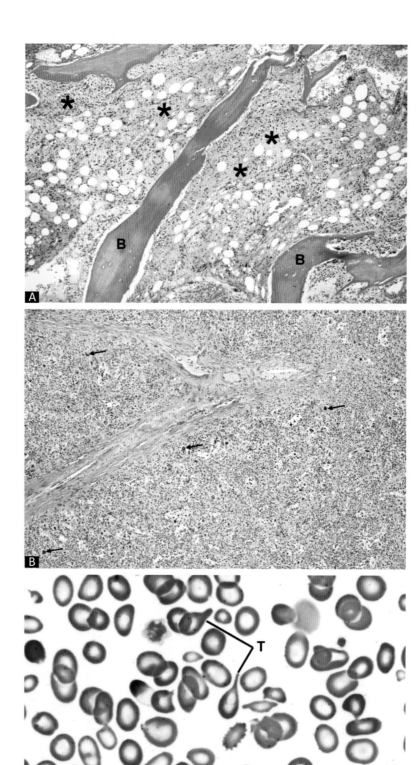

**Figs 3.8A to C:** Myelofibrosis

**A.** Parts of the hematopoietic bone marrow between the bone spicules (B) are replaced by fibrous tissue which appears eosinophilic (asterisks). **B.** The spleen shows signs of extramedullary hematopoiesis. Megakaryocytes are readily recognized even at low magnification due to their large nuclei (arrows). **C.** Peripheral blood contains tear drop-shaped RBCs (T).

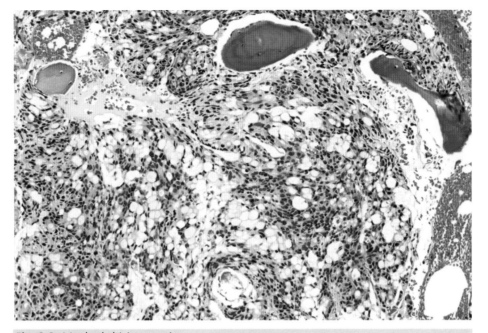

**Fig. 3.9:** Myelophthisic anemia
The hematopoietic bone marrow between the bone spicules has been replaced by adenocarcinoma cells.

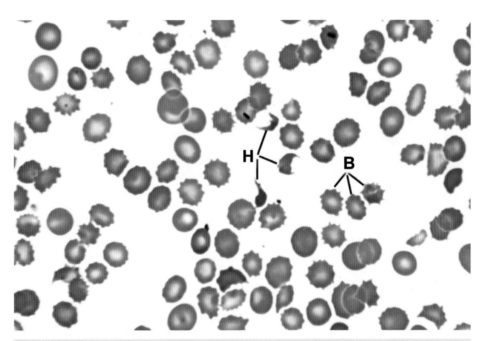

**Fig. 3.10:** Microangiopathic hemolytic anemia
Peripheral blood smear from a patient with DIC contains deformed RBC known as helmet cells (H) or burr cells (B).

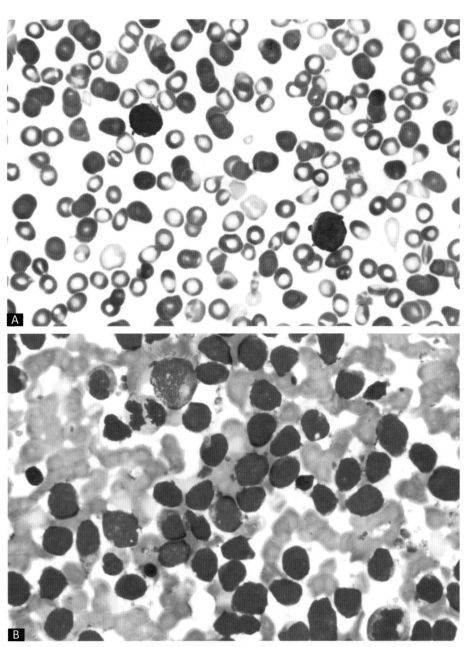

**Figs 3.11A and B:** Acute myeloid leukemia

**A.** The peripheral blood smear contains blasts with scanty cytoplasm and a prominent nucleoli. **B.** Bone marrow aspirate contains numerous blasts which have replaced normal hematopoietic cells.

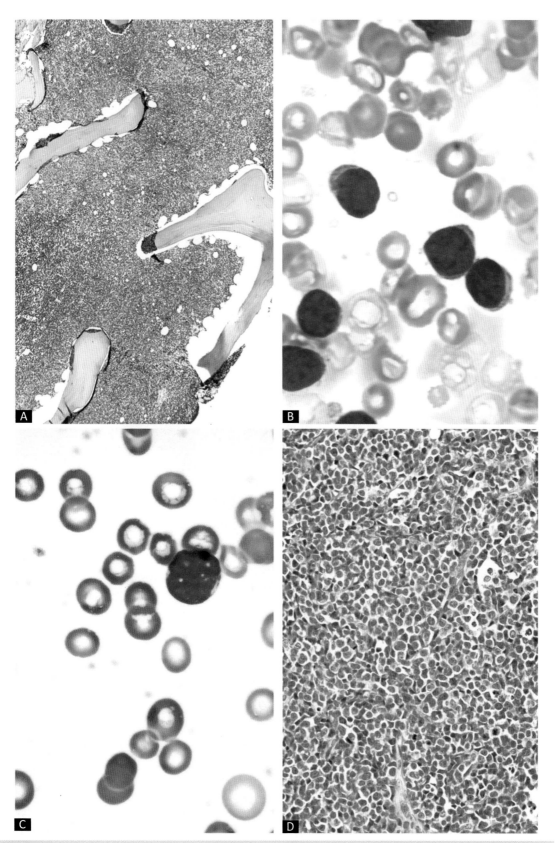

**Figs 3.12A to D:** Acute lymphoblastic leukemia/lymphoma
**A.** Bone marrow section is densely infiltrated with large lymphoid cells replacing normal hematopoietic cells. **B.** In ALL the bone marrow aspirate contains numerous immature lymphoid cells. **C.** The peripheral blood contains ALL blast with scanty cytoplasm. **D.** Lymph node in this case of ALL is diffusely infiltrated with large lymphoid cells classified as lymphoblasts.

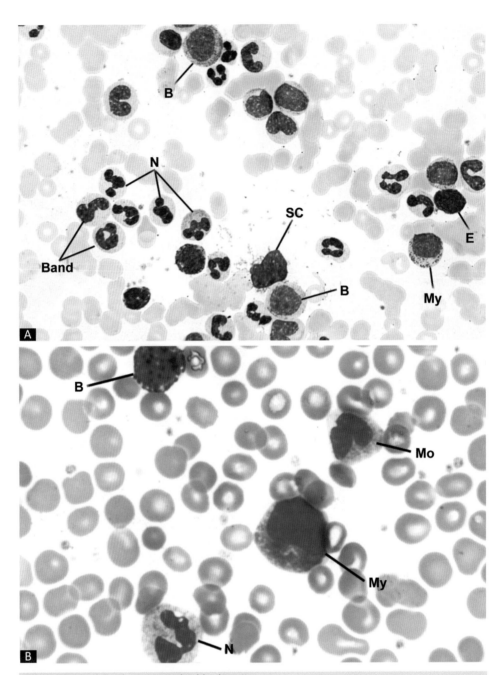

**Figs 3.13A and B:** Chronic myeloid leukemia

**A.** The peripheral blood smears show an increased number of WBCs including segmented neutrophils (N) and nonsegmented neutrophils (Bands), myeloblasts (My), basophils (B) and erythroid precursors (E), as well as smudge cells (SC). **B.** Higher magnification of a peripheral blood smear shows several cell types including a segmented neutrophil (N), a basophil (B), a monocyte (Mo) and a myeloblast (My).

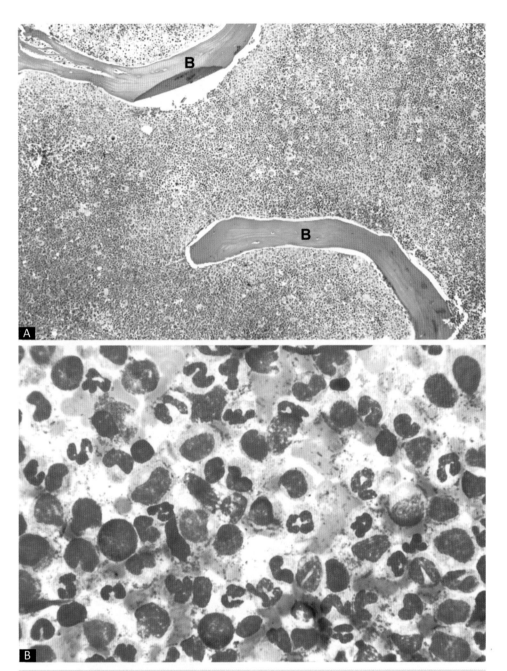

**Figs 3.14A and B:** Chronic myeloid leukemia

**A.** The hematopoietic bone marrow is hypercellular and the immature myeloid cell fills over 90% of the spaces between the bone spicules (B). **B.** Bone marrow aspirate reflects the hypercellularity of the bone marrow which contains blasts and myeloid cells at various stages of maturation.

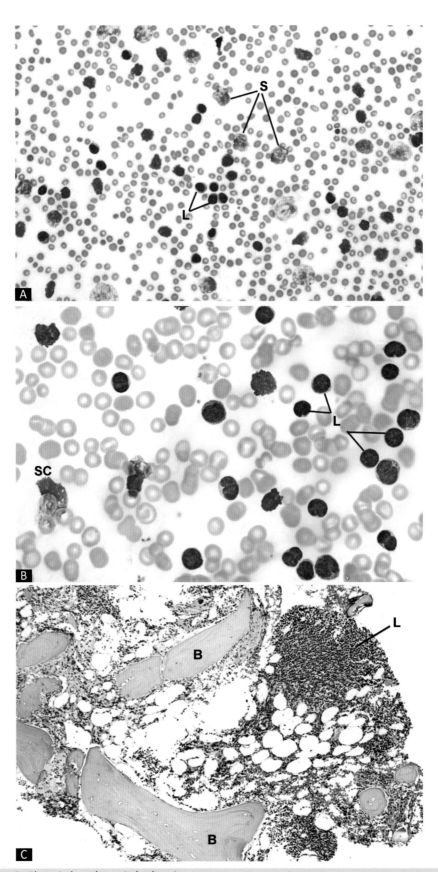

**Figs 3.15A to C:** Chronic lymphocytic leukemia

**A.** The peripheral blood contains numerous lymphocytes (L) and so-called "smudge cells" (SC). **B.** Higher magnification shows lymphocytes (L) and smudge cells (SC). **C.** The bone marrow between the bone spicules (B) is infiltrated with lymphocytes (L).

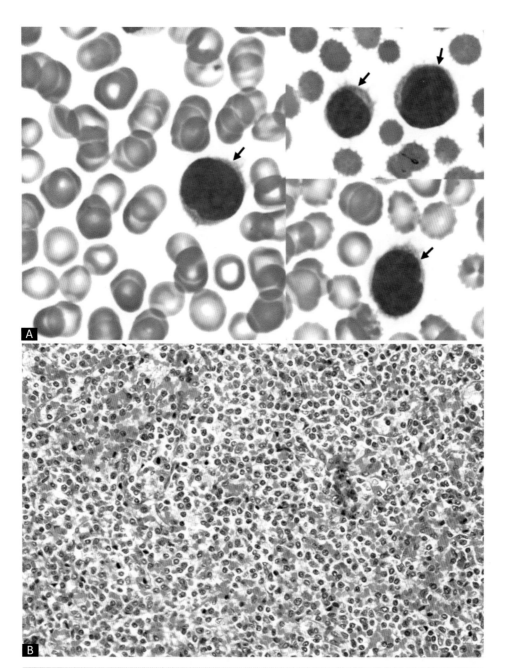

**Figs 3.16A and B:** Hairy cell leukemia

**A.** The peripheral blood contains neoplastic cells with round nuclei and well developed cytoplasm which has a ruffled surface extending into short villi (hairs) (arrows). **B.** The red pulp of the spleen is infiltrated with leukemic cells obliterating the white pulp, which is not visible.

HEMATOPOIETIC AND LYMPHOID SYSTEM

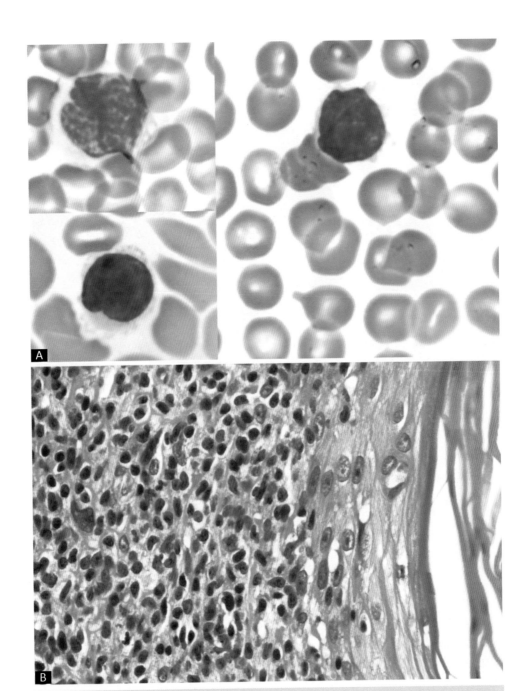

**Figs 3.17A and B:** Peripheral T-cell lymphoma

**A.** Peripheral blood smear in Sézary syndrome contains lymphocytes which have indented or lobulated nuclei and scant cytoplasm (Sézary cells). **B.** Mycosis fungoides presents with dermal infiltrates of T lymphocytes invading the epidermis. The keratin layer (on the right) is not infiltrated.

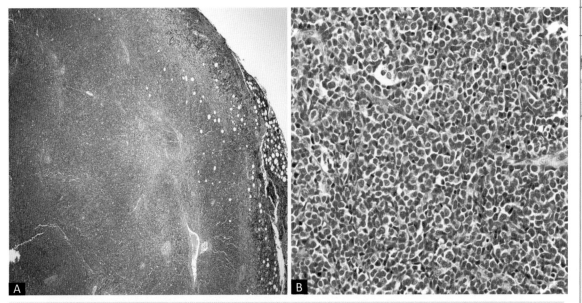

**Figs 3.18A and B:** Acute lymphoblastic lymphoma
**A.** The lymph node is diffusely infiltrated with lymphoid cells which also extend into the perinodal fat tissue
(F). **B.** At higher magnification one may see that the lymphoid cells have large nuclei and scant cytoplasm.

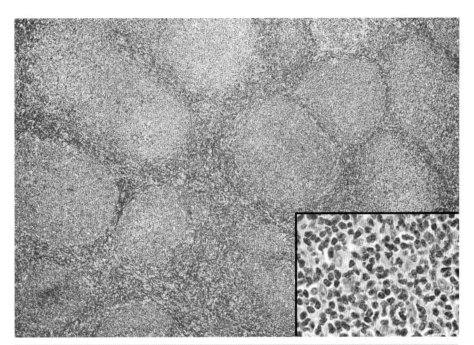

**Fig. 3.19:** Follicular lymphoma
The normal lymph node architecture has been replaced by follicles showing "back to back" arrangement and lacking marginal and mantle zones. Inset higher magnification of a neoplastic follicle composed of relatively uniform small cells with cleaved nuclei.

HEMATOPOIETIC AND LYMPHOID SYSTEM

CHAPTER

**3**

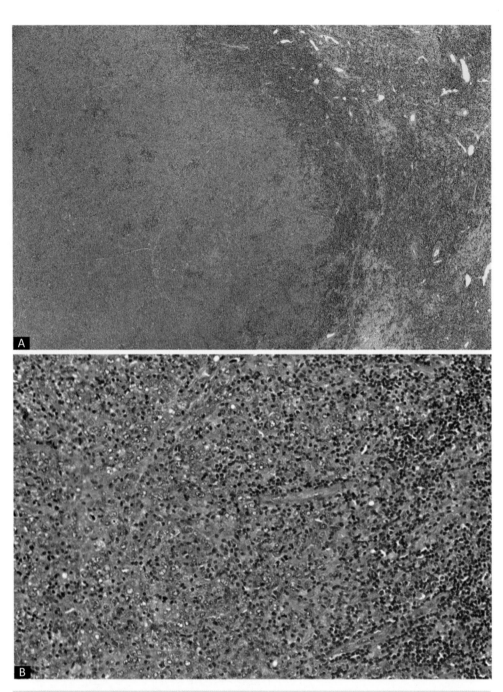

**Figs 3.20A and B:** Diffuse large B cell lymphoma

**A.** Relatively large lymphoid cells diffusely infiltrate the lymph node. **B.** At higher magnification one may see that the lymphoid cells have hyperchromatic nuclei which vary in shape from round and oval to cleaved and lobulated. The nuclei of lymphoma cells are 3-5 times larger than the nuclei of residual mature lymphocytes which may be still seen as small round cells between the neoplastic cells.

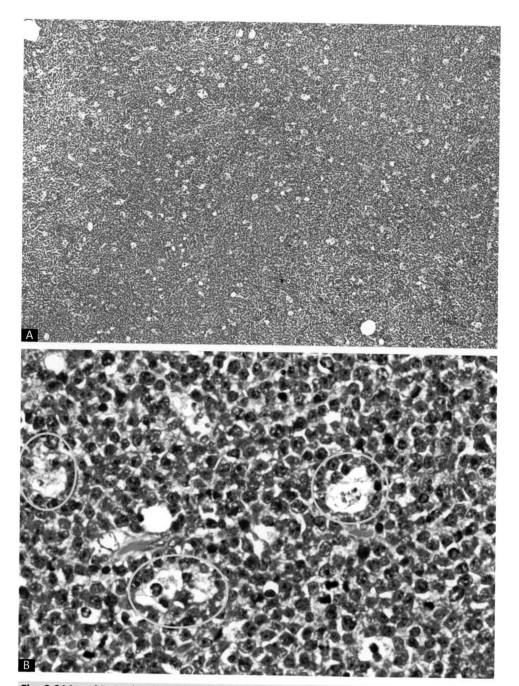

**Figs 3.21A and B:** Burkitt lymphoma
**A.** The lymph node is densely infiltrated with relatively uniform cells and clear spaces containing dead cells imparting the infiltrate a "starry sky" pattern. **B.** At higher magnification one may see that the clear spaces (encircled) contain remnants of dead cells taken up in part by macrophages.

ATLAS OF HISTOPATHOLOGY

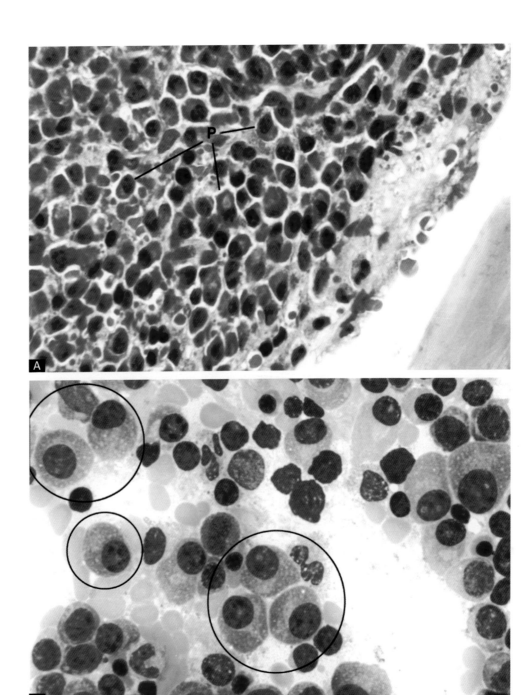

**Figs 3.22A and B:** Multiple myeloma

**A.** Bone marrow biopsy shows neoplastic plasma cells which have replaced normal hematopoietic bone marrow cells. **B.** Neoplastic plasma cells shown here in a bone marrow aspirate have eccentric nuclei in a well developed bluish tinged cytoplasm and thus resemble their normal counterparts.

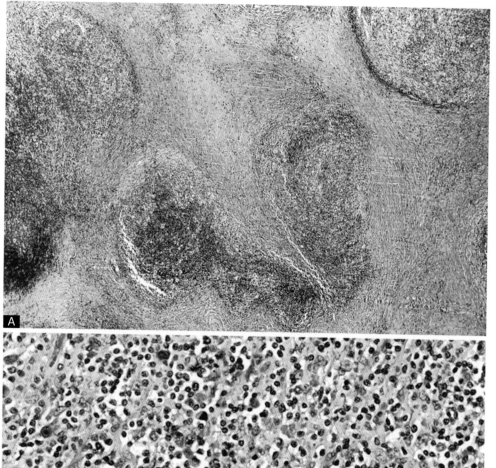

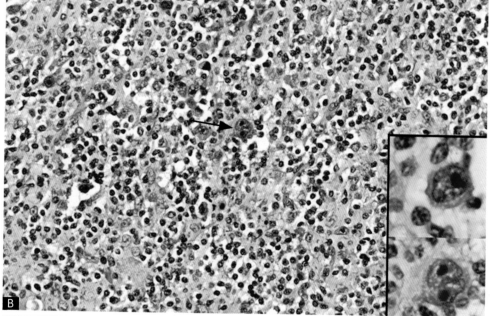

**Figs 3.23A and B:** Hodgkin lymphoma (classical type)
**A.** In nodular sclerosis the lymph node is subdivided by broad fibrous strands into smaller nodules. **B.** Higher magnification view shows a mixed infiltrate with prominent Reed-Sternberg cells (arrow). A mononuclear and a binuclear Reed-Sternberg cell, both of which have prominent nucleoli, are shown in the inset.

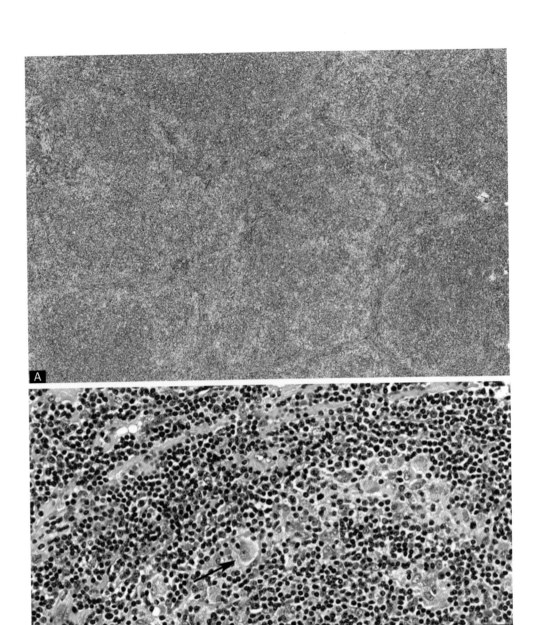

**Figs 3.24A and B:** Hodgkin lymphoma (nodular lymphocyte predominance type)
**A.** The normal architecture of the lymph node has been replaced by nodular infiltrates of lymphocytes and macrophages. **B.** Higher magnification view of the lymph node infiltrated with lymphocytes and macrophages which have a more abundant cytoplasm. The arrow and the inset show popcorn cells.

# 4 Digestive System

*Rashna Madan*

## Introduction

*The gastrointestinal tract comprises a series of roughly cylindrical muscular viscera which are lined by mucosa. Their lumina lie in successive continuity beginning with the esophagus, followed by the stomach, the three components of the small intestine (duodenum, jejunum and ileum) and the large gut (cecum, appendix, ascending, transverse, descending and sigmoid colon and rectum), culminating in the anus. This tract's primary role is to breakdown ingested food and liquid, absorb nutrients and egest waste. In this chapter, we will illustrate and review primarily the inflammatory/infectious and neoplastic conditions of various parts of the gastrointestinal system.*

## Esophagus

The esophagus is an expandable pipe that connects the pharynx to the stomach and propels swallowed matter toward the gastric lumen via the gastroesophageal junction (GEJ). Upper and lower esophageal sphincters are present at the proximal and distal ends of this viscus. Histologically the esophagus is made up of four layers, beginning with the mucosa which faces the lumen, the submucosa, muscularis propria and adventitia. The mucosa is composed of non-keratinized squamous epithelium, lying on a lamina propria composed of vascularized connective tissue with few scattered inflammatory cells and mucus glands, deep to which is the muscularis mucosa. Next is the submucosa which is composed of fibroadipose tissue with scattered mucus glands. The remaining layers are the thick muscularis propria (composed predominantly of smooth muscle with the addition of a skeletal muscle component in the proximal esophagus) and the adventitia (**Figs 4.1A to C**).

Abnormalities of the esophagus may be:
- Developmental anomalies.
- Inflammatory and infectious conditions.
- Preneoplastic conditions and neoplasms.

### Developmental Anomalies

*Atresia* and *fistulae* refer to deficient development and to an abnormal connection between two hollow viscera respectively. These are anomalies that usually present in the neonatal period with regurgitation on feeding. Often esophageal atresia is associated with a fistula between the esophagus and the trachea leading to severe complications when esophageal contents enter the respiratory tree. These pathologic conditions are not associated with specific histopathologic changes.

### Inflammatory and Infectious Conditions

Esophagitis may occur in several forms which may be related to: (a) chemical irritation caused by the reflux of the gastric juices; (b) infections; or (c) inflammation of unknown etiology, as in eosinophilic esophagitis.

### Reflux Esophagitis

*Reflux esophagitis* describes the microscopic findings in gastroesophageal reflux disease (GERD). The GERD refers to esophageal injury that occurs when gastric acid (or even duodenal bile when severe) regurgitates into the esophagus. This typically occurs when the lower esophageal sphincter is rendered incompetent and is associated with several factors including alcohol use, smoking, pregnancy and hiatal hernia. Patients usually manifest with heartburn and difficulty swallowing. Mucosal biopsies of the distal esophagus, accessed via endoscopy may be used to demonstrate these changes which include signs of epithelial proliferation, i.e. hyperplasia of the basal layers of the squamous epithelium (which extends above the lower 20% of the epithelium) and superficial located lamina propria papillae (that are present in the upper third of the epithelium). Some eosinophils within the epithelium are also suggestive of this diagnosis and with worsening disease; neutrophils and even ulceration may be present **(Fig. 4.2)**. Some patients with long standing GERD may develop Barrett's esophagus (discussed below).

### Eosinophilic Esophagitis

*Eosinophilic esophagitis* is a disorder characterized by abundant intraepithelial eosinophils in both the proximal and the distal portions of esophagus in patients who do not respond to anti-GERD therapy and have a normal pH on monitoring. The individuals often have allergies and may present with GERD-like symptoms. Morphologically numerous intraepithelial eosinophils are present, even forming collections (eosinophilic microabscesses) in the superficial epithelium **(Figs 4.3A and B)**.

### Infectious Esophagitis

Esophageal infections are most often caused by viruses or fungi. These infections may be isolated or may also occur in other regions of the gastrointestinal tract.

*Cytomegalovirus esophagitis* refers to the infection and subsequent ulceration produced by the cytomegalovirus (CMV), a member of the herpes family of viruses. It typically affects patients with compromised function of their immune systems. Stromal and endothelial cells in granulation tissue as well as columnar cells affected by the virus are enlarged (cytomegalo) and demonstrate pathognomonic basophilic or eosinophilic viral inclusions which are present in the nucleus (sometimes surrounded by a halo resembling an "owl eye") and in the cytoplasm **(Fig. 4.4)**. The presence of the virus may also be confirmed by a specific immunohistochemical stain.

*Herpes esophagitis* is an infection by the Herpes simplex virus (type I or II), another member of the herpes viral family which predominantly affects immunocompromised individuals, but may also occurs in otherwise healthy persons. Characteristically fluid filled vesicles are noted which progress to punched out ulcers. The viral effect is best appreciated in epithelial cells at the periphery of these ulcers. These epithelial cells may be single or multinucleated; in the case of the latter, there are several nuclei whose contours mould to one another. The nuclei are filled with an eosinophilic (Cowdry Type A) intranuclear inclusion which results in the margination of chromatin at the periphery of the nucleus **(Fig. 4.5)**. As above, a specific immunohistochemical stain for this virus is also available.

*Candida esophagitis* is a fungal infection by *Candida* species that classically produces whitish plaques (composed of fungal elements, inflammatory cells and keratin debris from the mucosa) that overlie erythematous or ulcerated mucosa. Fungal elements consist of yeast forms as well as pseudohyphae (which are elongated structures with indentations but lacking the true septations of hyphae), the latter should be seen within tissue to distinguish true infection from normal flora **(Figs 4.6A and B)**. A compromised immune system or prior antibiotic treatment increases the risk of this infection but are not absolute prerequisites.

## Preneoplastic Conditions and Neoplasms

### Barrett Esophagus

*Barrett esophagus*, which refers to intestinal metaplasia within esophageal mucosa, occurs as a consequence of long standing GERD. Both endoscopic and pathologic abnormalities are required for this diagnosis. An abnormal patch of "velvety red" columnar mucosa extending above the GEJ into the esophagus is noted endoscopically, which contrasts with the normal whitish squamous mucosa. This should correspond microscopically to the presence of intestinal type columnar epithelium which is characterized by the presence of goblet cells; the latter typically have a bulbous supranuclear mucin content that resembles a drinking goblet (Fig. 4.7A).

The clinical significance of this condition lies in being the chief risk factor for adenocarcinoma. Hence these patients require continued endoscopic surveillance with biopsies to evaluate for the development of dysplasia or carcinoma. Barrett's esophagus that is likely to progress to carcinoma, typically first develops dysplasia. *Dysplasia* may be *low grade* where the cells are mucin depleted and have stratified elongated nuclei that are present on the mucosal surface (Fig. 4.7B). On the other hand, *high grade* dysplasia is characterized by significant architectural abnormalities including crowded, branched and irregular glands, sometimes with cribriform patterns, and increasing cytologic atypia with higher nuclear-cytoplasmic ratios, prominent nucleoli and abnormal mitoses (Fig. 4.7C). Unlike adenocarcinoma, high grade dysplasia does not show invasion into the lamina propria or beyond.

### Carcinoma of the Esophagus

*Adenocarcinoma* accounts for half the esophageal malignancies in the United States and is the most frequent tumor in the distal esophagus. It is typically a tumor of older white males and as stated above is related, in the vast majority of cases, to Barrett's esophagus. The presence of GERD and the presence and extent of dysplasia contribute to the risk of carcinoma. The morphology ranges from well differentiated with extensive gland formation to poorly differentiated with limited to minimal evidence of glands (Figs 4.8A to C). The prognosis largely depends on the stage of the cancer with advanced stages showing poor survival.

*Squamous carcinoma* typically affects middle aged African-American males exposed to risk factors, such as alcohol and tobacco, although other factors including but not limited to caustic damage, achalasia and prior radiation have also been implicated. This carcinoma is more frequently located in the mid-portion of the esophagus and is usually well to moderately differentiated, being composed of nests of squamous cells with or without keratinization (Fig. 4.9). As with adenocarcinoma, survival is largely stage dependent.

## Stomach

The stomach is a mucosa lined distensible muscular sac which partly digests food by enzymatic action and propels its contents into the duodenum. Anatomically it extends from the GEJ to the duodenum and is divided from proximal to distal into the cardia, fundus, body, pyloric antrum and sphincter. Similar to the intestine, gastric histology reveals four layers: (1) the mucosa (comprising the epithelium, the lamina propria composed of connective tissue, vasculature and inflammatory elements and the muscularis mucosa, which is the slim smooth muscle that delineates this layer from the next); (2) the submucosa; (3) the muscularis propria (the main smooth muscle layer) and (4) the serosa which refers to the mesothelium that forms the outermost coat of the stomach that is exposed to the peritoneal cavity (Fig. 4.10A).

The mucosal surface is thrown into folds (rugae) that extend along the long axis of the stomach. At the microscopic level, the mucosal epithelium is invaginated into tubular structures which consist of the gastric foveolae that face the lumen and are continuous with the more deeply located gastric glands. The foveolae are lined by columnar mucous cells with basal nuclei and numerous mucin granules. Present further down are mucous neck cells also which have less mucin and are purported to be the source of other cell types (the mucosal lining is changed over a 2–6 day period). The gastric glands somewhat differ depending on the region of the stomach. Oxyntic glands predominate in the fundus and body, and consistent of acid secreting parietal cells with distinctive eosinophilic cytoplasm as well as the more basophilic chief cells that produce the protein digesting enzyme pepsin in proenzyme form (Fig. 4.10B). The acid aids in digestion. The mucosa is usually sheltered from the strongly acidic gastric content by the mucin and bicarbonate ions produced by the foveolar cells.

Additionally the vasculature supplies bicarbonate and oxygen and removes acid. The cardia and pylorus typically have mostly mucous glands with a few oxyntic elements (Fig. 4.10C). Also present are endocrine cells, which are significant for manufacturing histamine in the body and producing gastrin in the antrum (G cells).

Abnormalities of the stomach may be:
- Developmental anomalies
- Inflammatory/infectious conditions (gastritis) and gastropathies
- Polyps and neoplasms.

### Developmental Anomalies

*Pyloric stenosis* refers to the hyperplasia of pyloric muscle that interferes with the passage of gastric content into the small intestine and produces projectile emesis in the neonatal period. A similar condition may occur in adults as a consequence of gastritis or peptic ulceration or secondary to malignancy.

### Inflammatory and Infectious Conditions (Gastritis) and Gastropathies

Gastritis can clinically and pathologically be classified as acute or chronic. Gastric inflammation can have many causes including: (a) irritants and toxic substances in food and drugs; (b) infections and (c) autoimmune mechanisms. In many instances gastric chronic inflammation is multifactorial and may lead to peptic ulceration.

#### Acute Gastritis

*Acute gastritis* refer to disease of varying severity that occurs when the normal defensive mechanisms of the gastric mucosa are disrupted or overcome allowing access to the damaging effects of gastric acid or other corrosives. It is usually associated with mucosal erosions and shallow ulcerations. Etiologies include non-steroidal anti-inflammatory drugs (NSAIDs); alcohol; infections; systemic illnesses, such as uremia or sepsis; trauma; radiation; chemotherapy or corrosive ingestion. Hence these findings are not uncommon in intensive care unit patients. Some causes, alcohol or chemicals for example, directly damage the mucosa. The pathologic changes range from minor changes such as edema and congested blood vessels to active inflammation (with neutrophils within the epithelium), to erosion of the epithelial surface, to more extensive ulceration with or without hemorrhage and/or perforation.

#### Chronic Gastritis

*Chronic gastritis with Helicobacter pylori* accounts for the vast majority of cases of chronic gastritis. Chronic gastritis refers to prolonged inflammation in the stomach with lingering symptoms. Less frequent etiologies for chronic gastritis include autoimmune gastritis, bile reflux, radiation and systemic diseases among others.

H. pylori is a bacillus that typically affects individuals in regions with poor sanitation, poverty and crowding. This bacillus is held responsible for most duodenal ulcers, chronic gastritis and gastric ulcers. It preferentially affects the gastric antrum but may in some cases spread to involve the entire stomach. This organism is associated with hyperacidity. H. pylori mediates its effects via several factors including toxins (CagA), the urease enzyme and flagella among others.

On biopsy, the lamina propria is infiltrated by plasma cells and lymphocytes. There is often an active component with neutrophils within the epithelium or even collections within the gastric glands (pit microabscesses). Commonly there are lymphoid follicles with germinal centers which are an acquired form of mucosa associated lymphoid tissue (MALT) (Figs 4.11A and B). Over time, there may be mucosal atrophy which refers to the loss of glands (particularly oxyntic glands) as well as intestinal metaplasia (which is a change to an intestinal type epithelium with goblet cells).

While *H. pylori* can be seen using routine stains, they can be better visualized using special stains including silver stains such as the Steiner (Fig. 4.11C). The spiral bacilli are usually found in the mucus overlying the foveolar surface but occasionally can be found deeper. They are unlikely to be found in areas of intestinal metaplasia. An immunohistochemical stain is also available; this is useful to identify post-antibiotic therapy alterations in morphology.

Other methods of detection include a serologic test or detection of urease activity either in the patient's breath or in the gastric biopsy. *H. pylori* predisposes infected individuals to the development of peptic ulcers, gastric adenocarcinoma (atrophy is an antecedent) and lymphoma (including MALT lymphomas). *Helicobacter heilmannii* is a related species causing less severe disease in humans that is believed to be acquired from animals.

### Peptic Ulcer Disease

*Peptic ulcer disease (PUD)* refers to chronic, often solitary, ulcers that occur in the duodenum and stomach in a background of chronic gastritis. *H. pylori* is the most frequently implicated cause. Factors creating a hyperacidic environment while diminishing mucosal protection may result in PUD. *H. pylori* and Zollinger-Ellison syndrome lead to hyperacidity. The later refers to gastrin producing tumors, which stimulate acid production from the parietal cells. The NSAIDs and corticosteroids decrease prostaglandin synthesis which is necessary for mucosal protection. Smoking and stress are additive factors.

The ulcers are more common in the first part of the duodenum or the gastric antrum but are not restricted to these sites. The ulcer is classically described as a punched out defect whose margins are flush with the surrounding mucosa ("heaped-up" margins are seen in ulcerating carcinomas). The floor of the PUD ulcer is level and not too ragged owing to enzymatic digestion. On microscopy, the most superficial layer is composed of necrotic debris, deep to which is an exudate with numerous neutrophils that overlies inflamed granulation tissue (composed of fibroblasts and numerous small blood vessels), that lies on a scar composed of fibrous tissue (**Figs 4.12A and B**). The depth of the ulcer varies from absence of only the mucosa to loss of the full thickness gastric wall, resulting in a perforation. Hemorrhage and scarring are other possible complications.

### Autoimmune Gastritis

*Autoimmune gastritis* is a less common form of chronic gastritis where there is atrophy (or loss) of the oxyntic glands in the gastric body (contrasting with the antral predominant disease of *H. pylori*). There are circulating antibodies to parietal cells and their product intrinsic factor; although it is postulated that the parietal cell loss may be mediated by T cells. With diminishing parietal cells, there is loss of gastric acid (achlorhydria) which in turn impairs iron absorption leading to iron deficiency anemia. Vitamin $B_{12}$ cannot be absorbed without intrinsic factor and this deficiency results in a type of megaloblastic anemia (termed pernicious anemia). The low acid leads to markedly elevated gastrin levels and hyperplasia of the gastrin producing endocrine cells predisposing these patients to developing carcinoid tumors. There is also risk of developing hyperplastic and dysplastic polyps as well as adenocarcinoma.

Grossly the mucosa is thin with attenuated rugae. Biopsies demonstrate lymphocytes and plasma cells in the lamina propria, loss of oxyntic glands and intestinal metaplasia (**Fig. 4.13**). The endocrine cell hyperplasia is best appreciated with immunohistochemical stains.

### Other Forms of Gastritis

*Eosinophilic gastritis* is a rare condition where numerous eosinophils infiltrate the lamina propria and epithelium of the stomach (**Fig. 4.14**), and often multiple other gastrointestinal viscera (eosinophilic gastroenteritis). Primary food allergens are implicated and there may be elevated levels of food-specific IgE in the serum as well as peripheral eosinophilia. This histology may also be secondary to parasites or even *H. pylori* uncommonly.

*Reactive (chemical) gastropathy* applies to chemical damage to the gastric mucosa that is usually related to duodenopancreatic/bile reflux or NSAIDs. The mucosa shows foveolar hyperplasia (the foveolae appear elongated and tortuous) with mucin depleted lining epithelium and propagation of smooth muscle in the lamina propria (**Fig. 4.15**). Notably absent is *H. pylori*, and inflammation is usually not significant.

*Iron related gastropathy (iron pill gastritis)* refers to mucosal injury that may occur with therapeutic iron ingestion. Erosions or ulcers of the mucosa may be detected, not infrequently with overlying brown pigment **(Fig. 4.16A)**. The Perl's Prussian blue stain may be used to identify this as iron **(Fig. 4.16B)**.

*Ménétrier's disease* is a form of hypertrophic gastropathy. Hypertrophic gastropathies are characterized by hyperplasia of a mucosal epithelial component resulting in exaggerated rugal folds. In Ménétrier's disease, the foveolar mucous cells are affected leading to long tortuous foveolae with dilated underlying glands **(Figs 4.17A and B)**. On biopsy, this change is very similar to that seen in hyperplastic polyps (see below); however, in Ménétrier's disease, the change is diffuse with involvement of the entire gastric body. The underlying abnormality is increased transforming growth factor alpha. These mucosal abnormalities interfere with protein absorption (protein losing enteropathy), resulting in hypoproteinemia. There is an increased risk of developing adenocarcinoma. Zollinger-Ellison syndrome is another hypertrophic gastropathy where there is parietal cell hyperplasia.

## Polyps and Neoplasms

Polyps are protrusions that extend above the mucosal surface. Numerous lesions may produce this gross appearance, ranging from inflammation to hyperplasia to tumors.

### Hyperplastic Polyp

*Hyperplastic polyp* is the most frequent gastric polyp. It occurs in association with chronic gastritis (that may or may not be related to *H. pylori*) and is typically located in the antrum. Like fundic gland polyps, these have smooth contours. Microscopically, hyperplastic polyps show drawn out tortuous foveolae and dilated foveolar glands, an inflamed and edematous lamina propria and often erosions of the polyp surface **(Figs 4.18A and B)**. These polyps are benign but larger polyps are at risk for dysplasia.

### Fundic Gland Polyp

*Fundic gland polyp* is a fairly common endoscopic finding which may occur sporadically or in the background of familial adenomatous polyposis (FAP) or Zollinger-Ellison syndrome. The polyps contain dilated oxyntic glands with parietal and chief cells **(Figs 4.19A and B)**. They are benign but may rarely develop dysplasia.

### Inflammatory Fibroid Polyp

*Inflammatory fibroid polyp* refers to a benign proliferation of spindle cells with admixed inflammatory cells such as eosinophils and blood vessels **(Figs 4.20A and B)**. They typically occur in the submucosa of the stomach or small bowel. They are favored to represent a reactive rather than neoplastic process.

### Gastric Adenoma

*Adenoma* is a polyp composed of dysplastic epithelium. Adenomas may be sporadic or occur in patients with FAP. The favored location is the antrum. The stomach usually shows chronic gastritis with atrophy and intestinal metaplasia. The dysplastic epithelium is composed of mucin depleted cells with long hyperchromatic nuclei that are pseudostratified **(Fig. 4.21)**. The dysplasia may be low grade with relatively simple glandular architecture, or high grade, with advanced cytologic atypia and architectural abnormalities. These changes are confined within the pre-existing basement membrane and do not show invasion of the lamina propria. Invasion is a hallmark of adeno-carcinoma which also shows greater cytologic atypia. Adenomas over 2 cm in size harbor an elevated risk for adenocarcinoma. Adenocarcinoma may involve as much as 30% of gastric adenomas.

### Gastric Adenocarcinoma

*Adenocarcinoma* is by far the most frequent malignant tumor in the stomach, typically affecting middle aged individuals. Histologically, two main forms are recognized: (1) the *intestinal type* which is characterized by malignant glands **(Figs 4.22A and B)** and (2) the *diffuse type* which lacks glands but frequently shows signet ring cells. Signet ring cells are malignant epithelial cells whose cytoplasm is distended by mucin vacuoles which displace their nuclei (Fig. 4.22C). The intestinal type produces defined masses that are more frequent in the antrum while the diffuse type preferentially affects the gastric body. This latter type may produce a classical gross appearance where there is no discrete tumor but instead a widespread infiltration of the gastric wall (termed "linitis plastica" or leather bottle stomach).

There are several predisposing factors for the development of gastric adenocarcinoma and most of these apply to the intestinal type which is more common in Asia, South America and Central/ Eastern Europe. These include multifocal atrophy with intestinal metaplasia, familial adenomatous polyposis (FAP) and possibly diet-related carcinogens such as N-nitroso compounds. The pathogenesis of the diffuse type remains unclear but deficient function of E-cadherin (an intercellular adhesion protein) has been implicated.

Adenocarcinoma that extends no further than the submucosa is termed *early gastric cancer* and has a very good prognosis if amenable to resection. On the other hand, *advanced gastric cancer*, which refers to carcinoma infiltrating beyond the submucosa into the gastric wall (Fig. 4.22D), has a poor prognosis.

### Carcinoid Tumor

*Carcinoid tumor* is a well-differentiated neuroendocrine tumor that arises from the neuroendocrine cells of the gut wall. This tumor may behave like a low grade carcinoma and is capable of lymph node as well as distant metastasis. They are more frequently found in the small bowel and the lung. In the stomach, they may be associated with atrophic gastritis, Multiple Endocrine Neoplasia 1 (Zollinger-Ellison syndrome) or be sporadic. The latter are more aggressive. Histologically there are nests, trabeculae or glands of fairly uniform cells with granular "salt and pepper" nuclear chromatin (Figs 4.23A and B). Immunohistochemical stains, such as chromogranin and synaptophysin, may be used to highlight the neuroendocrine nature of these tumors. As in other sites in the gut, aggressive high grade neuroendocrine carcinomas may rarely occur; however, these are distinct from carcinoid tumors.

### Gastrointestinal Stromal Tumor

*Gastrointestinal stromal tumor (GIST)* is a mesenchymal neoplasm composed of cells that are related to the interstitial cells of Cajal. These cells of Cajal, a normally occurring component of the gut, coordinate peristalsis. GISTs are most frequently found in the stomach although other parts of the gut and the abdomen may be affected. These tumors have activating mutations in the *KIT* gene that encodes a tyrosine kinase (c-KIT) that may be detected in the tumor cells using an immuno-histochemical stain (CD117). A minority of GISTs have mutations in the gene for platelet derived growth factor receptor alpha. Rarely these tumors may be associated with Carney's triad or neurofibromatosis type 1.

Grossly these are typically well circumscribed tumors located in the submucosa or deeper. Histologically they are composed of fairly uniform spindle cells whose nuclei may be indented by perinuclear vacuoles (Figs 4.24A and B). A variant shows rounded to ovoid epithelioid cells (Fig. 4.24C). When spindled, the differential diagnosis for GISTs includes benign mesenchymal tumors such as leiomyomas (Fig. 4.24D) or schwannomas (Fig. 4.24E). Immunohistochemical markers will usually resolve this issue.

The risk of aggressive behavior (such as metastases) is stratified based on their size, mitotic rate and location. They are often responsive to specific tyrosine kinase inhibitors, which may be used in addition to surgery to manage these tumors.

### Lymphoma

*Lymphoma* of the stomach is most often a mature B-cell lymphoma of the extra-nodal marginal zone type. These are also called MALTomas (lymphomas of MALT) and are often related to *H. pylori* infection. In fact, elimination of this organism with antibiotic therapy typically results in remission. On biopsy, there is marked proliferation of B-lymphocytes and plasma cells in the lamina propria.

The lymphocytes extend into the glands to produce characteristic lymphoepithelial lesions. The lymphoid cells may contain more cytoplasm than usual and acquire a monocytoid appearance (Figs 4.25A and B). This low grade lymphoma is at risk for developing into the high grade diffuse large B-cell lymphoma (Fig. 4.25C).

## Small Intestine

The small intestine is a roughly 6 meter long mucosa lined muscular tube that digests food material, absorbs nutrients and propels luminal content to the colon via peristalsis. It comprises a proximal duodenum, a mid-jejunum and a distal ileum.

The small bowel shows the typical four layers of mucosa, submucosa, muscularis propria and serosa. The mucosa has a unique microscopic architecture wherein the luminal surface is thrown into innumerable finger-like structures with a core of lamina propria and overlying epithelium that are called villi. These vastly increase the surface for nutrient absorption. The villous epithelium predominantly shows columnar absorptive cells, goblet cells and infrequent endocrine cells. The villi invaginate into crypts of Lieberkühn that in turn contain endocrine cells, Paneth cells (which have supranuclear intense eosinophilic granules and a proposed role in innate immunity) and stem cells which repopulate the epithelium. Scattered inflammatory cells and small blood vessels, including lymphatics, are present in the lamina propria which is demarcated from the submucosa by the muscularis mucosa (Fig. 4.26A). Some regional variations exist, such as the presence of mucous glands in the submucosa of the duodenum (Fig. 4.26B). Aggregates of lymphoid tissue are present through the intestine. These are prominent enough to be grossly evident in the distal ileum and are termed Peyer's patches (Fig. 4.26C).

Abnormalities of the small intestine may be:
- Developmental anomalies
- Inflammatory/infectious conditions
- Polyps and neoplasms.

### Developmental Anomalies

*Meckel's diverticulum* is the remnant of the vitelline duct, a communication between the digestive tract and the yolk sac. It is a test-tube like projection extending out from bowel lumen and containing mucosa, submucosa and muscularis propria in its wall. The "rule of 2s" applies to this anomaly which affects roughly 2% of the population, is 2 times as frequent in men, measures approximately 2 inches in length and is located less than 2 feet from the ileocecal valve. Classically it is lined by small intestinal mucosa but when gastric mucosa is present, peptic ulcers may occur.

### Inflammatory and Infectious Conditions

Inflammatory conditions involving the intestine may have many causes, including infections and autoimmune inflammation. Here we shall illustrate only two conditions: (a) Gluten sensitive enteropathy and (b) Whipple disease.

#### Gluten-Sensitive Enteropathy

*Gluten-sensitive enteropathy (celiac disease/sprue)* is an immune mediated disease affecting the small intestine, which is provoked by exposure to gluten. This usually develops in genetically susceptible individuals who bear the HLA-DQ2 or HLA-DQ8 alleles. Gluten is found in several cereals, such as wheat and barley, and the gliadin component of gluten is implicated in this disease. This T-cell mediated process damages mucosal epithelial cells (enterocytes) and results in malabsorption. Dermatitis herpetiformis is a skin rash that often accompanies this disease. There are circulating antibodies to tissue transglutaminase, deamidated gliadin and endomysium which are important for the diagnosis of celiac disease. These patients are at increased risk for T-cell lymphoma and intestinal adenocarcinoma.

When fully developed, there is loss of the villous architecture resulting in a flattened mucosal surface and hyperplasia of the crypts **(Fig. 4.27A)**. Increase in intraepithelial lymphocytes may be seen **(Fig. 4.27B)** and this can be histologic pointer to this disease even before the villi are lost.

### Whipple Disease

*Whipple disease* is an infrequent multiorgan infection caused by *Tropheryma whippelii*, a Gram-positive actinobacterium. This affects the bowel, lymph nodes and joints. Macrophages filled with the micro-organism lead to blocked lymphatics, causing malabsorption and diarrhea. Grossly there are yellowish plaques on the mucosa and biopsy demonstrates broad villi filled with swollen macrophages that are filled with micro-organisms **(Figs 4.28A and B)**. These stain with the periodic acid-Schiff stain but are negative with the acid-fast stain for mycobacteria; the latter can mimic this histologic appearance.

## Polyps and Neoplasms

Polyps may be the result of numerous processes including hyperplasia, heterotopias, inflammation, dysplasia or tumors. Some of the polyps that occur in the small intestine (juvenile polyp, inflammatory polyp and adenoma) are described in the section on colon below. Adenocarcinomas of the small intestine are uncommon and will not be described here.

### Carcinoid Tumor

*Carcinoid tumor* is frequently seen in the small intestine (approximately 30–40% of all gut carcinoids). Carcinoids in jejunum and ileum (midgut carcinoids) are fairly aggressive, especially if large and involving the deeper bowel wall. Duodenal tumors tend to be less so. The most common site is the ileum and multiple tumors may be present.

Carcinoid syndrome results when vasoactive substances produced by these tumors (often ileal) reach the systemic circulation. The substances are subject to degradation in the liver (first pass metabolism) so the syndrome usually occurs when there are hepatic metastases. Elevated serotonin is typical. Clinical features include flushing, diarrhea, bronchospasm and tricuspid regurgitation.

The morphology is similar to that described above in the stomach. The cells typically have granular cytoplasm **(Figs 4.29A and B)**. Lymph node metastases **(Fig. 4.29C)** are present in over half the patients at first clinical recognition of the tumor.

Carcinoid tumors may also be identified in the large intestine, most often in the rectum.

### Gastrointestinal Stromal Tumor

*Gastrointestinal stromal tumor (GIST)* occurs in the small bowel next in frequency to the stomach. Morphologically they are similar to those in the stomach **(Figs 4.30A and B)**. Though there are some differences, epithelioid morphology is rare in the small bowel and some tumors show scattered small eosinophilic collagenous structures called skeinoid fibers. Again risk stratification for prediction of tumor behavior is based on tumor size, mitotic rate and location.

### Lymphoma

*Lymphoma* represents roughly a quarter of tumors in this part of the bowel. Types encountered in order of descending frequency are diffuse large B-cell lymphoma, marginal zone B-cell lymphoma and Burkitt's lymphoma **(Figs 4.31A and B)** among others.

## Colon

The colon is an approximately 1 meter long mucosa lined muscular tube that reabsorbs water and electrolytes from its luminal contents. It commences from the ileocecal valve with the cecum, followed by the ascending colon, via the hepatic flexure to the transverse colon, which in turn is continuous with the descending colon via the splenic flexure, the sigmoid colon and the rectum which then leads to the anal canal.

The colonic wall from the cecum to the rectum consists of the mucosa, submucosa, muscularis propria and serosa. The surface epithelium is covered by columnar absorptive cells and goblet cells; this dips into crypts lined by goblet cells, endocrine cells and Paneth cells (the latter are absent from the distal transverse colon onward) (Fig. 4.32). The outer layer of the muscularis propria is discontinuous and present as three equidistantly spaced tinea coli that extend along the length of the colon. The serosa is variably present as some portions are retroperitoneal.

Abnormalities of the colon may be:
- Developmental anomalies
- Inflammatory/infectious conditions
- Polyps and neoplasms.

## Developmental Anomalies

*Hirschsprung disease* is characterized by absent ganglion cells in the neural plexuses of the bowel wall (Meissner submucosal plexus and myenteric plexus of Auerbach). This results in impaired peristalsis. Genetic mutations (most frequently in the *RET* gene) are believed to impair the migration and survival of neural crest cells, the source of ganglion cells. The disease affects neonates. The sigmoid and rectum are often involved but the disease may affect proximal segments. The uninvolved bowel becomes hugely dilated (termed megacolon) and is at risk of perforation.

## Inflammatory and Infectious Conditions

Colitis may have many causes including: (a) infections; (b) ischemia and (c) inflammation of unknown etiology, as in inflammatory bowel disease, or lymphocytic colitis.

### Ischemic Colitis

*Ischemic colitis* may be acute (when there is a sudden compromise in blood flow) or chronic (when this develops over time). Some colon segments, such as the splenic flexure, sigmoid colon and rectum, are especially vulnerable to ischemia, as they are located near the ends of their arterial supplies (watershed zones). Causes for ischemia are numerous and include vascular disease (atherosclerosis, aneurysms, thromboemboli, radiation injury, etc.), states of low blood flow, mechanical compression of vascular supply as in volvulus (twisting of the bowel), intussusception (telescoping of the bowel) or secondary to adhesions. These conditions are common in older individuals.

In acute ischemic colitis, there is hemorrhagic necrosis of the mucosa while deeper portion of the crypts may persist, changes termed mucosal infarct (Fig. 4.33A). If the insult is severe, there may be a transmural infarct where the changes extend into the submucosa and the muscularis propria producing a dusky gross appearance. Serositis and perforation of the bowel may occur. Sepsis is another potential complication.

Chronic ischemic colitis is characterized by a fibrotic lamina propria and atrophic crypts (Fig. 4.33B).

### Pseudomembranous Colitis

*Pseudomembranous colitis* refers to infection by *Clostridium difficile* that classically occurs in patients who have received prior antibiotic therapy and often are hospitalized. The antibiotics probably alter the pre-existing bacterial environment in the bowel allowing emergence of this infection.

Grossly the mucosa is covered by pseudomembranes (which may also be seen in ischemic colitis). Microscopically there are ulcerations of the mucosa with overlying "volcano-like" pseudomembranes composed of neutrophils, fibrin and debris (Figs 4.34A and B).

### Amebic Colitis

*Amebic colitis* is an infection by the protozoan *Entamoeba histolytica*, more common in the developing world, that produces dysentery and liver abscesses. Ingestion of the acid resistant cysts results in the formation of trophozoites that damage the colonic mucosa. These produce flask-shaped ulcers

(Fig. 4.35A). The organisms may be visualized within the ulcers and often contain red blood cells (Fig. 4.35B).

### Inflammatory Bowel Disease

*Inflammatory bowel disease (IBD)* is a chronic relapsing inflammatory disorder of unclear etiology, although genetic predisposition, immune alterations, abnormal mucosal epithelium and interactions with gut micro-organisms have all been proposed. The IBD usually manifests as *Crohn's disease* which affects the small and large intestines or as *ulcerative colitis (UC)* which is mostly restricted to the colon. There are associations with joint disease, skin manifestations and hepatobiliary disease (primary sclerosing cholangitis). Both diseases have an elevated risk for adenocarcinoma, especially after a decade, and individuals with IBD often require surveillance for this.

Crohn's disease usually shows discontinuous involvement of the bowel (called skip lesions) affecting the colon, small bowel, both or any part of the gut. The inflammation extends through the bowel wall (transmural involvement) producing changes that include small superficial aphthous ulcers, cobblestone mucosa (a pattern produced by intermixed areas of affected and normal mucosa), deep fissure ulcers, markedly thickened fibrotic bowel walls, strictures or fistulae (the latter are connections between the bowel lumen and another viscus, often perianal). The characteristic microscopic finding is the presence of granulomas that are found in approximately a third of Crohn's disease biopsies but are absent in UC.

UC, on the other hand, shows continuous involvement of the superficial bowel wall (mucosa and submucosa), typically affecting the rectum (ulcerative proctitis), and involving the remaining colon partially or completely (pancolitis). The disease is largely restricted to the colon, although backwash ileitis (with limited distal ileal disease) may occur. Manifestations range from abnormal mucosa to broad based ulcers with intervening regenerating mucosa (pseudopolyps). Unlike Crohn's disease, effects of transmural disease, such as strictures or fistulae do not occur.

On biopsy, there are features of active inflammation superimposed on a chronic colitis. Chronic changes include mucosal architectural distortion with branched, short crypts and increased plasma cells within the lamina propria (**Figs 4.36A and B**). An additional finding is Paneth cell metaplasia (**Fig. 4.36C**), which refers to Paneth cells in the crypts of the distal colon (where they do not normally occur). Active inflammation is represented by cryptitis, where neutrophils are present in contact with the crypt epithelium and crypt abscesses, where collections of neutrophils aggregate within the crypt lumen (**Figs 4.36B and D**). In Crohn's disease, there may be granulomas, composed of epithelioid histiocytes and sometimes multinucleate giant cells (**Fig. 4.36C**).

Resection specimens more clearly demonstrate the transmural nature of Crohn's disease (**Fig. 4.36E**) in contrast to the mucosal and submucosal distribution of UC (**Fig. 4.36F**).

### Other Forms of Colitis

*Microscopic colitis* refers to colitis in patients with watery diarrhea, unimpressive endoscopic findings and microscopic abnormalities. It is of two classic types: (1) collagenous and (2) lymphocytic. *Collagenous colitis* typically affects middle aged women whose biopsies show a thick layer of collagen beneath the surface epithelium (**Figs 4.37A and B**) and greater numbers of lymphocytes within the epithelium. *Lymphocytic colitis* affects a broader range of individuals and does not demonstrate the abnormal collagen layer.

### Diverticular Disease

*Diverticular disease* is characterized by acquired diverticula which typically occur in the sigmoid colon of older individuals. Elevated pressure within the bowel lumen leads to herniation of the mucosa and submucosa through deficiencies in the muscularis propria producing diverticula (**Fig. 4.38A**). These points of weakness correspond to where nerves and vessels enter the muscularis. Blockage of the diverticula leads to inflammation and diverticulitis (**Fig. 4.38B**). Complications include wall fibrosis and strictures, pericolonic abscesses, sinus tracts or perforation.

### Graft versus Host Diseases

*Graft versus host disease* occurs in individuals who have been transplanted. The donor's immune cells that are present within the graft may occasionally attack the recipient's tissues, particularly the skin, gut and liver producing graft versus host disease. The microscopic appearance varies in severity from increased apoptotic epithelial cells in the colonic crypts (Fig. 4.39) to loss of crypts and ulceration.

## Polyps and Neoplasms

Polyps may be *pedunculated* where they are connected to the bowel wall by a stalk of mucosa covered tissue or *sessile* where they sit directly on the bowel mucosa.

### Juvenile Polyp

*Juvenile polyp* is a benign localized polypoid mucosal malformation that most often occurs in young children and affects the rectum. Typically these polyps have a stalk. Microscopically these polyps have distended crypts that contain mucin and inflammatory cells. The polyp surface is often eroded with underlying granulation tissue, and there is increased inflammation in the lamina propria (Figs 4.40A and B). These polyps may be sporadic, or when multiple, form part of the juvenile polyposis syndrome. The latter shows an elevated risk of colonic adenocarcinoma.

Juvenile polyps have more inflammation and lack the smooth muscle proliferation seen in the hamartomatous polyps of Peutz-Jeghers syndrome. This hereditary syndrome, an autosomal dominant disease produced by mutations in the *LKB1/STK11* gene, is characterized by numerous hamartomatous polyps of the gut, mucocutaneous pigmentation and an elevated risk for gut adenocarcinomas.

### Hyperplastic Polyp

*Hyperplastic polyp* is the most common colonic polyp, with a preference for the left colon and typically measuring less than 0.5 cm. It is a benign polyp that is postulated to occur as a consequence of decreased epithelial programmed cell death and decreased exfoliation of epithelial cells at the colonic surface. Hence mucinous epithelial cells accumulate and are thrown into uneven tufts or serrations. These changes are common in the upper portions of the crypts which are not dilated or branched (Figs 4.41A and B). When sparse in number, these polyps are currently not regarded to increase the risk of colon cancer.

### Sessile Serrated Polyp

*Sessile serrated polyp* is a recently recognized polyp with preference for occurring in the right colon. Although it bears a superficial resemblance to hyperplastic polyps, the sessile serrated polyp is larger and shows crypts that are lined by hypermucinous cells and are dilated and branched at their bases (Fig. 4.42). These polyps are prone to mutations in the *BRAF* gene and to DNA methylation. These polyps are at risk for the development of dysplasia and colonic adenocarcinoma.

### Serrated Adenoma

*Serrated adenoma* is a dysplastic polyp with papillary architecture, prominent crypt serration and epithelial cells with distinctive eosinophilic cytoplasm and stratified nuclei (Fig. 4.43). They typically present as pedunculated polyps in the left colon. They are at risk for the development of colonic adenocarcinoma.

### Adenoma

*Adenoma* is a common dysplastic polyp which may be sessile or pedunculated. Based on their microscopic architecture, adenomas are classified as tubular, tubulovillous or villous types reflecting their proportion of simple tubules and finger-like villi (Figs 4.44A and B). Adenomas at the very least show *low grade dysplasia* where the nuclei are longer and stratified and these cytologic alterations extend to the mucosal surface (Figs 4.44A to C). Some adenomas may show more advanced cytologic atypia and complex architecture with cribriforming and back to back glands, changes that are classified as *high grade dysplasia* (Fig. 4.44D).

Adenomas do not show invasion of the lamina propria. If there is invasion of lamina propria, but no extension into the submucosa, then a diagnosis of *intramucosal adenocarcinoma* is rendered. This tumor lacks the ability to metastasize and may be treated by polypectomy (unlike the invasive adenocarcinomas described below).

Adenomas are premalignant and it is recommended that patients undergo surveillance for this (usually commencing from 50 years of age). The risk of adenocarcinoma developing within an adenoma largely depends on the size of the lesion, with adenomas over 2 cm being especially at risk. High grade dysplasia is another risk factor. Villous lesions are more likely to be larger.

Adenomas may occur sporadically or as part of FAP which is an autosomal dominant disease occurring secondary to mutations in the adenomatous polyposis coli (*APC*) gene. The diagnosis is based on the presence of 100 or more adenomas but patients often present in excess of this. Unless a prophylactic colectomy is performed, virtually all patients will have colorectal adenocarcinomas by the end of their third decade. Variants of FAP include Gardner syndrome (associated with bony osteomas, desmoid and thyroid tumors) and Turcot syndrome (associated with central nervous tumors such as medulloblastomas and glioblastomas).

### Adenocarcinoma

*Adenocarcinoma of the colon*, the most frequent malignancy in the gastrointestinal tract, is a major cause of cancer death in the United States. This carcinoma is more often seen in developed countries, and dietary factors have been implicated. Affected individuals vary from late middle aged patients to elderly patients and there is a male preponderance. Inherited syndromes account for a small proportion of colon cancer. Hereditary non-polyposis colorectal cancer (Lynch syndrome) is characterized by inherited mutations in the genes responsible for the repair of DNA mismatch. This occurs during replication and affects microsatellite repeats, leading to microsatellite instability. Lynch syndrome is implicated in approximately 2–3% of colon cancer and preferentially affects the right colon in younger individuals; other viscera are also affected. Polyposis cancer syndromes (such as FAP) account for less than 0.5% of colorectal adenocarcinoma.

A few pathways have proposed for the genesis of colon cancer: the APC/beta-catenin pathway; the microsatellite instability pathway as well as methylation-induced gene silencing.

Adenocarcinomas of the right colon are more often large protruding masses while those of the left colon are more prone to obstruction producing a napkin-ring constriction. Histologically these adenocarcinomas invade into the submucosa or deeper. When low grade, they form irregular glands lined by fairly columnar malignant epithelial cells with high nuclear-cytoplasmic ratios and pleomorphic nuclei with nucleoli (Figs 4.45A and B). The stroma is altered (desmoplastic type). Poorly differentiated adenocarcinomas show limited gland formation. Several variants exist, such as mucinous adenocarcinoma where at least half of the tumor is mucin (Fig. 4.45C) or signet-ring adenocarcinoma where at least half the adenocarcinoma is composed of signet-ring cells (Figs 4.45D and E).

Prognosis is largely stage dependent. Some subtypes, such as the mucinous and signet-ring adenocarcinomas, tend to be first recognized at higher stages. The liver is the most frequent metastatic site.

## Appendix

The appendix is a vestigial blind ended cylindrical structure that arises from the cecum near the ileocecal valve. Typically its lumen is in continuity with that of the cecum. Histologically, the appendix is similar to the colon (Fig. 4.46) though mucosal lymphoid tissue is prominent here. The base of the appendix refers to the portion that connects to the cecum, while the free end of the appendix is called the tip.

Abnormalities of the appendix may be:
- Inflammatory/infectious conditions
- Neoplasms

## Inflammatory and Infectious Conditions

*Acute appendicitis* is a frequently encountered condition, especially in adolescents and young adults, where there is acute neutrophilic inflammation within the appendiceal wall. Increases in pressure within the lumen or obstruction of the same by fecaliths (which are inspissated concretions of stool) cause an ischemic insult. Also intraluminal bacteria propagate, all of which results in neutrophils coursing through the appendiceal wall. The process often begins with mucosal ulceration. Neutrophils within the muscularis propria establish the diagnosis. More severe disease traverses the entire wall to reach the serosa (**Figs 4.47A and B**). When associated with necrosis of the appendiceal tissue, this is termed *acute gangrenous appendicitis*. Without intervention, the appendiceal wall may give way or perforate which leads to peritonitis. Liver abscesses, pyelophlebitis or bacteremia are other possible complications.

### Neoplasms

Two most important neoplasms of the appendix are: (a) carcinoid tumors and (b) mucinous neoplasms.

### Carcinoid Tumor

*Carcinoid tumor* is a well differentiated neuroendocrine neoplasm. It is the most frequent tumor of the appendix and often it is found accidentally in appendices removed for other reasons or at autopsy. These tumors are usually small, have their greatest occurrence in young adults and preferentially involve the appendiceal tip. Histologically it is similar to other carcinoids of the bowel (**Fig. 4.48**). These carcinoids tend to be benign, particularly when less than 2 cm in size.

### Low Grade Appendiceal Mucinous Neoplasm

*Low grade appendiceal mucinous neoplasm (well differentiated mucinous adenocarcinoma)* is a low grade appendiceal neoplasm of debated nomenclature. Grossly the appendix frequently appears dilated and filled with mucin. The mucosa is replaced by mildly atypical mucinous epithelium arranged in simple villi, short papillae or even flattened. The process extends into the appendiceal wall (**Figs 4.49A and B**) which may rupture.

This appendiceal neoplasm is potentially capable of spreading to the peritoneal cavity and producing repeated and widespread accumulations of mucin (that often contain low grade mucinous epithelium) on the peritoneal surfaces of abdominal cavity and viscera (**Fig. 4.49C**). These accumulations are clinically termed pseudomyxoma peritonei (also sometimes called "jelly belly"). As this mucinous process often recurs after treatment and since it can ultimately be fatal because of intestinal obstruction, this peritoneal mucinous process is considered a low grade mucinous adenocarcinoma.

To summarize, the low grade appendiceal neoplasms may result in pseudomyxoma peritonei but are typically not associated with distant metastasis (a feature of conventional adenocarcinomas). As these tumors are not as aggressive as conventional adenocarcinomas, low grade appendiceal mucinous neoplasm is preferred terminology for some experts. Other experts prefer to use the term well differentiated mucinous adenocarcinoma for this same appendiceal tumor, because of its ability to cause pseudomyxoma peritonei.

Conventional frankly invasive adenocarcinomas resembling that in other gut sites may occasionally occur in the appendix.

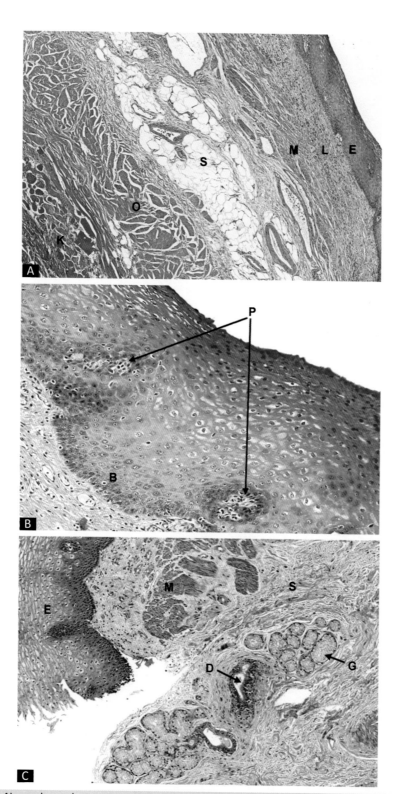

**Figs 4.1A to C:** Normal esophagus

**A.** The layers of the esophageal wall: (a) the mucosa lined by stratified squamous epithelium (E), resting on the lamina propria (L) and muscularis mucosa (M), (b) the submucosa (S) and (c) the muscularis propria which comprises both smooth muscle (O) and skeletal muscle (K) in the upper esophagus (the adventitia is not visualized in this photograph). **B.** The multilayered squamous epithelium consists of proliferative basal layers (B) which normally account for less than a third of the thickness of the epithelium. Finger-like projections of lamina propria (P) typically remain in the lower two-third of the epithelium. **C.** Mucus glands (G) with their accompanying duct (D) in the submucosa (S) of the esophagus; overlying unremarkable squamous epithelium (E) and muscularis mucosa (M) are also evident.

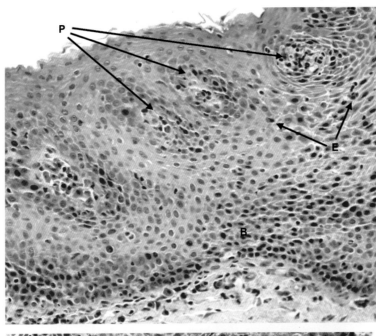

**Fig. 4.2:** Reflux esophagitis

The squamous epithelium shows basal layer hyperplasia (B) and the presence of lamina propria papillae (P) within the superficial epithelium. Only a few scattered intraepithelial eosinophils (E) are present in contrast to eosinophilic esophagitis.

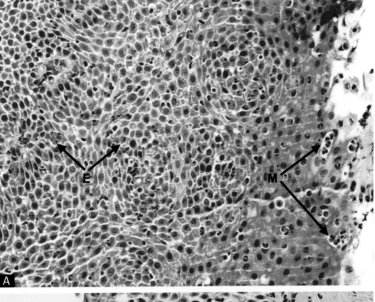

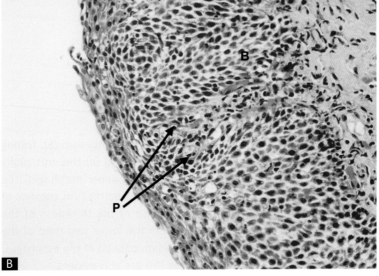

**Figs 4.3A and B:** Eosinophilic esophagitis

**A.** Here the squamous epithelium is characterized by a marked increase in intraepithelial eosinophils (E), greater than 25 per high power field, including collections of eosinophils known as microabscesses (M). **B.** This occurs in a background of changes that are similar to reflux esophagitis, i.e. basal layer hyperplasia (B) and superficially located lamina propria papillae (P).

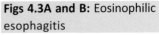

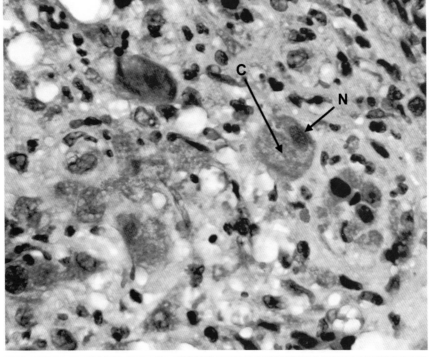

**Fig. 4.4:** Cytomegalovirus esophagitis
In this example several stromal cells within the granulation tissue of an ulcer demonstrate cellular enlargement with prominent basophilic intranuclear inclusions (N) and less well defined intracytoplasmic basophilic inclusions (C).

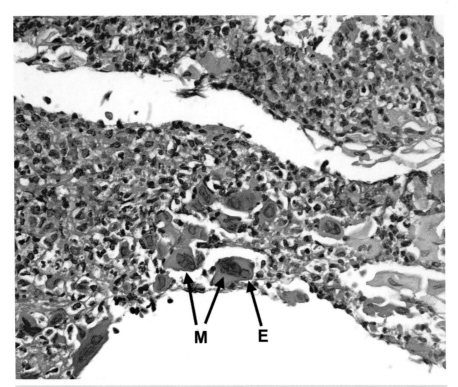

**Fig. 4.5:** Herpetic esophagitis
Several epithelial cells (E) demonstrate viral cytopathic changes with multiple nuclei (M) that are moulded to one another and showing marginated chromatin (as a result of displacement by the viral intranuclear eosinophilic inclusions).

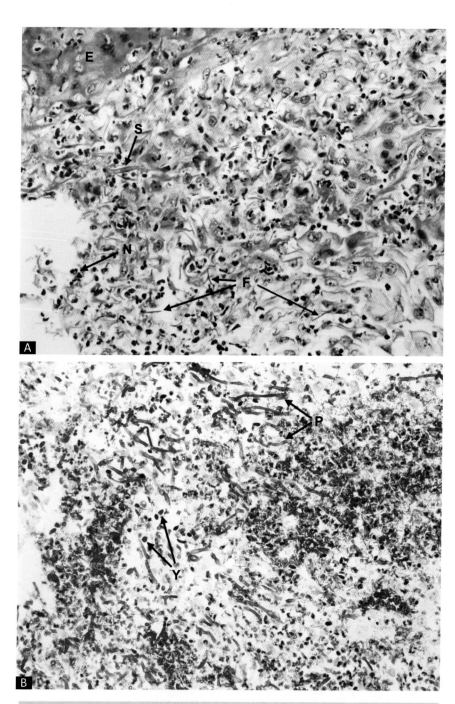

**Figs 4.6A and B:** Candida esophagitis

**A.** The squamous epithelium (E) is inflamed with numerous neutrophils (N). Fungal pseudohyphae (F) are noted admixed with superficial squamous cells (S) and neutrophils. **B.** The periodic acid-Schiff stain highlights the yeasts (Y) and pseudohyphae (P) of *Candida*.

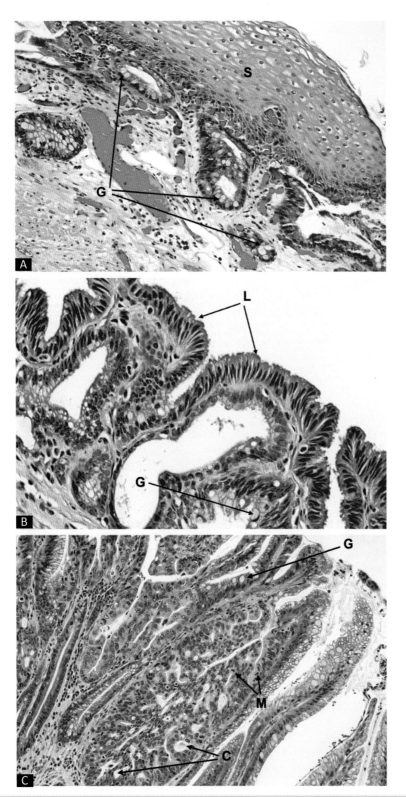

**Figs 4.7A to C:** Barrett esophagus

**A.** Underlying the squamous epithelium (S) of the esophagus, several glands are lined by columnar epithelium with mucin containing goblet cells (G). In conjunction with endoscopic findings, this histology is diagnostic of Barrett esophagus. **B.** *Low grade dysplasia* is characterized by epithelial cells with stratified, elongated nuclei (L) that are seen on the mucosal surface as well as in deeper portions of the glands. Glandular architecture remains fairly simple. Goblet cells (G) are also evident. **C.** *High grade dysplasia* has complex architecture with a cribriform pattern (C); this refers to fused glands with a sieve-like pattern. Increased cytologic atypia and several mitoses (M) are present. Goblet cells (G) are present.

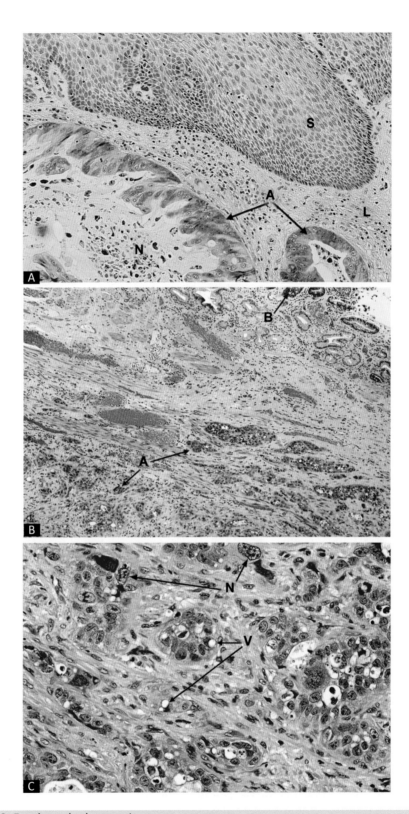

**Figs 4.8A to C:** Esophageal adenocarcinoma

**A.** Well differentiated adenocarcinoma is characterized by glands (A) that are lined by malignant epithelial cells and contain necrotic debris (N). These infiltrate the lamina propria (L). Overlying normal esophageal squamous epithelium (S) is noted. **B.** Poorly differentiated adenocarcinoma lacks the prominent gland formation seen in well differentiated adenocarcinomas. Instead nests of malignant epithelium (A) infiltrate into the muscle layer. Overlying Barrett esophagus (B) is present. **C.** At higher magnification, these cells demonstrate marked nuclear pleomorphism (N). The presence of cytoplasmic vacuoles (V) indicates that this is an adenocarcinoma.

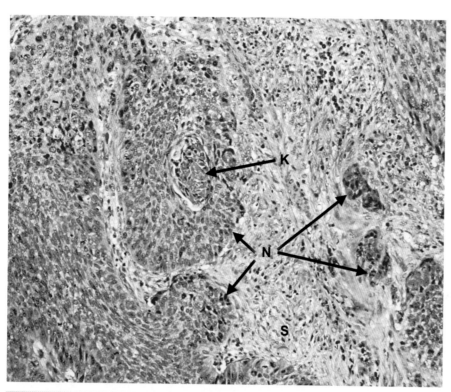

**Fig. 4.9**

*Esophageal squamous carcinoma* is composed of nests (N) of malignant squamous cells surrounded by a desmoplastic stroma (S). A focus of keratinization (K) is noted within one nest.

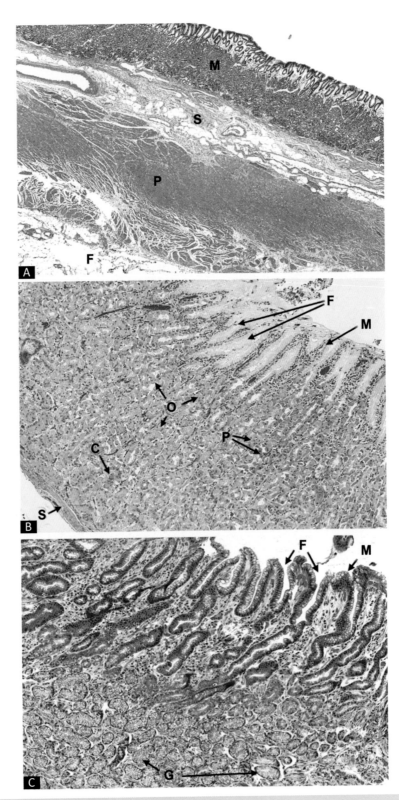

**Figs 4.10A to C:** Normal stomach

**A.** The gastric wall consists of the lumen facing mucosa (M), the submucosa (S), the muscularis propria (P), the subserosal adipose tissue (F) and the serosa which is not visualized in this image. **B.** Fundic/body mucosa comprises foveolae (F) lined by mucous cells (M) as well as oxyntic glands (O) which are lined by parietal (P) and chief (C) cells (S denotes the muscularis mucosa). **C.** Antral mucosa is composed again of foveolae (F) lined by mucous cells (M) as well as the deeper located mucous glands (G).

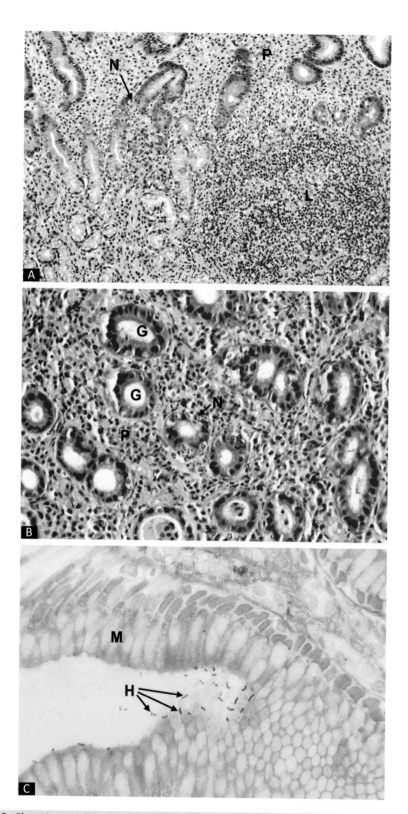

**Figs 4.11A to C:** Chronic gastritis caused by Helicobacter pylori
**A.** Chronic active gastritis with numerous plasma cells (P) and a lymphoid follicle (L) in the lamina propria as well as intraglandular neutrophils (N). **B.** At larger magnification, the lamina propria plasma cells (P) and neutrophils (N) with glands (G) are noted. **C.** The Steiner stain demonstrates the wavy to spiral bacilli (H) over the foveolar mucous cells (M).

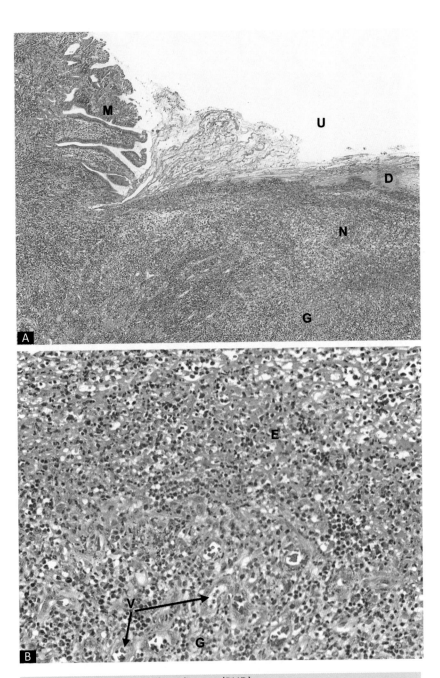

**Figs 4.12A and B:** Peptic ulcer disease (PUD)

**A.** The floor of the ulcer (U) shows the superficial fibrinous debris (D), deep to which is the necro-inflammatory exudate (N), that overlies the granulation tissue (G). The adjacent mucosa (M) shows reactive changes. **B.** A higher magnification image shows the exudate (E) composed of inflammatory cells and fibrin. The inflamed granulation tissue (G) has numerous small vessels (V).

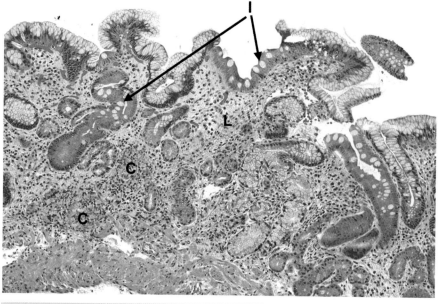

**Fig. 4.13:** Autoimmune gastritis
The mucosa shows loss of oxyntic glands, chronic inflammation (C) within the lamina propria (L) and intestinal metaplasia (I) with goblet cells.

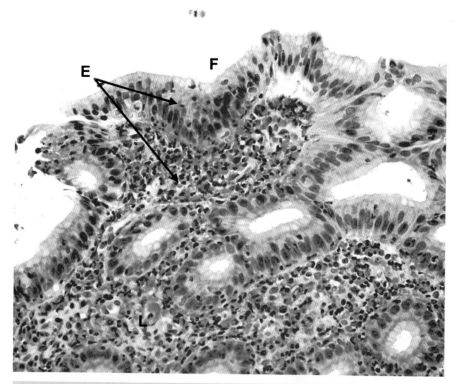

**Fig. 4.14:** Eosinophilic gastritis
Numerous eosinophils (E) are present within the lamina propria (L) and also within the epithelium (F denotes the surface foveolar epithelium).

DIGESTIVE SYSTEM

CHAPTER
**4**

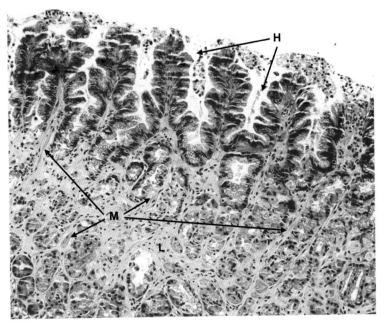

**Fig. 4.15:** Reactive (chemical) gastropathy

Mucin depleted epithelial cells line hyperplastic foveolae (H). There is smooth muscle (M) proliferation in the lamina propria (L) which lacks significant inflammation.

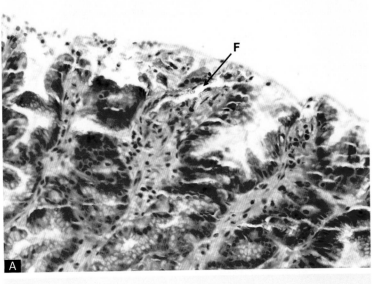

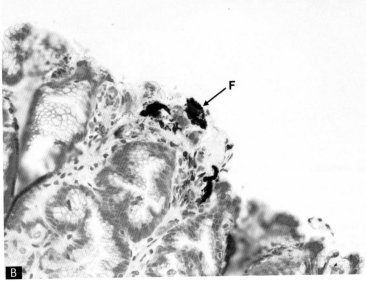

**Figs 4.16A and B:** Iron related gastropathy (iron pill gastritis)
**A.** Refractile brown pigment (F) is seen overlying reactive foveolar epithelium. **B.** The Perl's Prussian blue stain turns this pigment blue (F) confirming it to be iron.

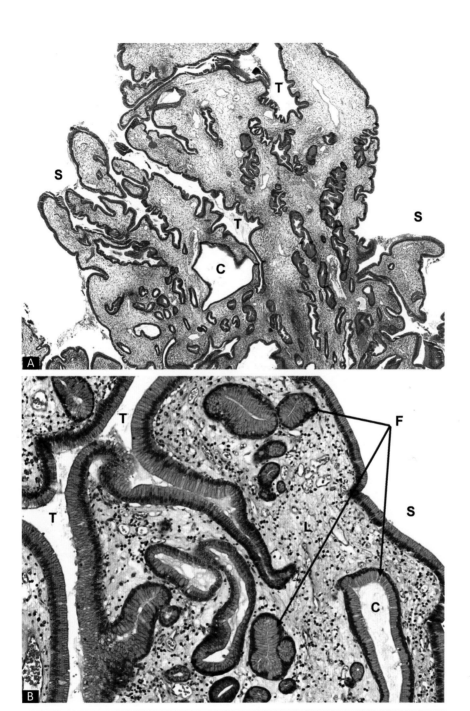

**Figs 4.17A and B:** Ménétrier disease of the stomach

**A.** These changes of hyperplastic tortuous foveolae (T) and cystic glands (C) occur diffusely throughout the gastric body (S denotes the mucosal surface) **B.** At larger magnification, the foveolar mucous cells (F) lining the tortuous foveolae (T) and glands (C) are evident. The lamina propria (L) shows mild inflammation (S denotes the mucosal surface).

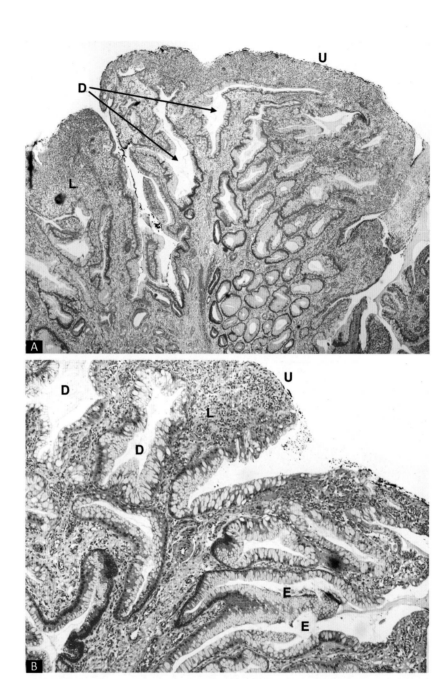

**Figs 4.18A and B:** Hyperplastic polyp of the stomach

**A.** This localized mucosal polyp is composed of dilated glands (D) and hyperplastic foveolae. The lamina propria (L) is inflamed and the surface is eroded (U). **B.** At greater magnification, the mucous cells lining the stretched out tortuous foveolae (E) and glands (D) are noted. There is granulation tissue composed of small blood vessels and fibroblasts underlying the eroded epithelial surface (U) and extending into the lamina propria.

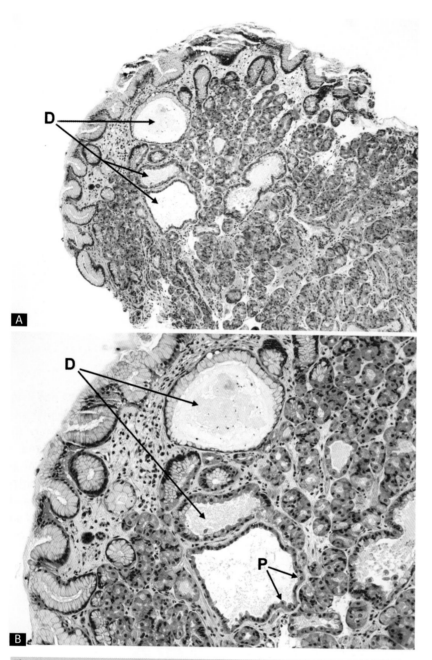

**Figs 4.19A and B:** Fundic gland polyp of the stomach

**A.** The mucosal polyp shows a number of dilated oxyntic glands (D).
**B.** A higher magnification image demonstrates several parietal cells (P) lining these dilated oxyntic glands (D).

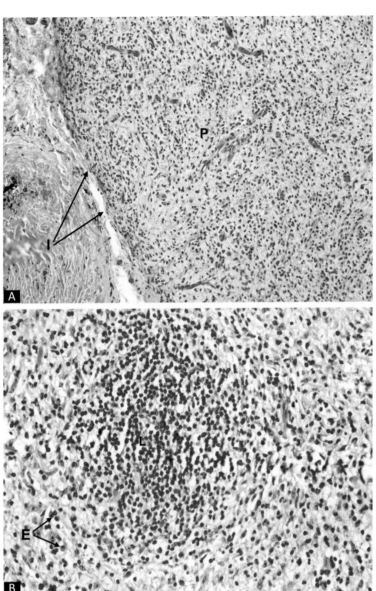

A

B

**Figs 4.20A and B:** Inflammatory fibroid polyp of the stomach
**A.** The interface (I) between the submucosa and polyp (P) is illustrated. **B.** At greater magnification, the polyp consists of eosinophils (E) and lymphocytes (L) superimposed on a background of bland spindle cells.

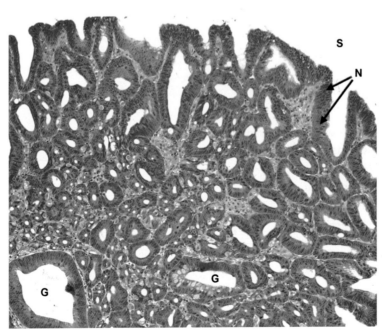

**Fig. 4.21:** Gastric adenoma
The tumor is composed of dysplastic mucin poor epithelial cells with lengthened, hyperchromatic nuclei (N). These changes not only involve the deeper glands (G) but also extend to the mucosal surface (S).

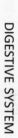

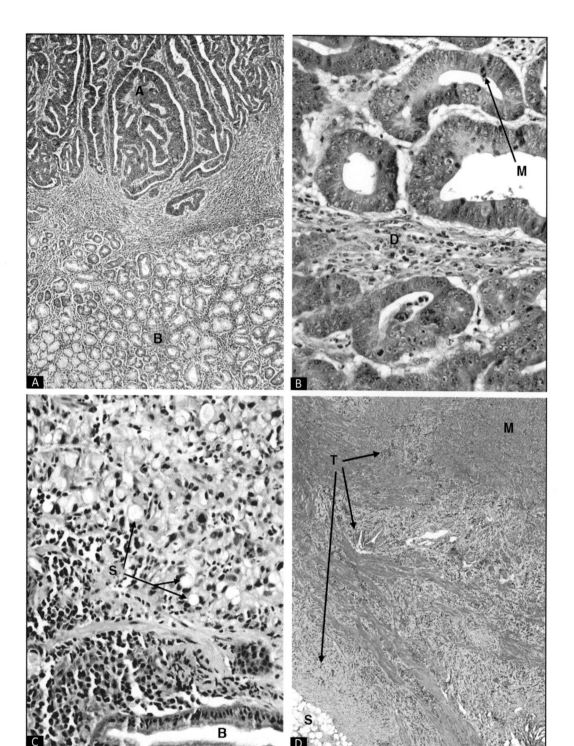

**Figs 4.22A to D:** Gastric adenocarcinoma

**A.** Intestinal type adenocarcinoma is composed of glands (A) lined by malignant epithelial cells that invade the gastric wall. This is in sharp contrast to the simple architecture and bland cytology of the adjacent benign mucosa (B). **B.** At larger magnification, the malignant cells have high nuclear to cytoplasmic ratios, marked variation in nuclear size and shape, prominent nucleoli and several mitotic figures (M). The glands are located within a desmoplastic stroma (D). **C.** Diffuse type adenocarcinoma lacks gland formation and often shows signet ring cells (S) whose cytoplasm is filled with mucin vacuoles that displace the nuclei to the outer edges of the cells (B marks an adjacent benign gland). **D.** Advanced gastric cancer is characterized by tumor cells (T) that have invaded beyond the submucosa—into the muscularis propria (M) and into the subserosal adipose tissue (S) (only the outer gastric wall is visualized in this image).

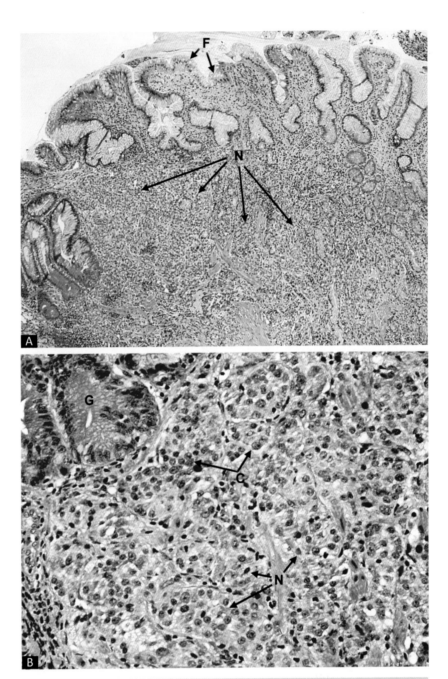

**Figs 4.23A and B:** Gastric carcinoid tumor

**A.** Nests (N) of tumor infiltrate the lamina propria and muscularis mucosae in this example (F denotes the surface foveolar epithelium). **B.** At greater magnification, the tumor nests (N) are composed of cells with stippled to granular "salt and pepper" chromatin (C) (G denotes overlying benign glands).

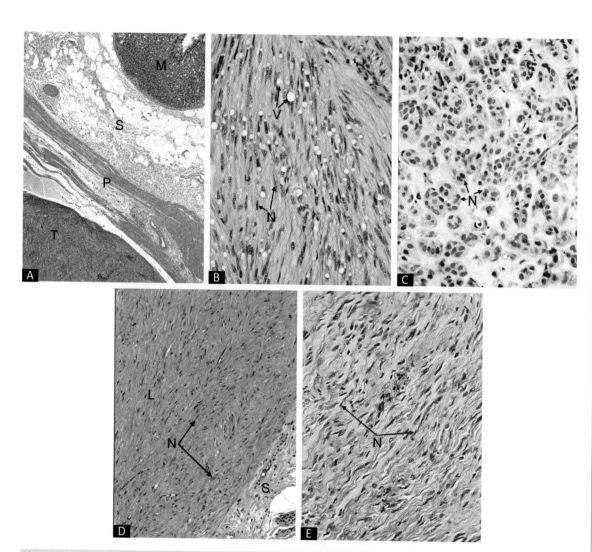

**Figs 4.24A to E:** Gastrointestinal stromal tumor (GIST) of the stomach

**A.** This image shows the well circumscribed GIST (T) located within the muscularis propria (P). The overlying submucosa (S) and mucosa (M) are also evident. **B.** At higher magnification, the tumor is composed of spindle cells with elongated nuclei (N). Several of the nuclei are indented by perinuclear vacuoles (V). **C.** Some gastric GISTs are composed of rounded epithelioid cells with round to ovoid nuclei (N) in this example. **D.** Leiomyoma is a benign tumor of smooth muscle that may mimic a GIST. In this image the leiomyoma (L) is located in the submucosa (S) and has spindle cells with cigar shaped nuclei (N). **E.** Schwannoma, a benign peripheral sheath tumor with characteristically wavy nuclei (N) is another potential mimic. Unlike GISTs, leiomyomas and schwannomas do not express CD117.

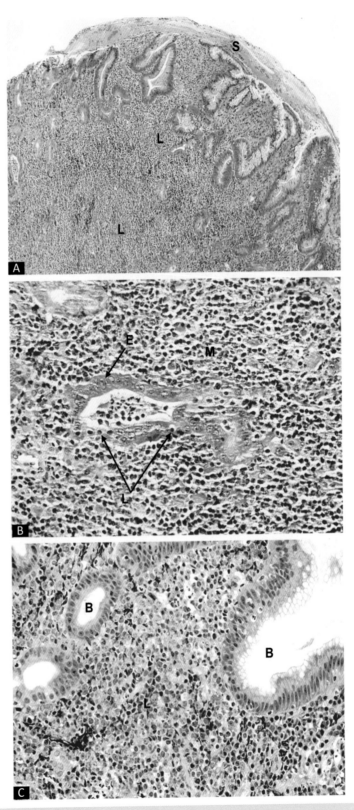

**Figs 4.25A to C:** Gastric lymphoma

**A.** Extranodal marginal zone lymphoma shows that the lamina propria is filled by an extensive infiltrate of lymphoid cells (L) (S denotes the mucosal surface). **B.** At higher magnification, these lymphoid cells (L) infiltrate into the glandular epithelium (E) to produce a lymphoepithelial lesion. The lymphoid cells have a considerable quantity of pale cytoplasm resembling monocytes; hence these are termed "monocytoid" cells (M). **C.** Diffuse large B-cell lymphoma shows sheets of large, overtly malignant lymphoid cells (L) virtually replacing the lamina propria (B marks intervening benign glands).

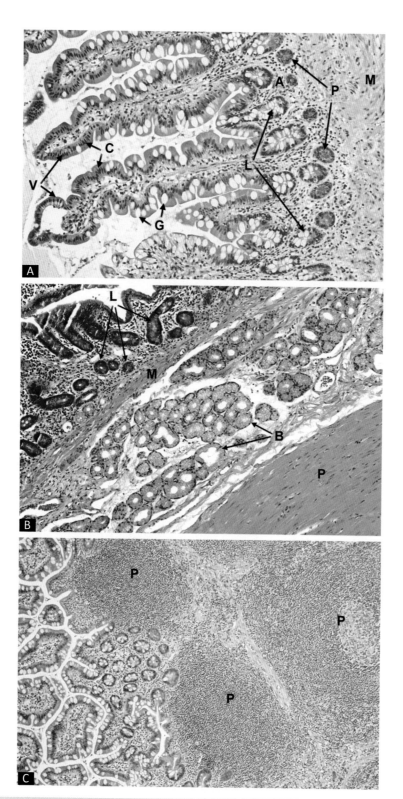

**Figs 4.26A to C:** Normal small intestine

**A.** Mucosa: The finger-like villi (V) are lined by columnar epithelial cells (C) and goblet cells (G). The villi dip down into the crypts of Lieberkühn (L). At the bases of these are Paneth cells (P) with eosinophilic supranuclear granules. The lamina propria (A) contains scattered inflammatory cells (M denotes the muscularis mucosa). **B.** Brunner's glands (B) are mucous glands present in the submucosa of the duodenum (L—crypts of Lieberkühn, M—muscularis mucosa, P—muscularis propria). **C.** Peyer's patches (P) refer to the prominent lymphoid tissue within the mucosa and submucosa. This is more frequently noted in the ileum.

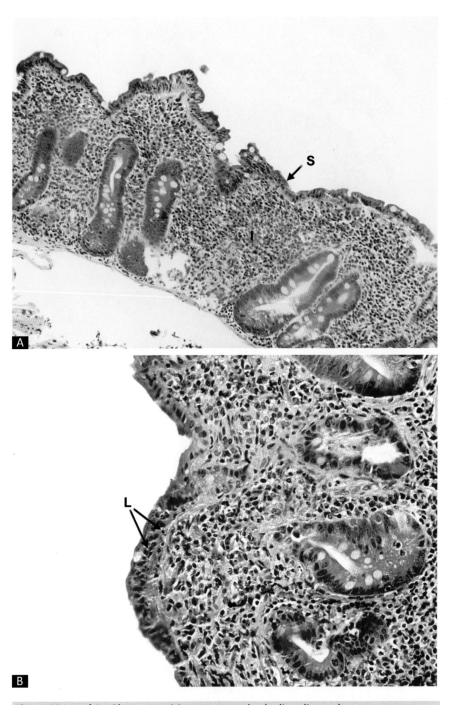

**Figs 4.27A and B:** Gluten-sensitive enteropathy (celiac disease)

**A.** The mucosal surface (S) shows loss of villi with corresponding crypt hyperplasia. The lamina propria is packed with inflammatory cells (I), particularly plasma cells. **B.** There are several intraepithelial lymphocytes (L).

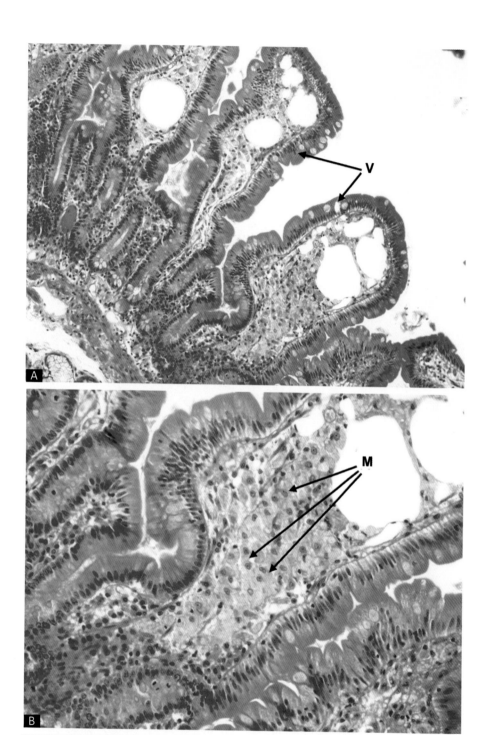

**Figs 4.28A and B:** Whipple disease

**A.** Several broad villi (V) with abnormal lamina propria are seen. **B.** At higher magnification, the lamina propria is packed with macrophages (M) that have abundant foamy cytoplasm.

DIGESTIVE SYSTEM

CHAPTER

**4**

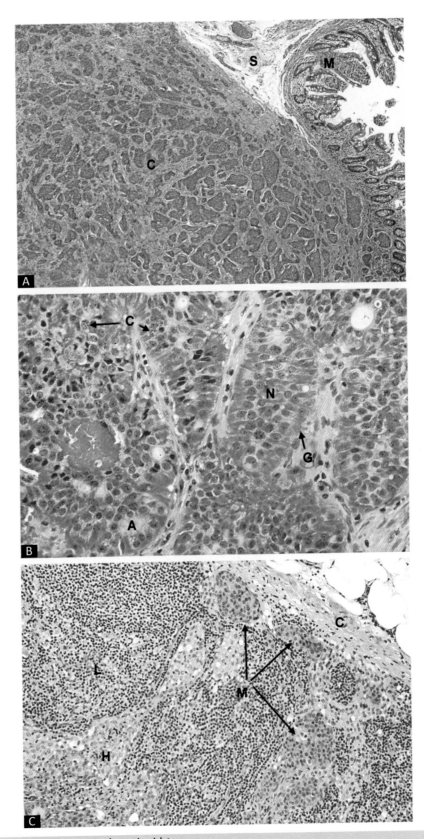

**Figs 4.29A to C:** Small intestinal carcinoid tumor
**A.** The carcinoid tumor (C) is clearly distinguished from the surrounding submucosa (S) and overlying mucosa (M). **B.** A greater magnification image demonstrates nests (N) and glands (A) of tumor cells which have "salt and pepper" chromatin (C) and eosinophilic granular cytoplasm (G). **C.** Lymph node metastasis. Underlying the lymph node capsule (C) are several groups of metastatic tumor cells (M). Adjacent non-neoplastic lymphocytes (L) and histiocytes (H) are also noted.

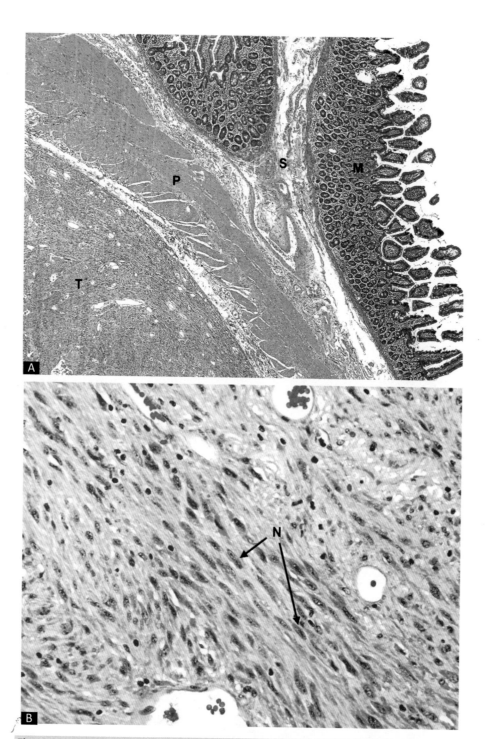

**Figs 4.30A and B:** Gastrointestinal stromal tumor (GIST) of the small intestine
**A.** The GIST (T) is noted within the muscularis propria (P); the overlying submucosa
(S) and mucosa (M) are uninvolved in this example. **B.** The spindle cell morphology
with relatively bland nuclei (N) are noted.

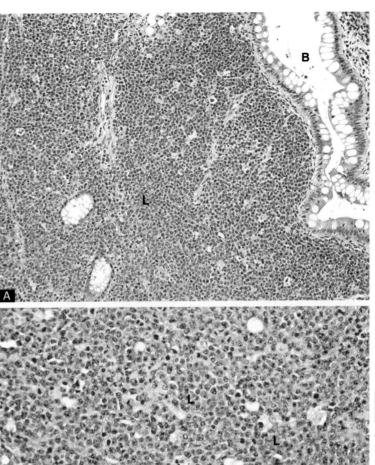

**Figs 4.31A and B:** Small intestinal lymphoma
**A.** Burkitt lymphoma. There is marked expansion of the lamina propria by an infiltrate of medium sized lymphoid cells (L) (B denotes benign intestinal crypts). **B.** Intervening between the malignant lymphoid cells (L) are several macrophages (M) producing the starry-sky appearance, often seen with this lymphoma.

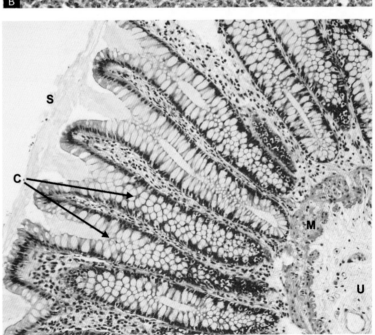

**Fig. 4.32:** Normal colonic mucosa
The colonic epithelial surface (S), which faces the gut lumen, is covered by columnar and goblet cells. This dips into regular tube-like crypts (C) which are lined by goblet cells. The mucosa is limited by muscularis mucosa (M), underlying which is the sub-mucosa (U).

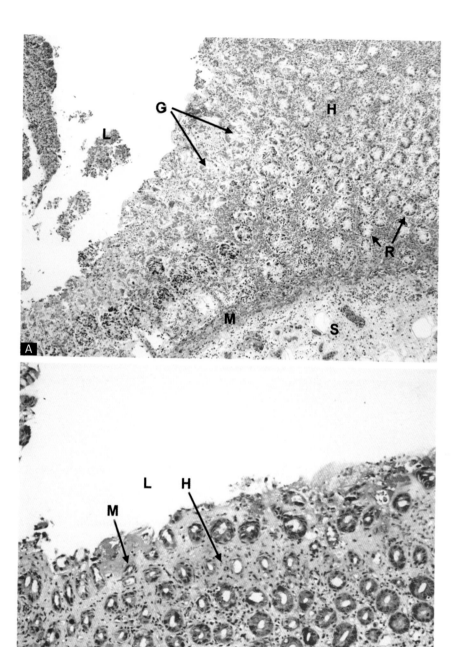

**Figs 4.33A and B:** Ischemic colitis

**A.** Acute ischemic colitis shows hemorrhagic necrosis (H) of the mucosa with the residual ghosts (G) of some necrotic crypts. Deeper crypts show regenerative changes (R) (M denotes the muscularis mucosa, S the submucosa and L the bowel lumen). **B.** Chronic ischemic changes include hyalinization (H) of the lamina propria with withered microcrypts (M) (L denotes the bowel lumen).

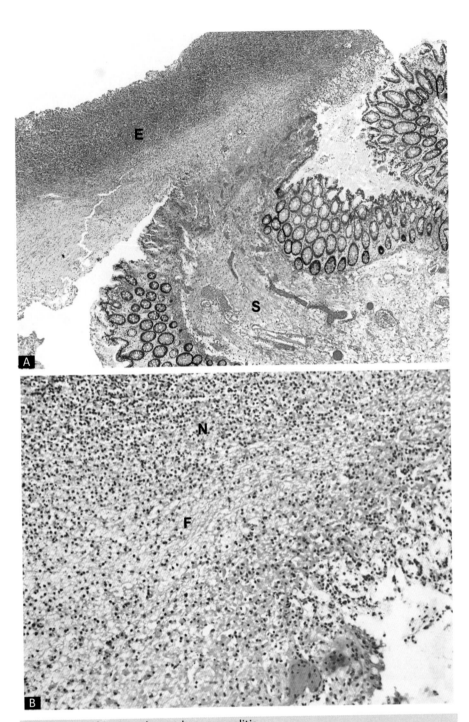

**Figs 4.34A and B:** Pseudomembranous colitis

**A.** The mucosa is ulcerated with an overlying volcano cloud of necroinflammatory exudate (E) (S denotes the submucosa). **B.** At greater magnification, the exudate consists of neutrophils (N) and fibrin (F).

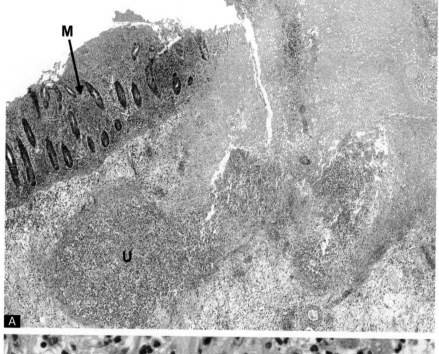

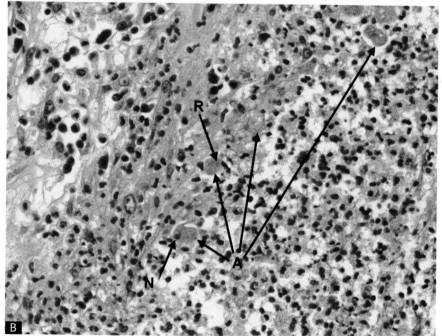

**Figs 4.35A and B:** Amebic colitis

**A.** The flask-shaped ulcer (U) has a wide base that undermines the mucosa (M). **B.** A larger magnification image demonstrates the trophozoites forms of amoeba (A) which have a peripheral nucleus (N) and often contain red blood cells (R).

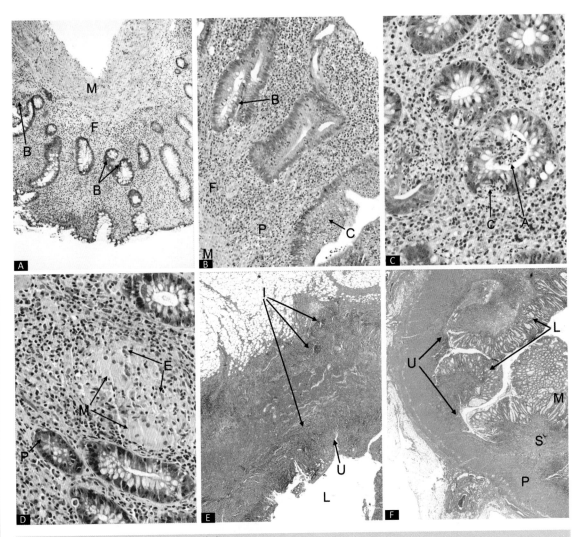

**Figs 4.36A to F:** Inflammatory bowel disease

**A.** The colonic crypts are branched (B) and foreshortened (F) as they do not reach the muscularis mucosa (M). **B.** Prominent cryptitis (C) with intracryptal neutrophils is present. The lamina propria is filled with plasma cells (P), crypt branching (B) and foreshortening (F) are present (M denotes the muscularis mucosa). **C.** In addition to cryptitis (C), crypt abscesses (A) with neutrophils within the crypt lumens are noted. **D.** Granulomas composed of epithelioid histiocytes (E) and sometimes multinucleate giant cells (M) are only found in Crohn's disease. Paneth cell metaplasia (P) may be seen in either type of inflammatory bowel disease. **E.** Crohn's disease shows fissure-like ulcers (U) and characteristically transmural inflammation with lymphoid aggregates (I) extending into the muscularis propria and subserosal fat (L denotes the bowel lumen). **F.** Ulcerative colitis has inflammation and ulceration (U) limited to the mucosa (M) and submucosa (S); the muscularis propria (P) is uninvolved. Regenerating mucosa between the ulcers form polypoid structures called pseudopolyps (L).

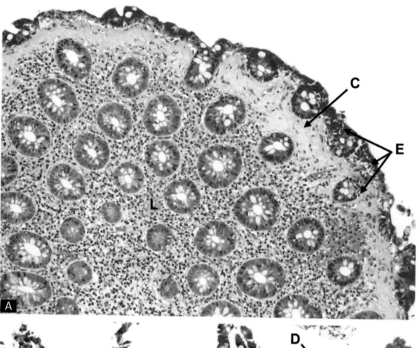

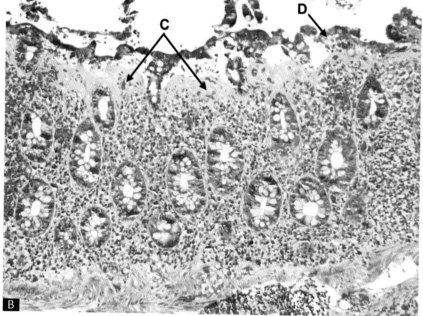

**Figs 4.37A and B:** Microscopic (collagenous) colitis
**A.** A thick collagen layer (C) is present beneath the surface epithelium (E) which contains an elevated amount of intraepithelial lymphocytes (L denotes the lamina propria). **B.** The trichrome stain highlights the abnormal collagen layer (C). The overlying epithelium may show tendency to detach (D) from the collagen in tissue sections.

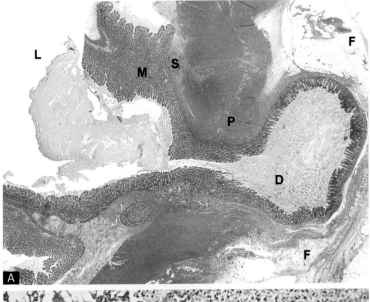

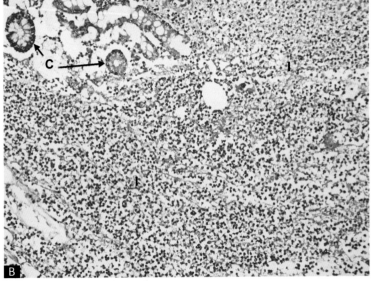

**Figs 4.38A and B:** Diverticulosis and diverticulitis of the colon
**A.** Diverticulosis. A diverticulum (D) of mucosa (M) and submucosa (S) protrudes through a weak area of the muscularis propria (P) into the pericolonic fat (F)(L denotes the lumen). **B.** Diverticulitis. A larger magnification image demonstrates numerous inflammatory cells (I) which indicates inflammation of the diverticulum (C denotes colonic crypts).

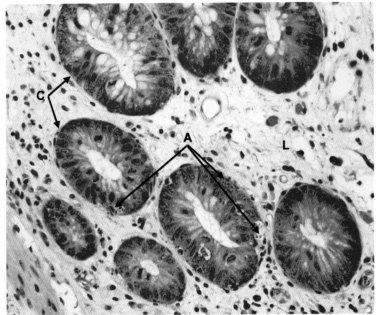

**Fig. 4.39:** Graft versus host disease
The disease typically causes apoptosis (A) of the epithelial cells of the colonic crypts (C). These dying cells appear to be exploding as they are replaced by cellular debris.

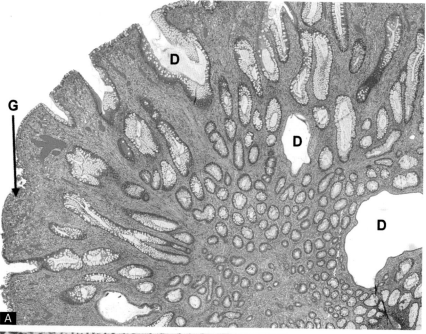

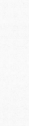

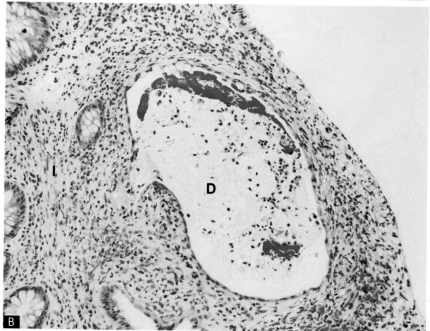

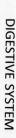

**Figs 4.40A and B:** Juvenile polyp

**A.** The polyp demonstrates several dilated glands (D). The surface is often eroded or ulcerated; hence granulation tissue (G) is a typical finding. **B.** At greater magnification, the dilated glands (D) contain mucus and inflammatory cells. The lamina propria also demonstrates an increased number of inflammatory cells (I).

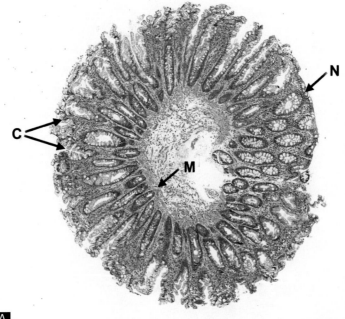

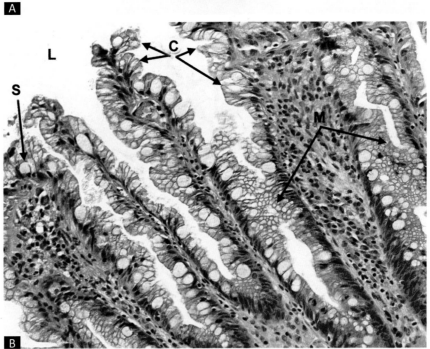

**Figs 4.41A and B:** Hyperplastic polyp

**A.** This cross-section demonstrates saw tooth-like crypts (C) lined by mucinous goblet and absorptive cells. These changes are predominantly in the upper portion of the mucosa. The crypt bases are not dilated or branched (M denotes the muscularis mucosa and N normal mucosa). **B.** At higher magnification, mucinous epithelial cells (M) line abnormal colonic crypts (C) with mildly serrated contours (S) around the lumen of the intestine (L).

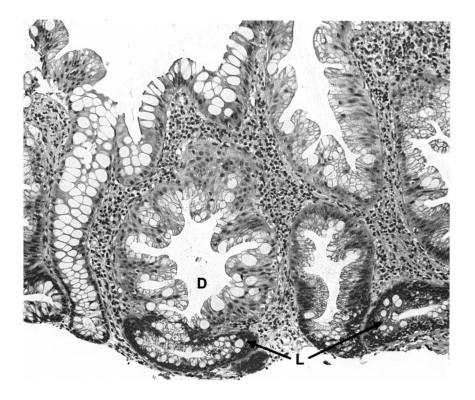

**Fig. 4.42:** Sessile serrated polyp

The polyp is composed of dilated crypts, often with a serrated contour (D) lined by hypermucinous epithelium. The changes extend to the crypt bases, which may also be branched, resembling the alphabet "L" or an inverted "T" (L).

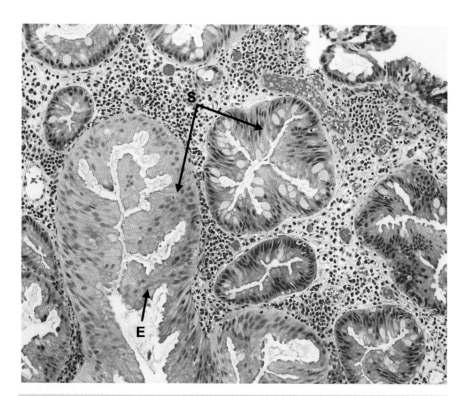

**Fig. 4.43:** Serrated adenoma

The tumor is composed of serrated glands (S), lined by dysplastic epithelium with eosinophilic cytoplasm (E) and stratified nuclei.

DIGESTIVE SYSTEM

CHAPTER

**4**

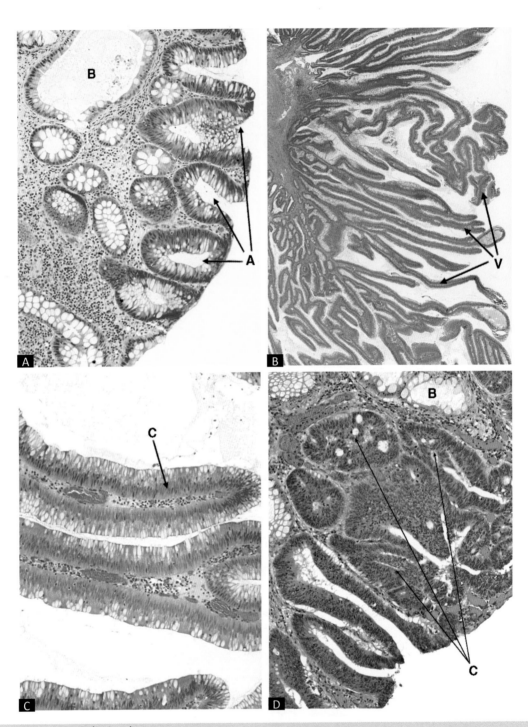

**Figs 4.44A to D:** Colonic adenoma

**A.** Tubular adenoma is composed of simple tubular glands (A), lined by stratified, elongated columnar nuclei which extend from the base of the adenomatous glands to the mucosal surface (B denotes adjacent benign crypts). **B.** Villous adenoma shows finger-like villi (V) with cores of lamina propria lined by adenomatous epithelium. **C.** At greater magnification, the stratified, elongated columnar nuclei (C) lining the villi are appreciated. **D.** Adenoma with high grade dysplasia demonstrates foci with complex cribriform architecture (C) as well as an increase in cytologic atypia. Unlike intramucosal adenocarcinoma, there is no invasion of the lamina propria (B denotes an adjacent benign colonic crypt).

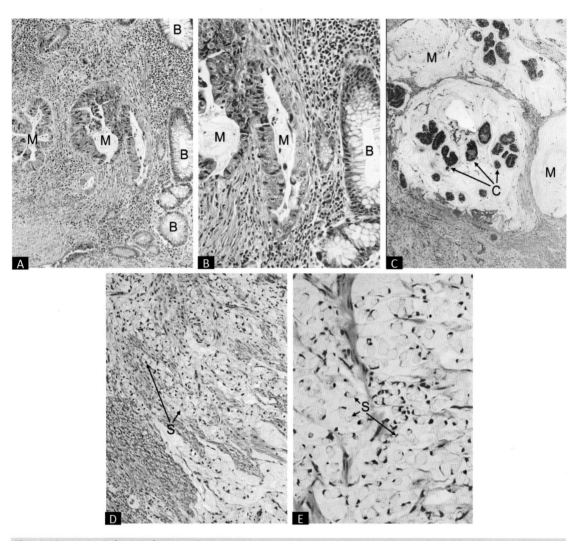

**Figs 4.45A to E:** Colonic adenocarcinoma

**A.** Well differentiated adenocarcinoma shows irregular malignant glands (M) that contrast with the adjacent benign glands (B). **B.** At higher magnification, the malignant glands (M) are lined by pleomorphic nuclei that contrast with those in the benign glands (B). **C.** Mucinous adenocarcinoma shows pools of mucin (M) containing clusters of carcinoma cells (C). **D.** Poorly differentiated (signet ring) adenocarcinoma lacks gland formation but instead demonstrates infiltration by signet ring cells (S). **E.** A larger magnification image demonstrates the mucin filled cytoplasm and peripherally located nuclei typical of signet ring cells (S).

DIGESTIVE SYSTEM

CHAPTER

**4**

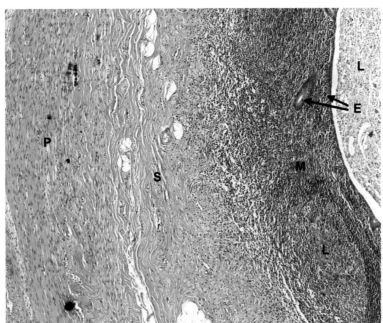

**Fig. 4.46:** Normal appendix
The mucosa (M) which faces the lumen (L) is composed of colonic type columnar epithelium (E) with prominent underlying lymphoid tissue (L) with germinal centers. The submucosa (S) and muscularis propria (P) are also appreciated.

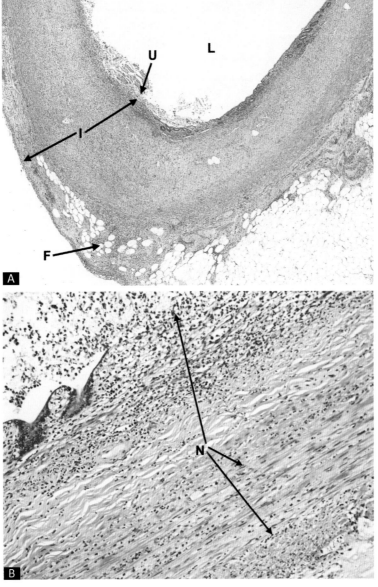

**Figs 4.47A and B:** Acute appendicitis
**A.** There is mucosal ulceration (U) and transmural acute inflammation (I) which extends into the periappendiceal fat (F) and to the serosa (serositis) (L denotes the lumen). **B.** At higher magnification, neutrophils (N) are the predominant inflammatory cell type.

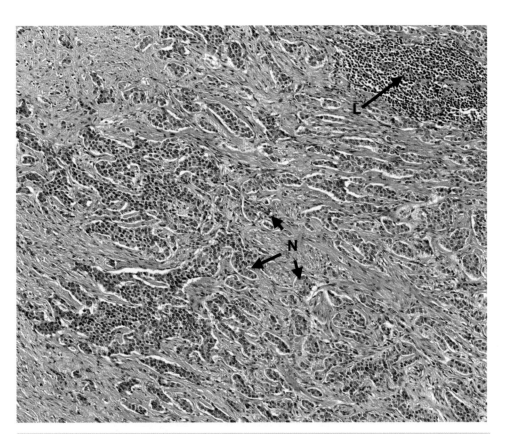

**Fig. 4.48:** Appendiceal carcinoid

Trabeculae and nests (N) of fairly uniform neuroendocrine cells are seen infiltrating the appendiceal wall (L denotes normal lymphoid tissue).

DIGESTIVE SYSTEM

CHAPTER

**4**

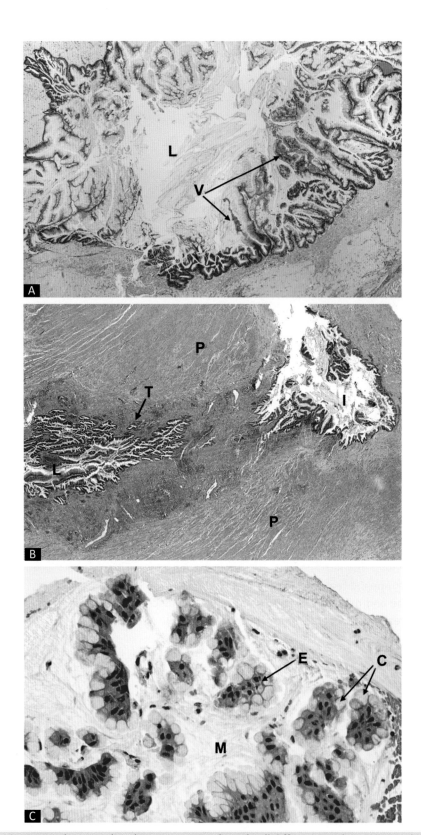

**Figs 4.49A to C:** Low grade appendiceal mucinous neoplasm (well differentiated mucinous adenocarcinoma) **A.** The appendix contains a tumor characterized by columnar mucinous epithelium arranged in villous architecture (V), occupying the appendiceal lumen (L). **B.** The tumor (T) extends from the lumen (L) to penetrate into the muscularis propria (P) of the appendix (I indicates the deeply located tumor). **C.** Peritoneal biopsy shows the typical features of a low grade mucinous adenocarcinoma: aggregates of mucin (M) and low grade columnar epithelium (E) with cytoplasmic mucin (C). These pathologic findings correspond clinically to pseudomyxoma peritonei.

# 5 Hepatobiliary System

*Maura O'Neil*

## Introduction

*The hepatobiliary system consists of the liver, gallbladder and the bile ducts. The liver performs many complex functions, the most important of which are metabolism of proteins, lipids and carbohydrates, bile acid synthesis and secretion, detoxification and biotransformation of drugs and toxins, and the storage of vitamins and lipids. The gallbladder stores bile and the biliary ducts transport bile from the liver to the gallbladder and from the gallbladder to the small intestine.*

## Liver

The liver is composed of hepatocytes, bile duct cells and cells lining the vascular spaces. The hepatocytes are arranged in hexagonal lobules which have in their center a terminal hepatic venule and at their periphery portal tracts (Figs 5.1A to C). Each portal tract (or point of the hexagon) contains terminal branches of the hepatic artery and hepatic portal vein and one or two interlobular bile ducts (Fig. 5.1C). The blood flows from the portal tract into the hepatic sinusoids, and leaves the lobule via the terminal hepatic venule.

A different way of looking at the architecture is to consider the functional unit of liver to be the area of liver parenchyma supplied by each terminal hepatic artery and hepatic portal vein. Thus, each functional acinus is bordered by terminal hepatic venules with plates of hepatocytes and sinusoids radiating out from a central portal tract core. Bile drains from the hepatic acinus to the bile duct within the portal tract.

The liver parenchyma is composed of cords of hepatocytes (Fig. 5.1C) one to two cells thick. In between the cords of hepatocytes are sinusoids which are lined by Kupffer cells, endothelial cells and stellate (Ito) cells. Kupffer cells are the tissue macrophages of the liver. Stellate or Ito cells are located within the space of Disse but are not readily identified in routine H&E stained slides.

The biliary network consists of bile canaliculi (intercellular spaces along the biliary side of hepatocytes), ducts of Hering, interlobular bile ducts, and main right and left hepatic ducts.

Diseases affecting the liver can present as an acute or chronic process. The most important diseases of the liver can be separated into the following broad categories:
- Inflammatory disease
- Metabolic disorders
- Cirrhosis
- Neoplasms.

### Inflammatory Diseases

*Hepatitis* is an acute or chronic inflammation of the liver which can be caused by: (a) viruses; (b) drugs and toxins; (c) autoimmune diseases and (d) diseases of unknown etiology. All forms of chronic hepatitis may be accompanied with hepatic fibrosis, which may progress to cirrhosis.

*Viral hepatitis* is the most common form of liver inflammation, which presents in an acute or chronic form. Most hepatic infections are caused by hepatotropic viruses (hepatitis viruses A, B, C, D and E); however, systemic viral diseases caused by cytomegalovirus, Epstein-Barr virus or yellow fever virus can also cause viral hepatitis.

*Acute viral hepatitis* is characterized by moderate to severe lobular inflammation, foci of necrosis and scattered apoptotic cells which have an acidophilic cytoplasm and pyknotic or fragmented nuclei (dead reds) **(Fig. 5.2)**. The viable hepatocytes may also show ballooning degeneration. The inflammatory cell infiltrate is predominantly composed of lymphocytes, a few macrophages, and occasional plasma cells. This lobular inflammation is most prominent in the centrilobular zones. The destruction and loss of hepatocytes leads to liver plate disarray and confluent, bridging or even massive liver cell necrosis. Portal tracts show varying degrees of inflammation. Complete resolution is likely in most acute viral hepatitis cases; however, in some cases viral hepatitis B, C and D may become chronic, which is especially true for viral hepatitis C.

*Chronic viral hepatitis* is clinically characterized by a persistent inflammation of the liver with more than 6 months of clinical signs and symptoms. Chronic viral hepatitis C is the most common necroinflammatory liver disease in North America and is the prototype for the morphology of all chronic hepatitides. The histopathologic changes seen include marked and patchy expansion of the portal tracts by predominantly lymphocytes with occasional interface hepatitis (or spilling over) into the adjacent lobule **(Fig. 5.3A)**. Prominent lymphoid nodules with germinal center formation may be present. Varying degrees of bile duct damage and steatosis are common. Lobular inflammation is important in terms of grading and prognosis and is characterized by individual cell apoptosis **(Fig. 5.3B)**, and cell dropout surrounded by aggregates of lymphocytes.

*Massive hepatic necrosis* caused by drugs or toxins is the most common cause of acute liver failure. Accidental or intentional ingestion of acetaminophen causes more than half of the cases of massive hepatic necrosis in the United States. Acetaminophen-induced injury is characterized by coagulative necrosis which is located predominantly in the perivenular (centrolobular) zone **(Fig. 5.4)**.

*Steatohepatitis* is a form of liver inflammation related to fatty change of hepatocytes, also known as steatosis. *Steatosis* is most often caused by obesity, diabetes, alcohol, drug-induced liver cell injury, and occasionally viral hepatitis C. Steatosis is characterized by an accumulation of fat in the cytoplasm of hepatocytes, which ultimately leads to a replacement of the cytoplasm with large fat droplets **(Fig. 5.5A)**. *Steatohepatitis* is often divided into alcoholic steatohepatitis and non-alcoholic steatohepatitis (NASH). Steatohepatitis consists of prominent steatosis and an inflammatory infiltrate consisting of both of neutrophils and lymphocytes **(Fig. 5.5B)**. Alcoholic steatohepatitis is characterized by steatosis, hepatocyte ballooning, Mallory hyaline and perivenular (chicken wire) fibrosis **(Fig. 5.5C)**. NASH is difficult to distinguish from alcoholic steatohepatitis. Subtle microscopic findings favoring the diagnosis of NASH include the presence of mixed and patchy macrovesicular and microvesicular steatosis, many glycogenated nuclei, and portal lympho-plasmacytic infiltrates.

*Autoimmune hepatitis* is a disease of unknown etiology characterized by the presence of circulating autoantibodies and liver inflammation. From the diagnostic point of view certain autoantibodies are especially useful such as anti-smooth muscle antibodies (SMA) and anti-liver kidney microsome 1 (ALKM-1). The liver biopsy findings are important for the diagnosis but are not specific. The most common microscopic feature of autoimmune hepatitis is a marked portal and periportal inflammation composed of lymphocytes and plasma cells **(Figs 5.6A and B)**. This inflammation may extend into the periportal areas of the lobules and may be accompanied by marked fibrosis.

*Primary biliary cirrhosis* (PBC) is an autoimmune destructive cholangitis affecting middle-aged women and characterized by high titers of antimitochondrial antibody (AMA) in serum and an elevated serum alkaline phosphatase. Early PBC is characterized by florid bile duct inflammation and injury **(Fig. 5.7A)**, sometimes accompanied by non-caseating epithelioid granulomas. Late PBC shows more extensive bile duct injury and expansion of portal tracts with lobular activity as well. As the disease

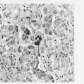

progresses there is a marked bile ductular reaction (proliferation) (Fig. 5.7B). Eventually fibrosis ensues and there is progressive bile duct loss.

*Primary sclerosing cholangitis (PSC)* is characterized by segmental stricturing along the biliary tree, caused by inflammation and fibrosis (Fig. 5.8A). The majority of patients with PSC also have ulcerative colitis. Cholangiographic findings are diagnostic and include alternating segments of extrahepatic bile duct stenosis and dilatation, giving the contrast filled bile ducts a "beaded" appearance. In the early stages of PSC the biopsy findings are non-specific. As the disease progresses, however, the characteristic periductal fibrosis or "onion skinning" become prominent (Fig. 5.8B).

*Hepatic abscess* is a localized suppurative liver infection. It is relatively rare in the United States but more common in developing countries. In the United States, hepatic abscesses are usually a complication of bacterial cholangitis, but in other parts of the world they may also be a manifestation of amebic or echinococcal infection. On gross and microscopic examination hepatic abscess presents as an accumulation of pus, often surrounding a central core of necrotic hepatocytes (Fig. 5.9). Chronic abscesses may have a fibrous capsule infiltrated with inflammatory cells.

*Schistosomiasis* in the liver is manifested by a granulomatous reaction to *Schistosoma* ova deposited in the portal tracts (Figs 5.10A and B). Surrounding the granulomas is lamellar fibrosis with bridging between portal tracts, but no regenerative nodule formation or progression to cirrhosis.

## Metabolic Disorders

Many metabolic and genetic disorders affect the liver but the microscopic changes produced by theses systemic diseases are usually nonspecific. Here we shall give only two examples to illustrate that some metabolic diseases may produce diagnostic microscopic changes.

*Alpha-1 antitrypsin ($\alpha_1$-AT) deficiency* is the most common genetic cause of liver disease in children and the most frequent genetic diagnosis requiring liver transplantation. The $\alpha_1$-AT molecule inhibits destructive neutrophil proteases and just a single amino acid substitution results in this disease. This single gene defect results in the protein's retention in the endoplasmic reticulum and subsequent accumulation. This accumulation of protein can be seen as globules in the hepatocytes and is demonstrated by a special stain, PAS, with diastase digestion (Fig. 5.11).

*Hereditary hemochromatosis* is an autosomal recessive disorder of iron metabolism. It is the most common genetic abnormality in the Caucasian population. The defect leads of inappropriate absorption of dietary iron leading to the deposition of massive amounts of iron in various organs. In the liver this manifests as massive accumulation of iron within hepatocytes (Figs 5.12A and B). This can eventually lead to cirrhosis and the development of hepatocellular carcinoma (HCC).

## Cirrhosis

*Cirrhosis* is the end result of many chronic inflammatory liver diseases. Although it may have many etiologies, the end stage of chronic liver disease is morphologically always the same and the diagnosis of cirrhosis can be readily made clinically, as well on gross and microscopic examination of the affected liver. Typically the normal liver architecture has been lost and replaced by fibrous strands and hepatocellular nodules. Microscopically, fibrous septa are seen encircling parenchymal nodules composed of hepatocytes (Figs 5.13A and B). These fibrous septa may contain chronic inflammatory cells and bile ducts. Hepatocytes resemble those in the normal liver, but often they may show bile accumulation and signs of regeneration.

## Neoplasms

Liver tumors can be histogenetically classified in three groups: (a) hepatocellular neoplasms; (b) bile duct neoplasms and (c) vascular neoplasms. Each of these three groups comprises both benign and malignant neoplasms.

*Hemangioma* is the most common benign tumor of the liver. Cavernous spaces are lined by a single layer of benign endothelial cells (Fig. 5.14). Large lesions can become fibrotic, hyalinized and calcified.

*Focal nodular hyperplasia (FNH)* is a common benign liver lesion, which occurs primarily in young women. The FNH is characterized by a central stellate scar (Figs 5.15A and B). Bile ductular proliferation at the margin of the fibrovascular zone is common; however true portal tracts are not found within the fibrous tissue.

*Hepatocellular adenoma* is a benign liver tumor composed of well differentiated hepatocytes arranged in liver plates two to three cells thick. The cells can have an increased nuclear to cytoplasmic ratio, resembling a well-differentiated HCC; however, the reticulin network (typical of normal liver parenchyma) is maintained in adenoma and usually lost in HCC. Adenomas lack portal tract structures and terminal hepatic venules (Fig. 5.16), which is helpful in distinguishing adenoma from FNH.

*Hepatoblastoma* is a liver cell tumor affecting young children and is rarely seen in adults. Hepatoblastomas is predominantly composed of immature liver cells, classified as fetal or embryonal, with an admixture of various mesenchymal cells. Tumors displaying the fetal phenotype are composed of small polygonal cells arranged in irregular trabecular cords (Fig. 5.17). The embryonal type consists of sheets of small cells with dark nuclei and scant cytoplasm and arranged in rosettes, cords and ribbons.

*Hepatocellular carcinoma (HCC)* is the most common primary malignant tumor of the liver. Most tumors develop in a background of cirrhosis, which may be a consequence of viral infection, chronic alcoholism or metabolic diseases such as hemochromatosis or $\alpha_1$-AT deficiency. Microscopically, HCC cells resemble normal hepatocytes to variable extents, but have an increased nuclear to cytoplasmic ratio with prominent nucleoli (Figs 5.18A and B). The tumor cells usually have distinct cell membranes with eosinophilic cytoplasm. Most often the tumor grows in a trabecular pattern with thickened cords of hepatocytes, greater than two hepatocytes thick. Other common architectural patterns of HCC include acinar and ductular patterns.

*Fibrolamellar HCC* is a variant of HCC with distinct clinical and histologic features. Unlike other types of HCC, fibrolamellar HCC is not associated with chronic liver disease or cirrhosis and occurs in a much younger age group (mean age 23). Fibrolamellar HCC is characterized by nests of eosinophilic cells embedded in a prominent fibrous stroma (Fig. 5.19). The tumor cells have abundant eosinophilic cytoplasm and may contain hyaline globular cytoplasmic inclusions.

*Cholangiocarcinoma* is a primary malignant tumor of the liver arising from bile ducts. Microscopically, it is composed of cuboidal or flattened epithelial cells forming irregular duct and gland like structures surrounded by prominent fibrous tissue (Fig. 5.20).

## Gallbladder

The gallbladder stores and concentrates bile made by the liver. Important diseases of the gallbladder can be separated into the following broad categories:
- Inflammation
- Neoplasms

### Inflammation

Inflammation of the gallbladder can be acute or chronic and is most often associated with gallstones (cholelithiasis).

*Acute cholecystitis* is characterized by exudation of neutrophils, fibrin and hemorrhage in the gallbladder wall (Fig. 5.21). The inflammation may be limited to the mucosa, but may penetrate the entire wall of the gallbladder and extend to the serosa.

*Chronic cholecystitis* is probably the result of repeated episodes of acute cholecytitis. Chronic cholecystitis is characterized by a variably thickened wall, scattered chronic inflammatory cells and Rokitansky-Aschoff sinuses **(Figs 5.22A and B)**. Rokitansky-Aschoff sinuses are buried crypts within the gallbladder wall resulting from reactive proliferation of the mucosa and subsequent fusion of the mucosal folds.

*Cholesterolosis* is a common asymptomatic finding in the gallbladder due to the accumulation of cholesterol in the subepithelial macrophages and epithelium. Foamy macrophages are most prominent in the lamina propria at the tips of the villi **(Fig. 5.23)**.

## Neoplasms

*Adenocarcinoma* of the gallbladder is the most common malignancy in the extrahepatic biliary system. The carcinoma can be exophytic or infiltrating. The infiltrating pattern is the most common and is characterized by malignant glands within a markedly dense/desmoplastic stroma **(Figs 5.24A and B)**.

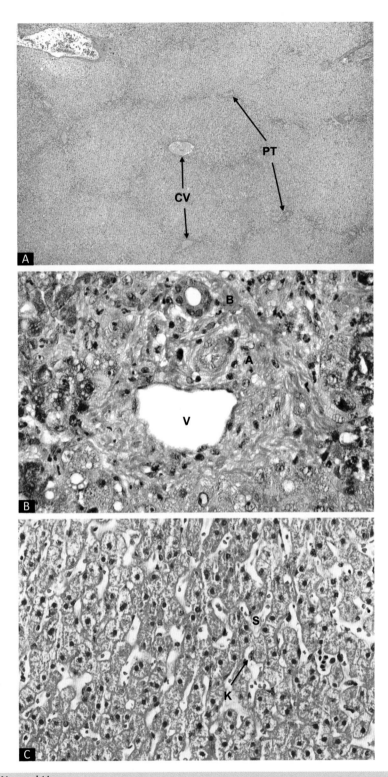

**Figs 5.1A to C:** Normal Liver

**A.** Hepatic lobule. Hepatocytes are arranged in hexagonal lobules with a central hepatic venule (CV) and rimmed by portal tracts (PT). Each portal tract represents a point of the hexagon and blood flows from the portal vein and hepatic artery in the portal tract to the vein in the center of the hexagon. **B.** Portal tract. Each portal tract contains a hepatic arteriole (A), portal venule (V) and one or two interlobular bile ducts (B). Normally these structures are surrounded by fibroconnective tissue and scant numbers of lymphocytes. **C.** Hepatocytes. The liver parenchyma is composed of cords of hepatocytes, each one or two cells thick. Sinusoids (S) are lined by endothelial cells and Kupffer cells (K). The central round nucleus of each hepatocyte is surrounded by abundant pink cytoplasm.

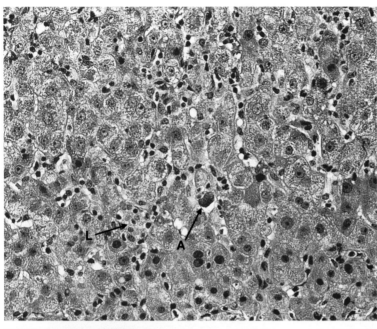

**Fig. 5.2:** Acute viral hepatitis Lobular inflammation and an acidophilic apoptotic cell (A) are seen here. The inflammatory infiltrate is composed primarily of lymphocytes (L).

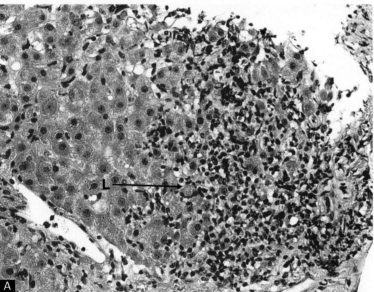

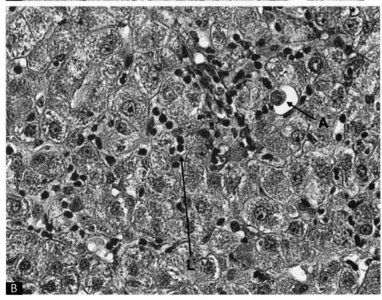

**Figs 5.3A and B:** Chronic viral hepatitis

**A.** Interface activity. Lymphocytes spill out from the portal tract into the periportal hepatocytes. The lymphocytes (L) surround individual or groups of hepatocytes. **B.** Active hepatitis is characterized by lobular necroinflammatory activity and individual cell necrosis or apoptosis (A) (dead reds). The inflammation is composed primarily of lymphocytes (L).

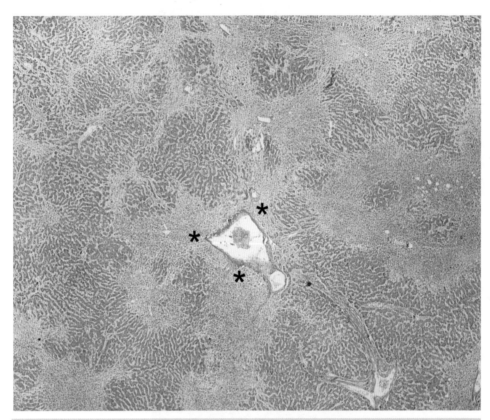

**Fig. 5.4:**
Massive hepatic necrosis caused by drugs or toxins is characterized by coagulative necrosis which is located predominantly in the perivenular zone (**). At low power the broad bands of necrosis appear pale in contrast to the non-necrotic zone of eosinophilic hepatocytes.

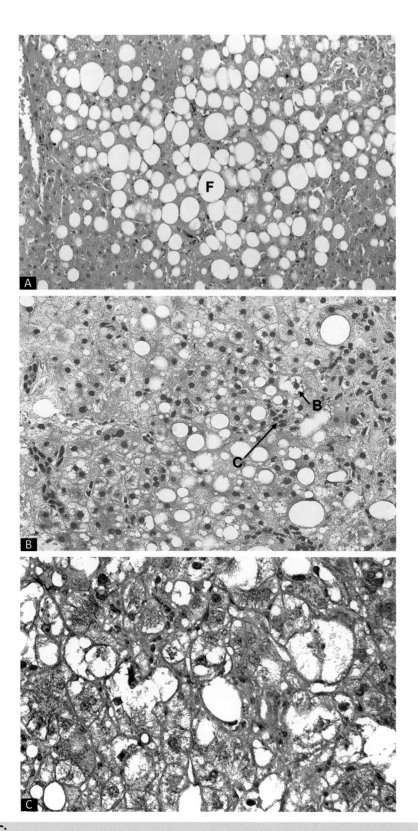

**Figs 5.5A to C:**
**A.** Steatosis. Steatosis or fatty change is characterized by replacement of the hepatocyte cytoplasm with fat droplets (F). **B.** Steatohepatitis. Variable degrees of microsteatosis and macrosteatosis are seen. Ballooning degeneration of hepatocytes (B) and chronic inflammation (C) also accompany the steatosis. **C.** Steatohepatitis. "Chicken wire" fibrosis is prominent and is characterized by distinct pericellular and perisinusoidal collagen deposition.

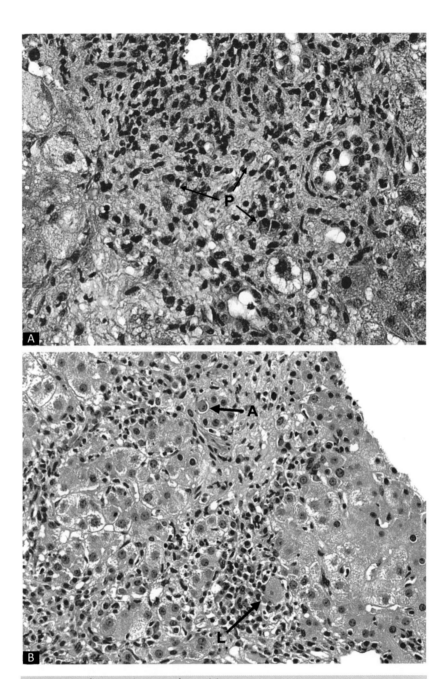

**Figs 5.6A and B:** Autoimmune hepatitis

**A.** A lymphoplasmacytic interface hepatitis is seen. The plasma cells (P) are readily identified. **B.** Similar to viral hepatitis, autoimmune hepatitis is characterized by a lymphocytic (L) interface hepatitis and individual apoptotic (A) hepatocytes.

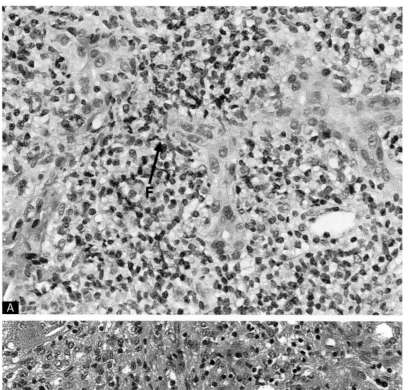

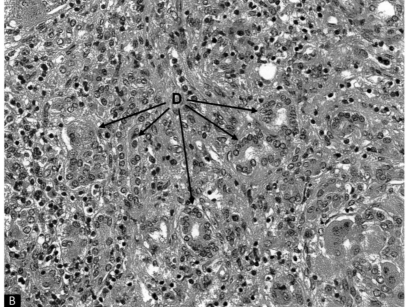

**Figs 5.7A and B:** Primary biliary cirrhosis

**A.** Early primary biliary cirrhosis (PBC) is characterized by florid bile duct inflammation (F) and injury. Late PBC shows more extensive bile duct injury and expansion of portal tracts with lobular activity as well. **B.** As the disease progresses there is a marked bile ductular proliferation (D).

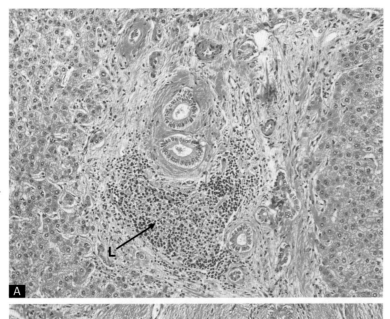

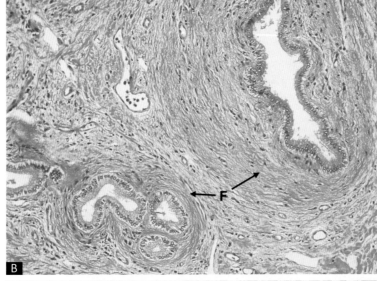

**Figs 5.8A and B:** Primary sclerosing cholangitis
**A.** The later stages of PSC show characteristic periductal fibrosis with a lymphocytic infiltrate (L) surrounding the duct. **B.** In other cases, the periductal fibrosis (F) may be quite striking, with a lack of associated inflammation.

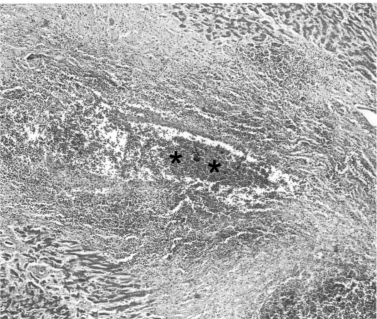

**Fig. 5.9:** Hepatic abscess
The abscess has a central necrotic core (**) surrounded by abundant acute inflammatory cells.

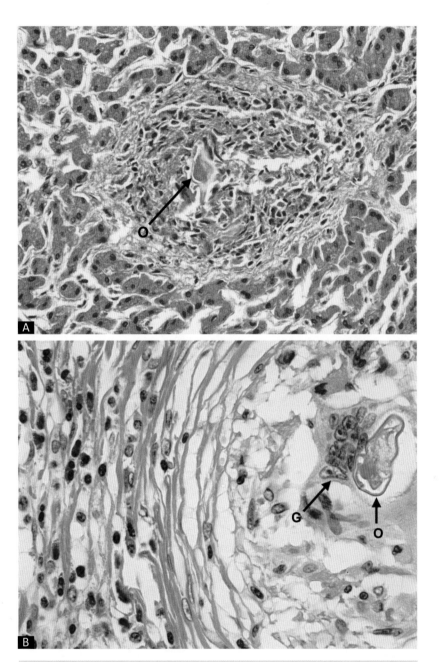

**Figs 5.10A and B:** Schistosomiasis

**A.** A granulomatous reaction to the Schistosoma ova (O) is present. **B.** The perigranulomatous lamellar fibrous reaction can be seen surrounding the centrally located ova (O) which is adjacent to a multinucleated giant cell (G).

HEPATOBILIARY SYSTEM

CHAPTER

**5**

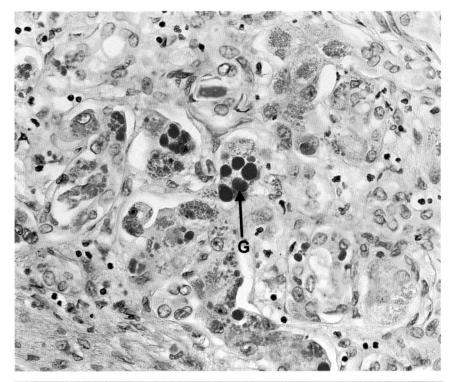

**Fig. 5.11:** Alpha-1-antitrypsin deficiency

The globules/inclusions (G) show strong pink staining (PAS staining after diastase digestion).

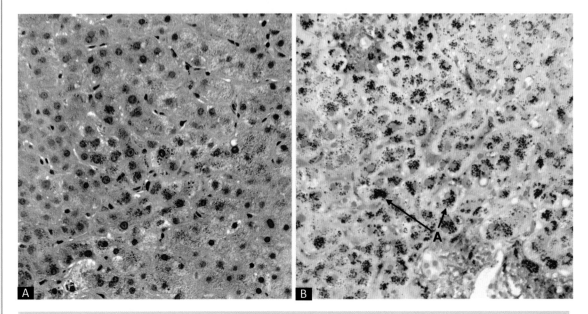

**Figs 5.12A and B:** Hereditary hemochromatosis

**A.** Abundant iron accumulation (A) in the hepatocytes. **B.** Hemosiderin which contains iron gives the typical Prussian blue reaction in the Perl iron stain.

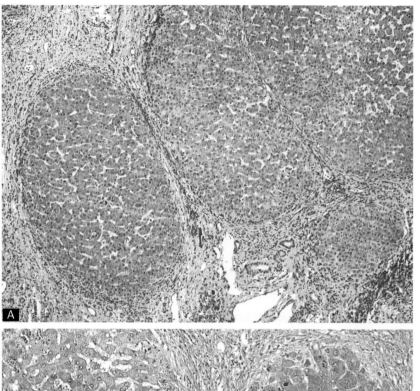

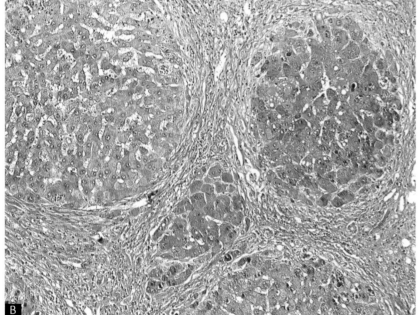

**Figs 5.13A and B:** Cirrhosis
**A.** Bridging fibrous septa completely encircle liver parenchymal nodules.
**B.** The bridging fibrosis is highlighted by a trichrome stain.

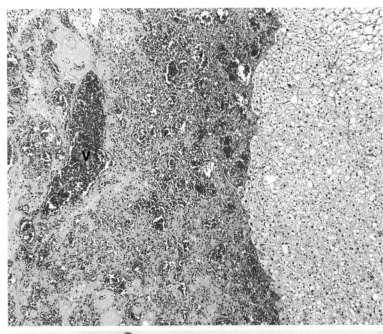

**Fig. 5.14:** Hemangioma
Large irregularly shaped vascular spaces (V) define this lesion. The vascular channels are lined by a single layer of benign endothelial cells.

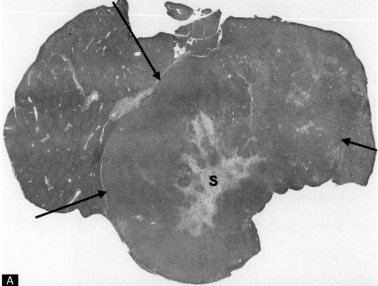

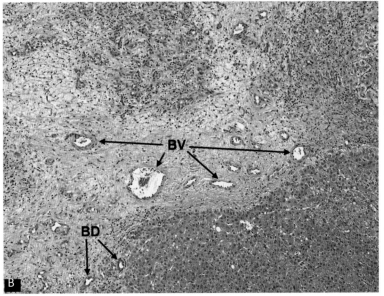

**Figs 5.15A and B:** Focal nodular hyperplasia
**A.** The central stellate scar (S) seen in FNH (demarcated with arrows) is composed of a large band of fibrosis with prominent blood vessels. **B.** Bile ductular proliferation (BD) can sometimes be seen at the margin of the fibrovascular zone of the central scar, however, true portal tracts are not found within the fibrous tissue.

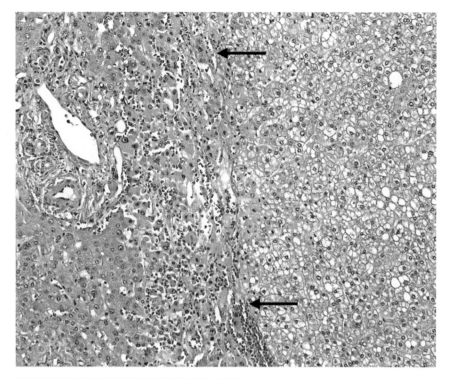

**Fig. 5.16:** Adenoma

Bland hepatocytes comprise this benign tumor. Within the tumor, portal tract structures and terminal hepatic venules are notably absent. The border between tumor and normal is marked with arrows at the bottom and top of the photograph.

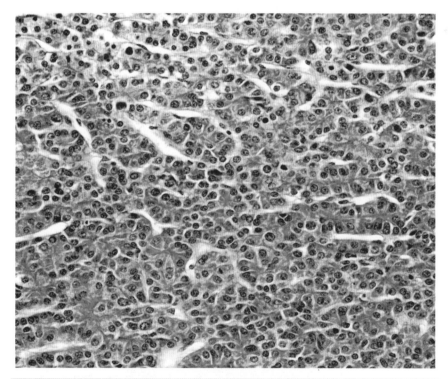

**Fig. 5.17:** Hepatoblastoma

This hepatoblastoma is classified as having a fetal epithelial pattern and is composed of trabeculae of cells which resemble fetal hepatocytes. The cells with small round nuclei and finely granular cytoplasm with scattered clear cells.

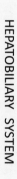

HEPATOBILIARY SYSTEM

CHAPTER

**5**

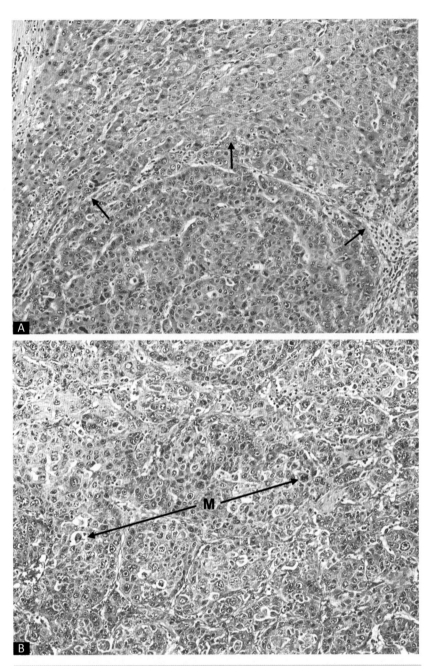

**Figs 5.18A and B:** Hepatocellular carcinoma (HCC)
**A.** HCC cells resemble normal hepatocytes, but have an increased nuclear to cytoplasmic ratio and prominent nucleoli. The sharp demarcation between normal liver and tumor can be seen here (arrows). **B.** Pleomorphic nuclei with prominent nucleoli and mitoses (M) are often present.

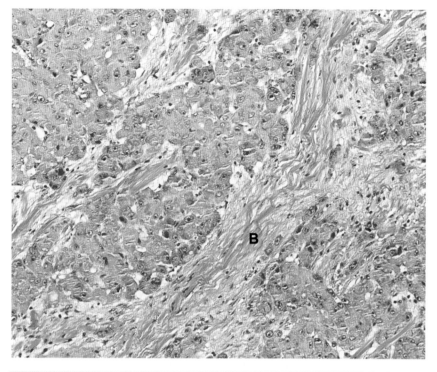

**Fig. 5.19:** Fibrolamellar hepatocellular carcinoma
Large polygonal cells are seen with abundant eosinophilic cytoplasm and prominent nucleoli. Collagen is present in parallel (lamellar) bands (B) which separate the islands of tumor cells.

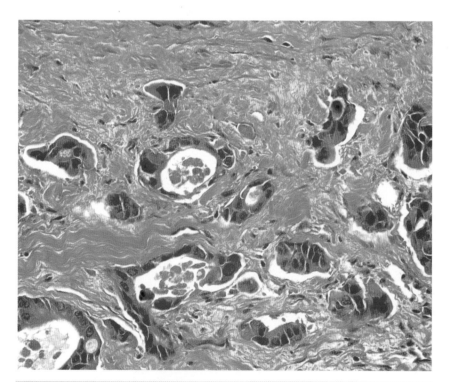

**Fig. 5.20:** Cholangiocarcinoma
Malignant glands are present within a fibrous stroma. The malignant glands have an irregular architecture with markedly pleomorphic nuclei.

HEPATOBILIARY SYSTEM

CHAPTER
**5**

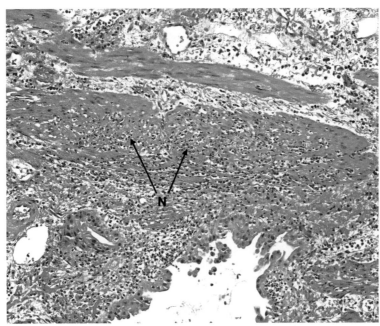

**Fig. 5.21:** Acute cholecystitis
Acute inflammation is characterized by the presence of neutrophils (N), fibrin and hemorrhage in the gallbladder wall. Neutrophils are seen here involving the mucosa as well as the muscle layer of the gallbladder.

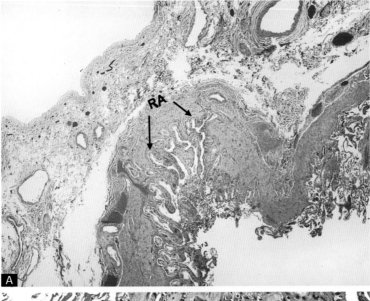

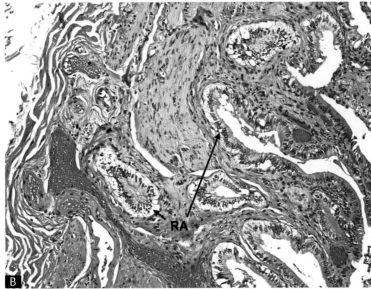

**Figs 5.22A and B:** Chronic cholecystitis
**A.** The gallbladder wall appears thickened. **B.** Buried crypts (Rokitansky-Aschoff sinuses) (RA) are seen within the muscular wall of the gallbladder.

ATLAS OF HISTOPATHOLOGY

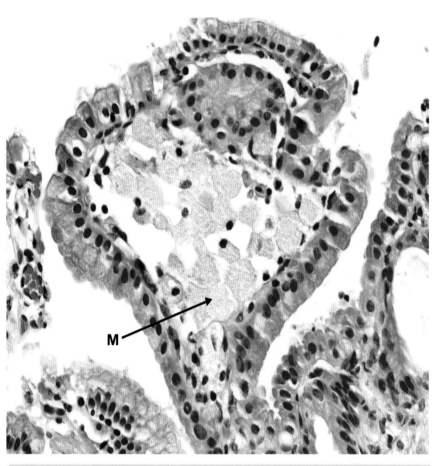

**Fig. 5.23:** Cholesterolosis

Accumulated cholesterol can be seen in foamy macrophages (M) which are present in the lamina propria at the tip of the villous.

HEPATOBILIARY SYSTEM

CHAPTER

**5**

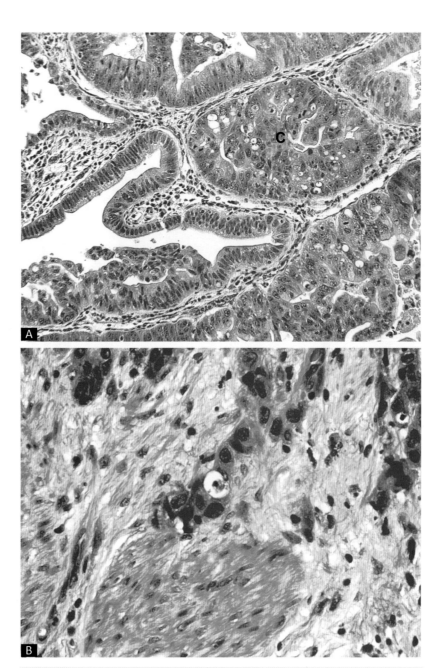

**Figs 5.24A and B:** Adenocarcinoma

**A.** The malignant glands are arranged in a cribriform (C) "back-to-back" manner replacing the normal mucosa and are infiltrating deep within the thick muscular wall. **B.** Marked nuclear atypia, a hallmark of malignancy, can be appreciated at higher magnification.

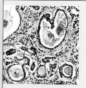

# 6 Pancreas

*Rashna Madan, Ivan Damjanov*

## Introduction

*The pancreas is a mixed endocrine-exocrine organ weighing 85–90 gm. It is located retroperitoneally and divided into a head with uncinate process, neck, body and tail.*

*The exocrine portion of the pancreas consists of acini and ducts (Fig. 6.1). Acinar cells secrete digestive enzymes, such as amylase, lipase or trypsin, often in proenzyme form, excreting them through the pancreatic ducts into the duodenum.*

*The endocrine portion of the pancreas comprises the islets of Langerhans composed of typical neuroendocrine cells resembling those in the intestines or the bronchi. Immunohistochemically these islet cells can be classified according to the hormones they secrete into the following groups: glucagon producing alpha cells, insulin producing beta cells, somatostatin secreting delta cells and the pancreatic polypeptide (PP) secreting cells.*

*Abnormalities of the pancreas may be grouped into the following categories:*
- *Congenital and inherited conditions*
- *Inflammatory diseases*
- *Neoplasms.*

## Congenital and Inherited Conditions

This category of diseases includes several rare pathologic entities such as agenesis of pancreas, pancreas divisum, annular pancreas, heterotopic pancreas and cystic fibrosis. Most of these conditions do not present with distinct histopathologic changes, and are uncommon or of limited clinical significance. Hence we shall limit our presentation only to cystic fibrosis.

*Cystic fibrosis* is an autosomal recessive inherited disorder that occurs predominantly in the Caucasian population. It is due to a mutation in the cystic fibrosis transmembrane conductance regulator (*CFTR*) gene located on the long arm of chromosome 7 (7q) that affects the transfer of chloride and bicarbonate ions into lumina lined by epithelial cells. There is a resultant lowering in water content. In the pancreas, this leads to thick secretions that block ducts with their ensuing dilatation as well as atrophy of the exocrine elements and secondary fibrosis (Fig. 6.2). Clinically the disease presents with malabsorption due to pancreatic insufficiency. Other organs affected include the lungs, liver, sweat glands and vas deferens.

## Inflammatory Diseases

Inflammation of the pancreas may be acute or chronic. In most instances the inflammation is limited to the pancreas and adjacent fat tissues.

*Acute pancreatitis* is, in most instances, caused by the abuse of alcohol or an obstruction of the common pancreatico-biliary ducts by calculi. Additional etiologic factors implicated in this disease, in approximately 20% of all cases, include drugs, metabolic disorders, trauma, infections and inherited mutations of trypsinogen and trypsin inhibitor genes. The latter may cause pancreatitis even in childhood. The acute inflammation is typically related to autodigestion of the organ by its own enzymes which are activated inside the pancreas. Pathologic findings include edema, acute inflammation, necrosis, hemorrhage and saponification of peripancreatic fat (Figs 6.3A to C). The latter refers to "soap formation" which results from calcium reacting with free fatty acids cleaved from triglycerides in damaged fat cells. Calcium soaps may serve as nuclei for additional calcification which may be microscopically and even grossly visible.

*Chronic pancreatitis* is a long standing condition characterized by fibrosis, chronic inflammation, variable involvement of the gland and variable loss of pancreatic function. Alcohol abuse, obstruction of ducts with biliary calculi, and recurrent bouts of acute pancreatitis play an important role in the pathogenesis of this disease. Cytokines that promote fibrosis are implicated. Areas of chronic pancreatitis are also frequently noted in specimens excised for neoplasms.

Microscopically, this condition is characterized by a loss of acinar elements which are replaced by fibrous tissue and foci of chronic inflammation (Figs 6.4A and B). The ducts and islets of Langerhans are less affected and persist longer. In fact relative prominence of the islets, termed islet cell aggregation, is often noted. The ducts may be focally narrowed or dilated and filled with inspissated secretions.

*Pancreatic pseudocyst* is a lesion frequently seen in patients who suffer attacks of acute pancreatitis and have localized enzyme mediated necrosis of tissue. In contrast to true cysts, which have an epithelial lining, the pseudocysts are lined on their internal side by a collection of cell debris, inflammatory cells, and granulation tissue (Figs 6.5A and B). Older lesions have a fibrous capsule which also may be infiltrated with chronic inflammatory cells.

*Lymphoplasmacytic sclerosing pancreatitis* is a relatively recently described chronic autoimmune disease characterized by marked ductal and periductal inflammation, fibrosis and venulitis (Figs 6.6A and B). The inflammatory infiltrate typically contains numerous plasma cells that secrete IgG subtype 4. This condition frequently presents as a mass lesion and on imaging may mimic cancer. Steroid therapy can usually reverse this process.

## Neoplasms

Pancreatic tumors may originate from the exocrine portion of the pancreas, i.e. ducts and acini, or the endocrine portion of pancreas, i.e. islets of Langerhans. Most tumors arise from the exocrine pancreas and originate from ducts, and many malignant tumors may originate from a preinvasive *in situ* lesion called pancreatic intraepithelial neoplasia.

On gross examination pancreatic tumors may be solid or cystic. Most tumors are solid, although some solid neoplasms may undergo cystic degeneration. Cystic tumors typically contain clear fluid or viscous mucinous material. Tumors undergoing cystic degeneration contain necrotic material in the cystic portion of the tumor mass.

Clinically, pancreatic tumors may be benign or malignant. Malignant tumors are considerably more common than benign tumors. Malignant tumors may be primary or metastatic. Primary malignant tumors are much more common than metastases.

### Tumors of the Exocrine Pancreas

*Pancreatic intraepithelial neoplasia (PanIN)* refers to intraductal epithelial alterations considered to represent precursors of invasive ductal carcinomas. PanIN is graded from I (minimally abnormal tall mucinous epithelium) to III (marked atypia) (Figs 6.7A and B). Higher grades of PanIN are frequently noted in transition to ductal adenocarcinoma and indeed they have several molecular alterations in common with that diagnosis.

*Ductal adenocarcinoma of the pancreas* is the most common malignant tumor of the pancreas. It typically affects the elderly patients, and clinically it has a bad prognosis. Microscopically, these adenocarcinomas are composed of cuboidal or columnar cells arranged into glandular structures which often secrete mucin (Figs 6.8A to E). Tumors forming ducts or glandular structures are

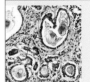

considered to be well-differentiated, and those that form few glands and are composed of solid growth of cells are classified as poorly to undifferentiated.

Several features are helpful in separating a well-differentiated adenocarcinoma from chronic pancreatitis. The presence of glands inconsistent with normal architecture is indicative of adenocarcinoma, i.e. neoplastic glands may be seen away from the center of lobules and be noted within or replacing vascular spaces, surrounding nerve bundles (perineural invasion) or invading peripancreatic fat. The presence of marked variation in nuclear size, prominent nucleoli, frequent and abnormal mitoses are features increasingly noted with less differentiated carcinomas.

Other microscopic types of carcinoma are less common and include colloid/mucinous carcinoma (which is associated with abundant mucin production), signet-ring carcinoma, adenosquamous carcinoma, anaplastic carcinoma and undifferentiated carcinoma with osteoclast-like giant cells.

*Microcystic serous cystadenoma* is the prototypic benign serous cystic neoplasm of the pancreas. It has a characteristic radiologic and gross appearance wherein it bears a close resemblance to a sponge, not uncommonly with a central scar. Microscopically this corresponds to numerous microscopic cysts which are lined by bland low cuboidal cells with clear cytoplasm that contains glycogen (Figs 6.9A and B).

*Mucinous cystic neoplasm (MCN)* and *intraductal papillary mucinous neoplasm (IPMN)* have different presentations but have the following features in common: they are both mucinous epithelium lined cysts and may range from being benign/low grade dysplastic to having severe dysplasia/carcinoma in situ or even invasive adenocarcinoma. Malignant findings may be focal and so necessitate having the cystic tumor resected and completely assessed histologically. Completely excised MCN and IPMN, even with carcinoma in situ, have a good prognosis; however, if an invasive adenocarcinoma is present, then the prognosis is guarded though typically better than for a de novo invasive ductal adenocarcinoma.

*Mucinous cystic neoplasm* is a tumor showing a very strong female preponderance. It occurs mostly in the body and tail of the pancreas and is not connected to the ductal system. A characteristic histologic feature is the presence of a distinctive stroma underlying the mucinous epithelium—"ovarian-type stroma", called so because it strongly resembles that seen in the ovary (Figs 6.10A and B).

*Intraductal papillary mucinous neoplasm* is a tumor of the proximal pancreas connected to the ductal system, either to the main pancreatic duct or to one of its branches. These tumors may be multifocal and may be seen in both sexes. Microscopically, they are composed of mucin secreting cells lining papillae (Figs 6.11A to D) and lack the ovarian type stroma of MCNs. A minority will have an associated adenocarcinoma, more frequently of the colloid type.

*Solid pseudopapillary neoplasm* presents as a partly solid and partly cystic mass in a young adult female. The solid areas are composed of densely packed papillae, lined by fairly bland round to oval cells of uniform appearance with nuclear grooves. Some cells contain hyaline globules within their cytoplasm. Hemorrhage is often present in the cystic portions of the tumor (Figs 6.12A to C). The tumor is readily resectable, and, with a few exceptions, it has a very good prognosis.

*Acinar cell carcinoma* is far less common than ductal adenocarcinoma but it has also an aggressive clinical course. These tumors are mostly seen in the middle aged to elderly persons, but may occur at any age and even in children, albeit rarely. The neoplastic cells have well developed granular cytoplasm and are arranged into acini, thus resembling pancreatic acinar cells (Fig. 6.13). They may produce enzymes which can be detected immunohistochemically to confirm this diagnosis. Occasionally, the production of lipase may reach the blood stream and result in multiple sites of fat necrosis.

## Tumors of the Endocrine Pancreas

*Pancreatic neuroendocrine tumor (PanNET)*, previously known as *islet cell tumor*, originates from the islets of Langerhans. The endocrine nature of the tumor cells can be demonstrated immunohistochemically with the antibodies to synaptophysin and chromogranin, which react with all neuroendocrine cells, benign or malignant. Tumors may be functional when they produce hormones that result in clinical syndromes. With the use of specific immunohistochemical techniques, these tumors may be classified clinically and pathologically as insulinomas, glucagonomas or somatostatinomas. Some pancreatic endocrine tumors secrete gastrin and are classified as gastrinomas, even though normal islets do not contain gastrin secreting cells. Some tumors do not secrete hormones or produce ineffectual hormones that do not result in clinical syndromes, and are classified as non-functional. Some PanNETs occur in the context of multiple endocrine neoplasia (MEN) I or von Hippel Lindau syndrome.

Most PanNETs are well differentiated neuroendocrine tumors. They may be solitary or multifocal and range in behavior from relatively indolent to malignant, though most tumors should be considered to have malignant potential. Small functional tumors, especially insulinomas tend to be cured by excision. On the basis of microscopic features, it is usually challenging to predict whether a tumor will clinically behave aggressively, though tumor grade (based on mitotic rate/proliferative rate) and stage are of prognostic significance. The presence of infiltrative growth and metastases are evidence for malignancy. PanNETs, even when malignant, may have a prolonged course.

Microscopically, PanNETs may have several growth patterns and thus form either solid sheets, acini, nests or trabeculae (Figs 6.14A to D). Neoplastic cells of PanNETs resemble normal islet cells. The chromatin in their nuclei is coarsely dispersed, usually described as "salt and pepper" pattern of chromatin distribution. The same nuclear features are typically seen in carcinoid tumors of the gastrointestinal and respiratory systems. Amyloid deposition, if present, is typically seen in the stroma of insulinomas.

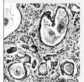

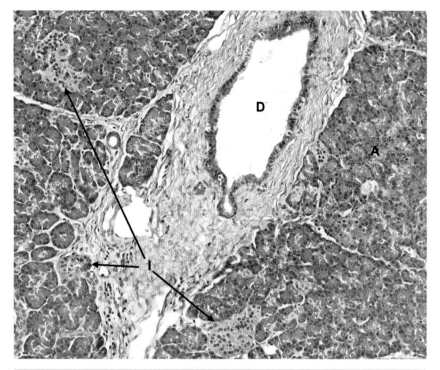

**Fig. 6.1:** Normal pancreas

An interlobular duct (D) lined by cuboidal epithelium is surrounded by lobules of acinar cells (A) which have small basal nuclei and granular eosinophilic or slightly basophilic cytoplasm. Islets of Langerhans (I) appear as groups of small cells with lightly stained cytoplasm.

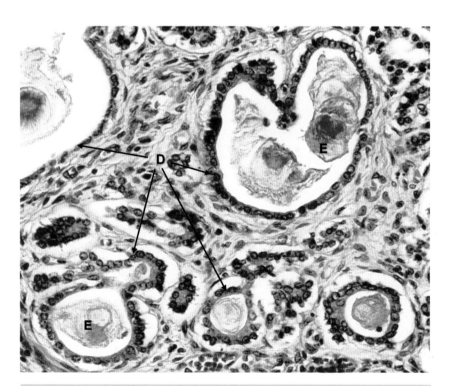

**Fig. 6.2:** Cystic fibrosis

Ducts (D) are dilated and filled with inspissated eosinophilic secretions (E).

PANCREAS

CHAPTER

**6**

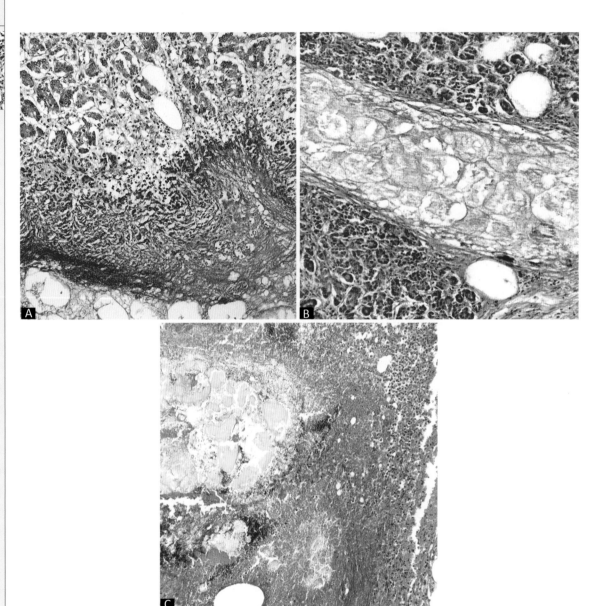

**Figs 6.3A to C:** Acute pancreatitis

**A.** The pancreas in the upper part of the figure appears edematous, whereas in the lower part of the figure the normal tissue architecture has been lost due to necrosis which also involves the adjacent fat tissue. At the interface with the area of necrosis the pancreas is infiltrated with neutrophils. **B.** Early fat necrosis is recognized by a loss of fat cell outlines and the amorphous amphophilic staining of the entire interlobular area. **C.** Late fat necrosis is characterized by a loss of cell outlines that have been replaced by amorphous amphophilic material. The aggregates of bluish material correspond to deposits of calcium soaps. On the right side of the figure there is acute inflammation that has destroyed the pancreatic acini.

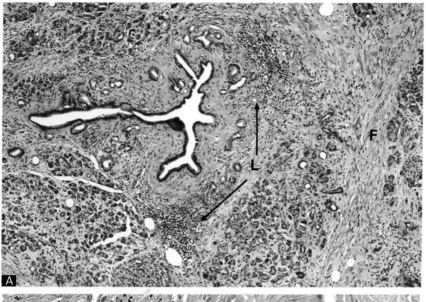

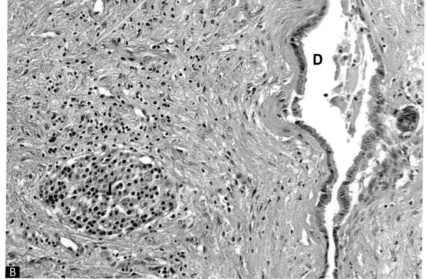

**Figs 6.4A and B:** Chronic pancreatitis

**A.** In early stages of chronic pancreatitis the overall lobular architecture is maintained although there is partial loss of acinar cells, increased fibrosis (F) and chronic inflammation with lymphocytes (L). **B.** Later stage with near complete acinar loss, only the duct (D) and islets (I) remain.

PANCREAS

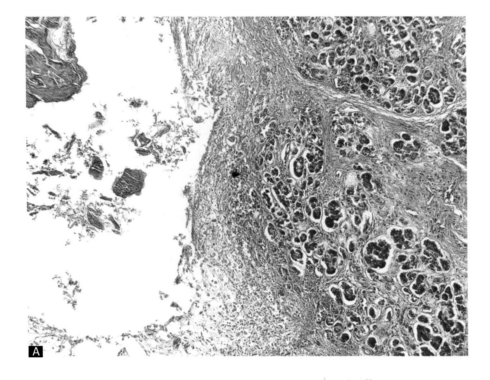

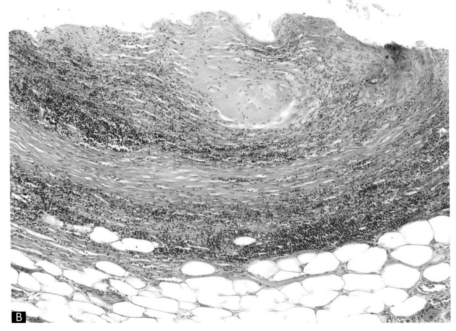

**Figs 6.5A and B:** Pancreatic pseudocyst

**A.** The internal luminal side is covered by cell debris and amorphous material and separated from the pancreas by fibrous tissue. **B.** Capsule of the chronic pseudocyst consists of dense fibrous tissue and scattered chronic inflammatory cells.

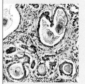

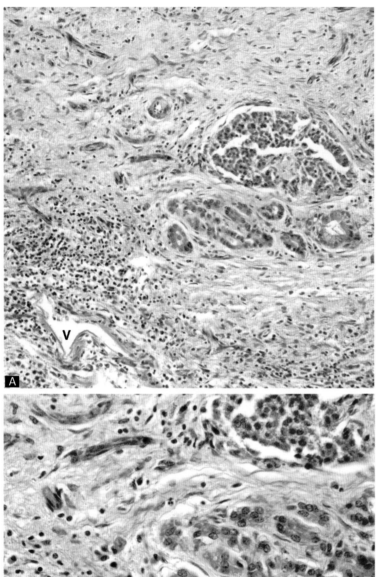

**Figs 6.6A and B:** Lymphoplasmacytic sclerosing pancreatitis
**A.** Fibrous tissue and chronic inflammatory infiltrates are seen replacing the pancreatic acini. There is also venulitis (V). **B.** Higher magnification shows that the inflammatory infiltrate consists of lymphocytes and plasma cells (arrow).

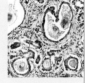

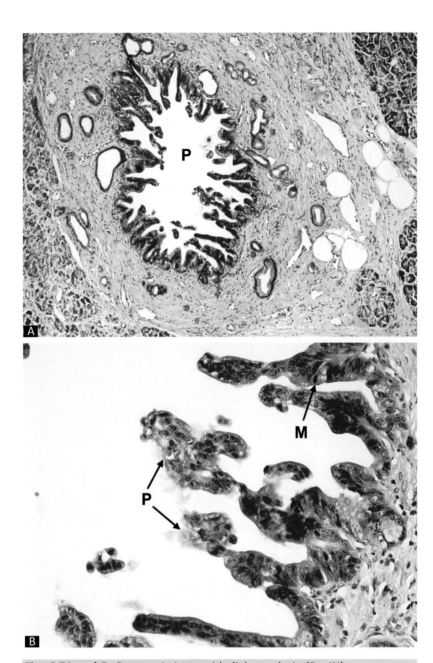

**Figs 6.7A and B:** Pancreatic intraepithelial neoplasia (PanIN)
**A.** PanIN (P) is a microscopic finding of dysplasia within the native pancreatic ductal system without itself forming a tumor. **B.** PanIN III demonstrates papillary architecture (P) lined by markedly atypical epithelial cells which show high nuclear to cytoplasmic ratios, loss of orientation and mitosis (M).

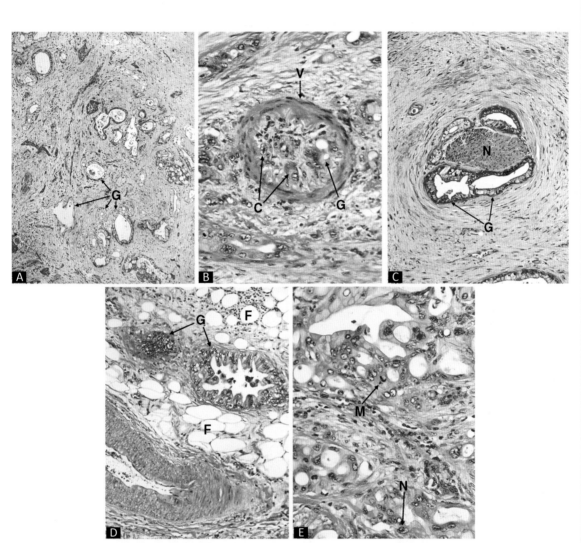

**Figs 6.8A to E:** Ductal adenocarcinoma
**A.** Haphazard arrangement of malignant glands (G) is accompanied by a loss of normal lobular architecture. **B.** Malignant glands (G) and cells (C) are present within a blood vessel (V). **C.** Perineural invasion where malignant glands (G) surround a nerve bundle (N). **D.** Malignant glands (G) infiltrating peripancreatic fat (F). **E.** Cytologic features include variation in nuclear size and prominent nucleoli (N). An abnormal mitosis (M) is also noted.

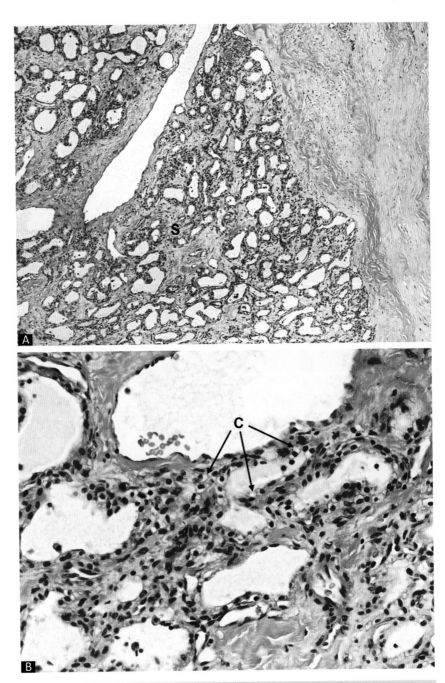

**Figs 6.9A and B:** Microcystic serous cystadenoma

**A.** A low magnification view illustrates the spongy/microcystic nature of the tumor (S). **B.** Numerous tiny cysts are lined by low cuboidal epithelium with uniform round nuclei and clear cytoplasm (C).

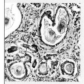

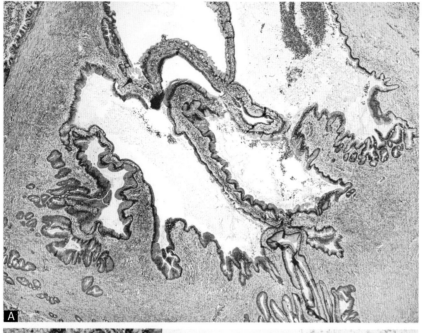

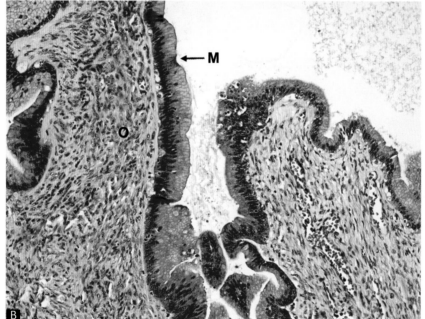

**Figs 6.10A and B:** Mucinous cystic neoplasm (MCN)
**A.** At low magnification a cystic tumor is evident. **B.** MCNs are lined by mucinous epithelium (M), underlying which is a dense ovarian-type stroma (O) that is typical of this neoplasm.

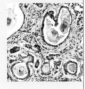

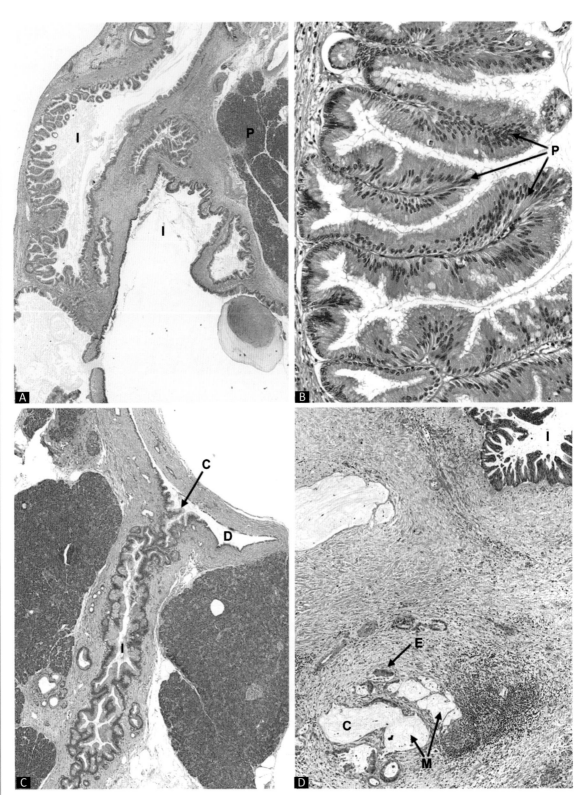

**Figs 6.11A to D:** Intraductal papillary mucinous neoplasm (IPMN)

**A.** The interface between the non-neoplastic pancreas (P) and the cystic IPMN (I). **B.** Finger-like papillae (P) of the tumor are lined by mucinous epithelium that is fairly uniform in this example. **C.** A communication (C) is present between a branch of the pancreatic duct (D) and the IPMN (I) is typical of this tumor. This connection is usually appreciated when macroscopically assessing the pancreatic resection. **D.** An IPMN (I) with high grade dysplasia is associated with an invasive colloid carcinoma (C) which is composed of mucin (M) and malignant epithelium (E).

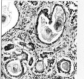

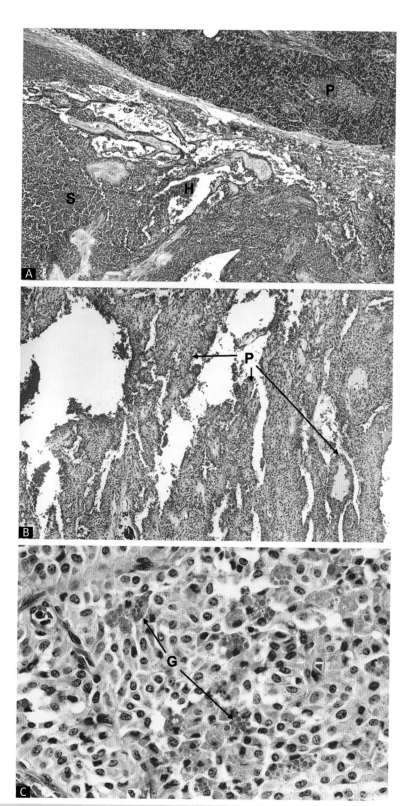

**Figs 6.12A to C:** Solid pseudopapillary neoplasm
**A.** The interface between the non-neoplastic pancreas (P) and the solid pseudopapillary neoplasm (S) is sharp. Note the hemorrhage (H) within the cystic areas of the tumor. **B.** The solid areas are composed of finger-like papillary structures (P) several of which appear adherent to one another. **C.** The neoplastic cells have bland nuclei and eosinophilic hyaline globules (G) within the cytoplasm.

PANCREAS

CHAPTER

**6**

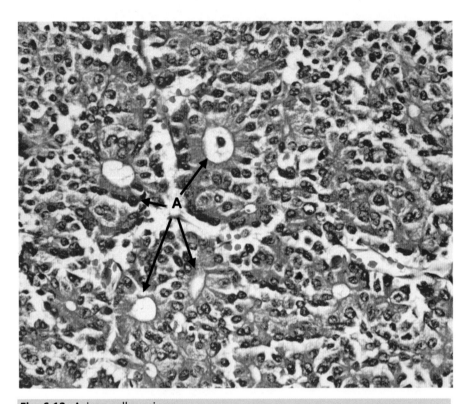

**Fig. 6.13:** Acinar cell carcinoma

The malignant cells resemble acinar cells with granular eosinophilic cytoplasm. Several acinar (gland-like) structures (A) are also present (Fig. *Courtesy:* Dr. Nora Katabi).

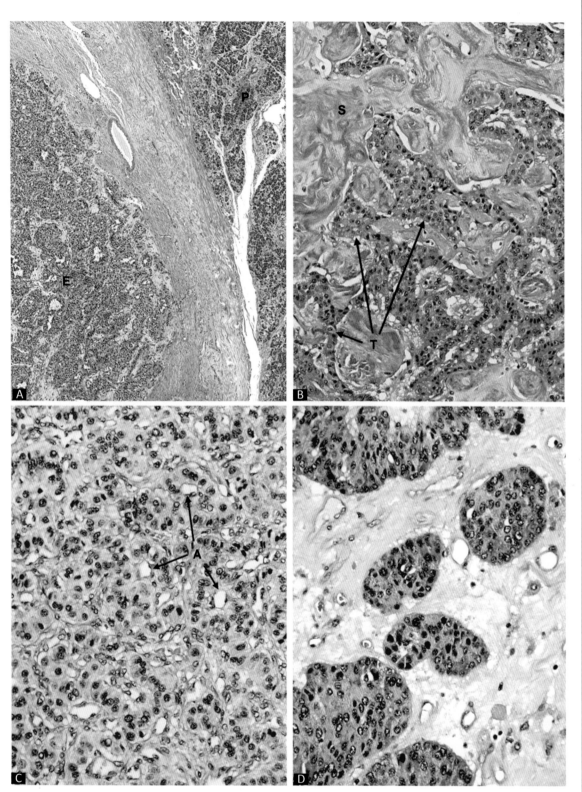

**Figs 6.14A to D:** Pancreatic neuroendocrine tumor

**A.** The well differentiated PanNET (E) is sharply demarcated from the normal pancreas (P). **B.** Fairly uniform cells are arranged in anastomosing trabeculae (T) within a sclerotic stroma (S). **C.** The neoplastic cells show a diffuse growth with a few acinar like structures (A). Classical salt and pepper nuclear chromatin is present. **D.** The tumor cells are arranged in a nested pattern.

# 7 The Urinary System

*Da Zhang, Ivan Damjanov*

## Introduction

*The urinary system includes kidneys, renal calices and pelves, ureters, urinary bladder and urethra. The primary function of the urinary system is to produce the urine, eliminate water and metabolic waste products, and thus contribute to the homeostasis of fluids, minerals and acid base balance. In this chapter we will deal primarily with the pathologic changes of the kidneys and the urinary bladder.*

## Normal Histology

*The kidney* is a complex organ composed functional units called nephrons **(Figs 7.1A and B)**. Each nephron consists of a glomerulus, proximal and distal tubules, a loop of Henle and collecting ducts. Nephrons are surrounded by an interstitium that contains capillaries, veins and arteries. Nephrons form the urine which flows through the collecting ducts into the renal calices and renal pelvis, from which it enters into the ureters, bladder and urethra.

*The ureters, urinary bladder and the urethra* are simple organs which contain a prominent smooth muscle layer, allowing them to contract or expand, and thus propel, store or extrude urine. Except for the terminal part of the urethra, which is lined by squamous epithelium, the remaining parts of the lower urinary system are lined by urothelial (transitional) epithelium.

## Overview of Pathology

The most important diseases of the urinary system are as follows:
- Developmental disorders
- Glomerular diseases
- Vascular kidney diseases
- Infectious diseases
- Neoplasms.

### Developmental Disorders

The most important developmental disorders of the kidney that produce typical histopathologic changes are: (a) polycystic kidney disease and (b) multicystic renal dysplasia.

*Polycystic kidney disease* is an autosomal dominant developmental disorder accounting for approximately 10% of all cases of end stage kidney disease in nephrology or renal dialysis and renal transplantation departments. The kidneys are enlarged, contain numerous cysts filled with clear fluid. Microscopically the cysts are lined by nondescript cuboidal or simple flat epithelium derived from dilated renal tubules and ducts **(Figs 7.2A and B)**.

*Multicystic renal dysplasia* is a developmental disorder that usually affects only one kidney, but may be bilateral as well. It presents a multicystic enlargement of the kidney, with numerous cysts replacing the normal parenchyma of the kidney. The solid tissue between the cysts consists of dysplastic tubules that cannot be properly classified, and stromal tissue that may contain heterologous elements such as bone, skeletal muscle or cartilage (Fig. 7.3).

## Glomerular Diseases

Glomerular diseases may result from: (a) proven or presumed immunological injury (e.g. poststreptococcal glomerulonephritis or membranous nephropathy); (b) metabolic disorders (e.g. diabetic nephropathy); (c) circulatory disorders (e.g. hypertension). Immunologic diseases of the kidney may occur in an isolated form (e.g. acute poststreptococcal glomerulonephritis), as part of a pulmonary renal syndrome (e.g. Goodpasture syndrome or Wegener granulomatosis) or as part of a systemic disease (e.g. lupus nephritis, which occurs in systemic lupus erythematosus).

*Acute poststreptococcal glomerulonephritis* is an immunologically mediated disease that occurs typically 10–14 days after an upper respiratory tract streptococcal infection. Immune complexes composed of streptococcal antigens and antibodies desposit or form in the glomeruli and are seen along the glomerular basement membranes. The glomeruli are enlarged, hypercellular and their capillary lumina are obliterated by inflammatory cells or proliferating endothelial and mesangial cells (Figs 7.4A to C). Immunofluorescence microscopy studies show widespread deposits of immune complexes in the glomerular basement membrane and mesangial areas. By electron microscopy there are typical deposits of immune complexes in the form of subepithelial "humps"; the smaller immune complexes seen by immunofluorescence microscopy are presumably not evident by electron microscopy. The disease occurs mostly in children and heals spontaneously in over 90% of cases. The remaining 9% patients may have protracted disease, and in 1% of all patients the disease may progress to chronic glomerulonephritis and end stage kidney disease. Acute poststreptococcal glomerulonephritis of adults has a less favorable outcome than the same disease in children and one-third of patients have chronic consequences.

*Rapidly progressive glomerulonephritis (RPGN)*, also known as subacute glomerulonephritis, is a severe form of glomerular injury characterized by focal fibrinoid necrosis of glomerular loops and formation of crescents in the urinary space between the capillary loops and the Bowman capsule (Figs 7.5A and B). The prototypical disease presenting as crescentic glomerulonephritis is Goodpasture syndrome, a pulmonary-renal syndrome mediated by cytotoxic antibodies against the globular part of collagen type IV in the glomerular and pulmonary basement membranes. Crescentic glomerulonephritis may also be a feature of Wegener granulomatosis and in many cases its pathogenesis remains unknown. In all these patients immunofluorescence microscopy will reveal no immune deposits in the glomeruli and it is thus customary to call such cases "pauci-immune crescentic glomerulonephritis". Timely treatment may prevent the progression of the disease, which without treatment has a tendency to destroy glomeruli and cause progressive renal failure within a matter of several weeks.

*IgA nephropathy* is a milder form of chronic glomerulonephritis in which the changes are limited to mesangial areas. Microscopically, it presents with widening of mesangial areas, which contain deposits of IgA and proliferating mesangial cells (Figs 7.6A and B). The tissues present with microscopic hematuria and proteinuria and few other clinical symptoms. Although it has presumptively an immunologic pathogenesis, it usually does not respond to corticosteroids and immunotherapy. Overall IgA nephropathy has a good prognosis, although in a minority of cases it may progress to end-stage kidney disease.

*Lupus nephritis* is a common feature of systemic lupus erythematosus. Although all parts of the kidney may be involved, glomerular changes predominate. Glomerulonephritis may present in several forms, and it is customary to classify them in six categories, reflecting the severity of the disease. For example, in class III lupus nephritis there is focal and segmental mesangial proliferation, whereas in class IV most glomeruli are involved and show proliferative and exudative glomerulonephritis (Figs 7.7A and B). The deposits of immune complexes on the subepithelial and subendothelial side of the glomerular basement membranes and in the mesangial areas may be demonstrated by immunofluorescence microscopy and electron microscopy. There is also proliferation of mesangial and endothelial cells, and in severe cases even formation of epithelial cell crescents. Inflammatory cells are also seen in the glomeruli and include neutrophils or macrophages. Lupus nephritis usually responds favorably to corticosteroids and immunomodulatory therapy, but if untreated it will cause kidney failure.

*Membranous nephropathy* is an immunologically mediated disease characterized by diffuse "membranous" thickening of the glomerular basement membranes without cellular proliferation or exudation of inflammatory cells in the glomeruli **(Figs 7.8A to D)**. This thickening results from the widespread deposition and/or formation of the immune complexes along the subepithelial side of the glomerular basement membranes. By immunofluorescence microscopy immune deposits appear granular (lumpy-bumpy). By electron microscopy one may see that these dense deposits are separated one from another by uninvolved basement membrane. Membranous nephropathy presents with nephrotic syndrome which does not respond to steroid therapy. It is a slowly progressive disease and, over a period of approximately 10 years, it will usually cause renal failure.

*Minimal change disease* (nil disease) is a disease of unknown etiology, thought to be immunologically mediated by cytokines secreted by T lymphocytes and macrophages. By light microscopy the glomeruli appear normal **(Figs 7.9A and B)**. There are no immune deposits visible by immunofluorescence microscopy or electron microscopy. The only change is seen by electron microscopy and it involves fusion of the foot processes of glomerular epithelial cells (podocytes). Minimal change disease presents clinically with nephrotic syndrome, which typically responds well to steroid treatment.

*Focal glomerulosclerosis (FGS)* is a name for a heterogeneous group of renal diseases that presents with sclerosis and hyalinization of some capillary loops in some glomeruli **(Figs 7.10A and B)**. Clinically FGS presents with nephrotic syndrome that does not respond to steroid treatment. Currently FGS is the most common cause of nephrotic syndrome in adults, most likely because it is one of the renal features of AIDS and, among others, it is a well known may be a complication of intravenous drug abuse. The FGS is resistant to therapy and has a tendency to progress to end stage kidney disease.

*Diabetic glomerulopathy* may present in two forms: (a) diffuse glomerular basement membrane and (b) nodular mesangial glomerulosclerosis (Kimmelstiel-Wilson disease) **(Fig. 7.11)**. In all forms of diabetic renal disease there is also hyalinization of arterioles and fibrosis of the intima and media of renal arteries. Glomerular and vascular changes are in part caused by hypertension which is almost invariably present in OST patients. Diabetic glomerulopathy presents with proteinuria which may progress to nephrotic syndrome. In later stages of the disease there is also tubular atrophy and loss which combined with glomerular and vascular lesions leads to renal failure.

*Renal amyloidosis* may develop due to the deposition of amyloid fibrils in the glomeruli, in the glomerular basement membranes and in the mesangial matrix **(Figs 7.12A and B)**. The deposits of amyloid cause thickening of the glomerular basement membranes and expansion of mesangial areas leading to complete hyalinization of glomeruli and ultimately to renal failure. In addition to glomeruli amyloid deposits may be found in arterioles, arteries and tubular basement membranes and interstitial spaces. Amyloid may be of the AA type (derived from the serum amyloid associated (SAA) protein, or of the AL type (derived from light chain of immunoglobulins). Amyloidosis is an incurable disease.

*Chronic glomerulonephritis* is the outcome of many glomerular diseases. Microscopically it presents with hyalinization of glomeruli **(Fig. 7.13)**. Loss of glomeruli is accompanied by an atrophy and a loss of tubules, interstitial fibrosis and secondary obliterative (endarteritic) changes in the arteries and arterioles. Clinically chronic glomerulonephritis is equivalent to end stage renal disease manifesting itself as renal failure and uremia. The disease requires renal dialysis or renal transplantation.

### Vascular Kidney Diseases

*Hypertension* represents the most common causes of renal injury and renal failure in the elderly. The renal changes are included under the term of *nephroangiosclerosis* which includes fibrosis of arteries, hyalinization of arterioles, hyalinization of glomeruli, atrophy and a loss of tubules, accompanied by interstitial fibrosis **(Fig. 7.14)**. Vascular changes of hypertension may be superimposed on many other renal diseases. Hypertension is most often combined with diabetes mellitus.

*Acute tubular necrosis* is common complication of renal hypoperfusion typically found in shock. Inadequate blood supply may lead to hypoxic necrosis, which most prominently affects the proximal tubules **(Fig. 7.15)**. If the patients survive and the blood supply is reestablished the tubules may regenerate. It is worth mentioning that similar tubular necrosis may be caused by numerous nephrotoxins, heavy metals or cytotoxic drugs.

### Infectious Diseases

*Pyelonephritis* is a generic term used for renal infections, most often caused by bacteria. Bacteria may reach the kidney hematogenously (*descending infection*) or through the ureters (*ascending infection*).

*Acute pyelonephritis* presents with bacterial spread to the kidneys and a subsequent suppurative inflammation which involves the tubules and spreads to the renal interstitium **(Figs 7.16A and B)**.

*Chronic pyelonephritis* is a complication of acute infection that has not been cured. It presents with chronic tubulointerstitial inflammation and destruction of tubules. The remaining tubules undergo atrophy and contain eosinophilic casts, which give them the appearance of the thyroid (thyroidization of the renal parenchyma), whereas the blood vessels show secondary narrowing and thickening of their walls, similar to the changes of nephroangiosclerosis **(Fig. 7.17)**.

*Cystitis*, i.e. the inflammation of the urinary bladder, is a very common bacterial infection.

*Acute cystitis* presents microscopically with mucosal infiltrates neutrophils **(Figs 7.18A and B)**. Infection may be accompanied by ulceration of the urothelium and hemorrhage.

*Chronic cystitis* is usually associated with infiltrates of lymphocytes, plasma cells and macrophages in the lamina propria. Longstanding inflammation may be associated with deposition of fibrous tissue in the lamina propria and muscularis.

### Neoplasms

*Benign neoplasms* of the kidney and the urinary system in general are much less common than the malignant tumors.

*Oncocytoma* is the most common benign renal tumor. It is composed of uniform cells which have small round nuclei and abundant eosinophilic cytoplasm **(Fig. 7.19)**. The tumor has an excellent prognosis and rarely, if ever, undergoes malignant transformation.

*Malignant neoplasms* of the kidneys and the lower urinary system are common. The most important neoplasms are: (a) renal cell carcinoma; (b) Wilms' tumor and (c) urothelial carcinoma of the calices, renal pelvis, ureters, urinary bladder and urethra.

*Renal cell carcinoma* is a malignant tumor most often originating from the proximal renal tubules. Microscopically it presents most often as a clear cell carcinoma **(Figs 7.20A and B)**. Papillary renal cell carcinomas are less common, but have a better prognosis than clear cell carcinoma.

*Wilms' tumor* (nephroblastoma) is malignant neoplasm of infancy and childhood. The tumor is composed of immature cells resembling those found in normal nephrogenesis. Three paterns, known as blastemal, stromal and epithelial, are most often recognized **(Fig. 7.21)**.

*Urothelial carcinomas* most often occur in the urinary bladder but they may originate from any part of the urinary tract lined by urothelium of the kidney to the urethra. Most tumors present as papillary outgrowth, which can be microscopically subdivided into two groups: (a) low grade papillary carcinomas and (b) high grade papillary carcinomas **(Figs 7.22A to C)**. These tumors are initially limited in growth but may become invasive; high grade tumors have a tendency to become invasive carcinomas more often than the low grade tumors.

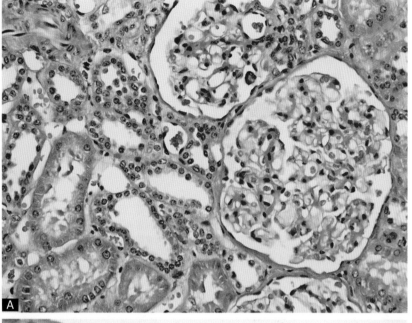

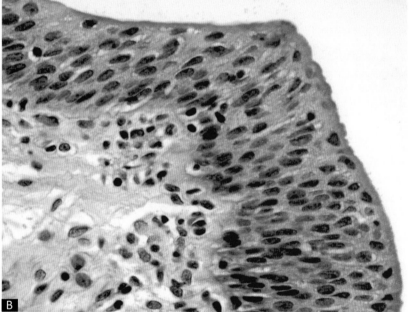

**Figs 7.1A and B:** Normal urinary system
**A.** Kidney consists of glomeruli, tubules, stroma and blood vessels. **B.** Urothelial epithelium. Also known as transitional epithelium, it consists of several layers, including a surface layer of umbrella cells. The thickness of the epithelium varies: it is thick in contracted organs and thin in expanded organs.

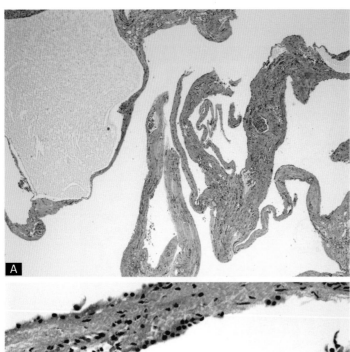

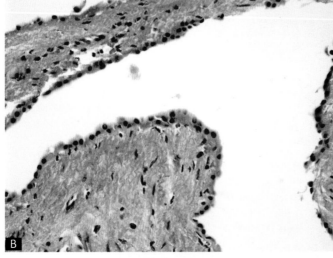

**Figs 7.2A and B:** Polycystic kidney disease
**A.** Normal renal parenchyma has been replaced by cysts lined by nondescript simple epithelium derived from dilated tubules and ducts. **B.** Higher power view shows nondescript cuboidal cells lining the cysts.

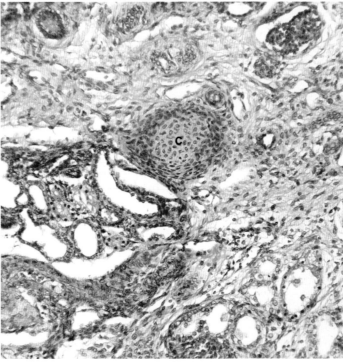

**Fig. 7.3:** Multicystic renal dysplasia
The solid tissue taken out around the nondescript cysts contains atrophic tubules, fetal glomeruli, stromal connective tissue and cartilage (C).

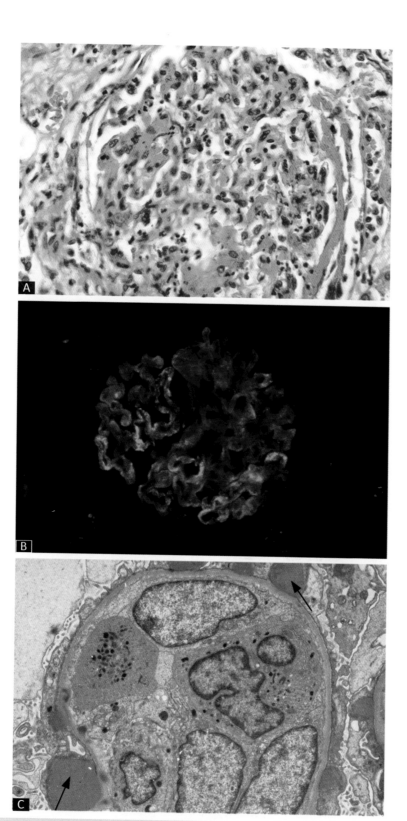

**Figs 7.4A to C:** Acute poststreptococcal glomerulonephritis
**A.** The glomerulus is hypercellular and contains numerous neutrophils as well as proliferating mesangial and endothelial cells. **B.** Immunofluorescence microscopy shows widespread immune complex deposits in the glomerulus. **C.** By electron microscopy the capillary lumen is obliterated by proliferated cells. On the subepithelial surface of the glomerular basement membrane there are deposits of immune complexes forming typical humps (arrows).

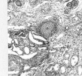

ATLAS OF HISTOPATHOLOGY

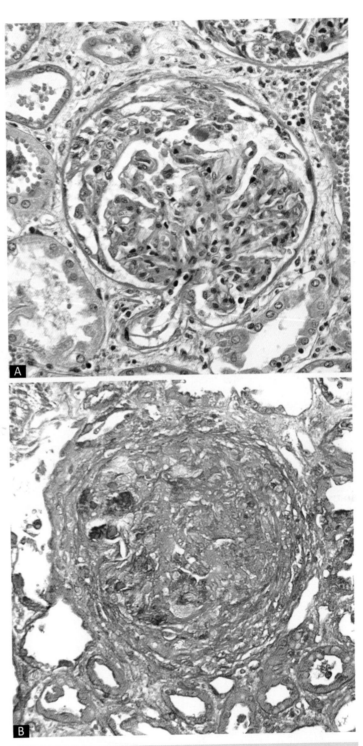

**Figs 7.5A and B:** Crescentic glomerulonephritis

**A.** The urinary space between the collapsed capillary loops and the Bowman's capsules contains inflammatory cells admixed to proliferating epithelial cells and strands of fibrin. **B.** The disease leads to rapid destruction of glomeruli which become replaced by fibrous connective tissue (shown here as blue with the trichrome stain).

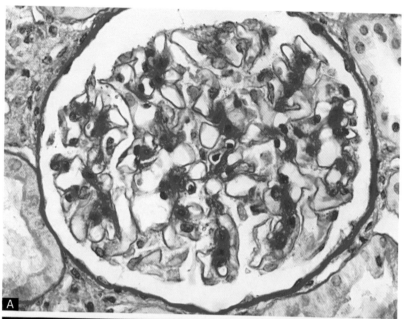

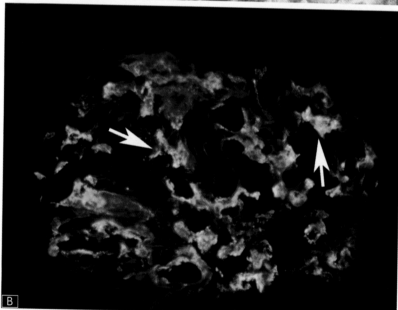

**Figs 7.6A and B:** IgA nephropathy

**A.** The glomerulus shows widening of mesangial areas which contain an increased number of mesangial cells. **B.** Immunofluorescence microscopy shows deposits of IgA in the mesangial areas (arrows).

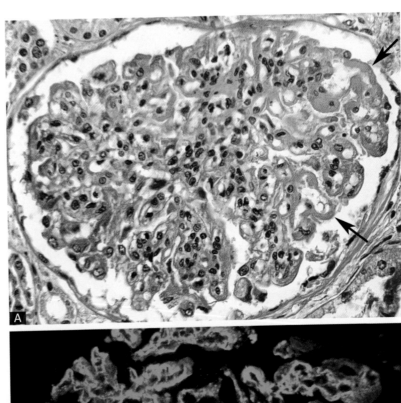

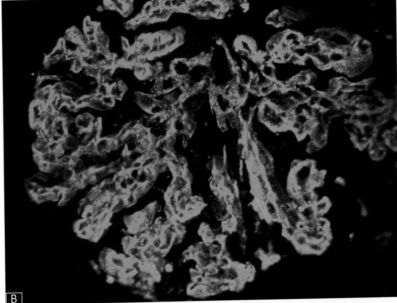

**Figs 7.7A and B:** Lupus nephritis

**A.** The glomerulus is hypercellular and also segmentally shows thickening of the glomerular basement membranes in the form of so-called "wire loops" (arrows). **B.** Immunofluorescence microscopy shows widespread deposits of immune complexes along the glomerular basement membranes and in the mesangial areas.

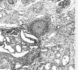

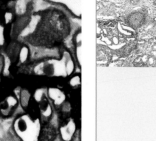

**Figs 7.8A to D:** Membranous nephropathy

**A.** Light microscopy shows diffuse thickening of the glomerular basement membranes without increased cellularity of the glomerulus. **B.** Deposits of immune complexes along the glomerular basement membrane are accompanied by projections of the basement membrane which is best demonstrated by silver impregnation. **C.** Immunofluorescence microscopy shows granular (lumpy-bumpy) deposits along the glomerular basement membranes. **D.** Electron microscopy shows evenly spaced deposits of dense immune complexes on the epithelial side of the basement membrane.

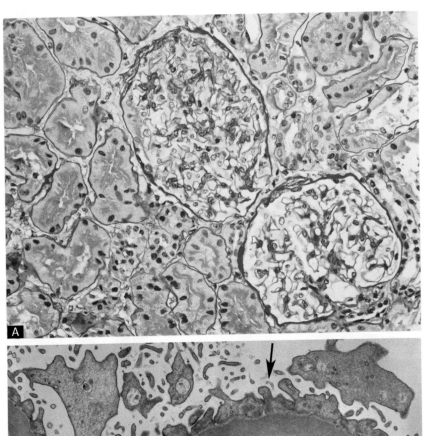

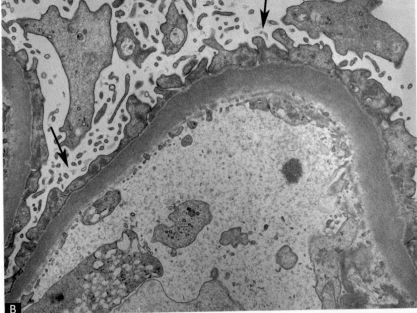

**Figs 7.9A and B:** Minimal change disease
**A.** By light microscopy the glomeruli appear essentially normal, and the glomerular basement membranes are of normal thickness (PAS staining). **B.** By electron microscopy the only visible change is the fusion of the foot processes of the epithelial cells (arrows).

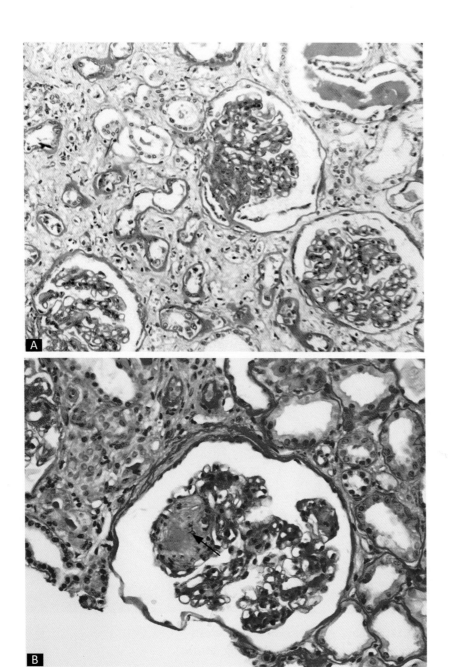

**Figs 7.10A and B:** Focal segmental glomerulosclerosis
**A.** The middle of the three glomeruli shows sclerosis of the capillary loops at 6 o'clock, whereas the other two glomeruli are essentially normal (PAS stain). **B.** A portion of the glomerular capillaries is hyalinized (arrow).

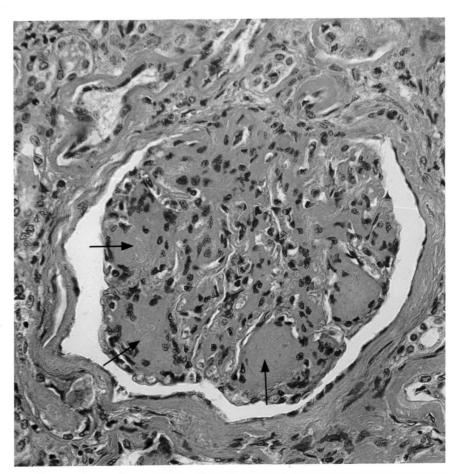

**Fig. 7.11:** Diabetic nodular glomerulosclerosis
Mesangial areas show nodular widening (arrows).

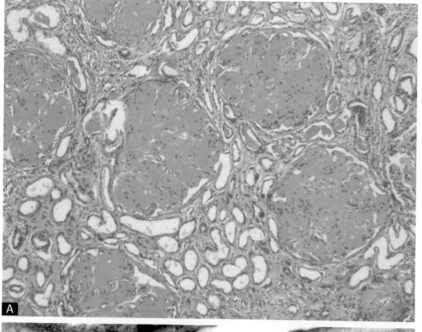

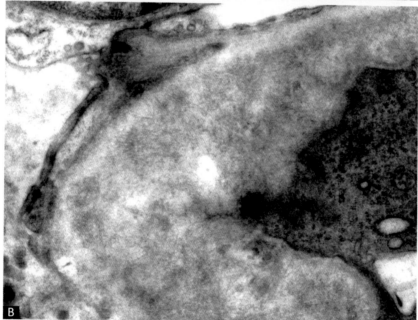

**Figs 7.12A and B:** Amyloidosis
**A.** Eosinophilic deposits of amyloid have obliterated the normal capillary structure of the glomerulus. **B.** Electron microscopy shows that amyloid has a fibrillar beaded structure.

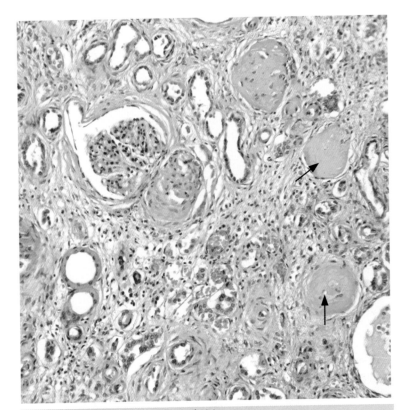

**Fig. 7.13:** Chronic glomerulonephritis

Only one of the five glomeruli depicted here is still preserved whereas the other four are almost completely hyalinized (arrows). Fibrous tissue is replacing most of the tubules and the remaining tubules are atrophic.

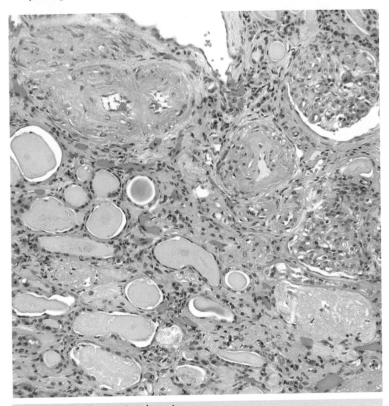

**Fig. 7.14:** Nephroangiosclerosis

Hypertension causes vascular changes such as thickening of the arterial walls and narrowing their lumina and atrophy of the tubules.

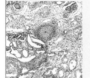

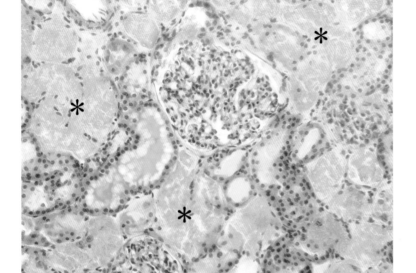

**Fig. 7.15:** Acute tubular necrosis
Necrotic proximal tubules have lost their nuclei and have finely granular amorphous eosinophilic cytoplasm (asterisk). The remaining distal tubules and glomeruli have preserved nuclei.

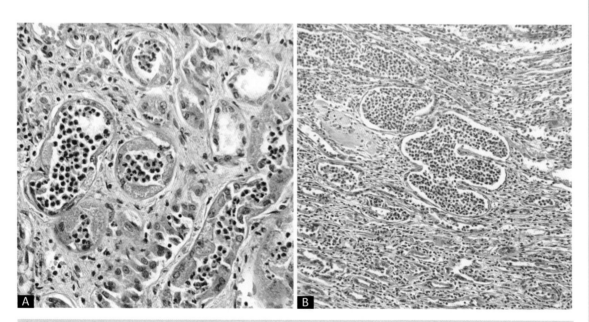

**Figs 7.16A and B:** Acute pyelonephritis
**A.** In early stages of the ascending infection the tubules contain neutrophils in their lumen. **B.** In advance stages of the infection the intratubular pus has caused dilatation of tubules and atrophy of the tubular cells. Inflammatory cells are also found in the interstitial spaces.

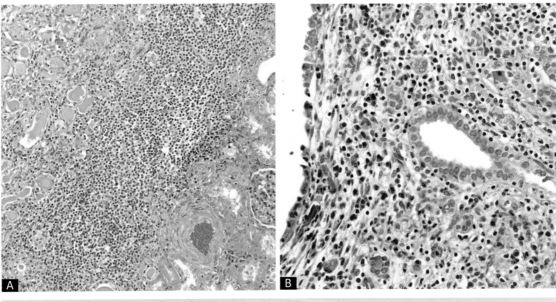

**Figs 7.17A and B:** Chronic pyelonephritis

**A.** Chronic inflammation has caused destruction of the tubules in the midozone. In the upper part of the figure one may see atrophic tubules filled with proteinaceous casts (thyroidization of the kidney). In the lower part of the figure one may see the preserved glomerulus and tubules which have been spared of destruction. **B.** At higher magnification one may see that the inflammatory infiltrate consists predominantly of lymphocytes and plasma cells. On the left side one may see the epithelium lining the pyelon.

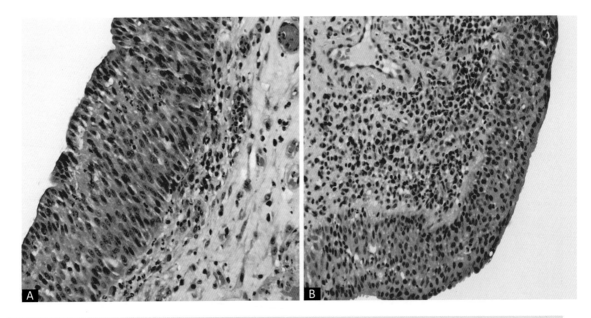

**Figs 7.18A and B:** Cystitis

**A.** Acute cystitis is evidence by the infiltrates of neutrophils transmigrating through the urothelium. **B.** Chronic cystitis is characterized by infiltrates of lymphocytes, plasma cells and macrophages in the lamina propria of the urinary bladder.

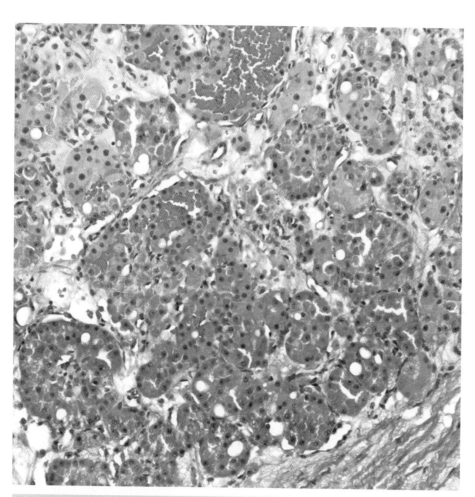

**Fig. 7.19:** Renal oncocytoma

The tumor is composed of oncocytes, i.e. cells that have abundant eosinophilic cytoplasm, and relatively uniform nuclei.

THE URINARY SYSTEM

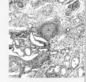

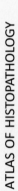

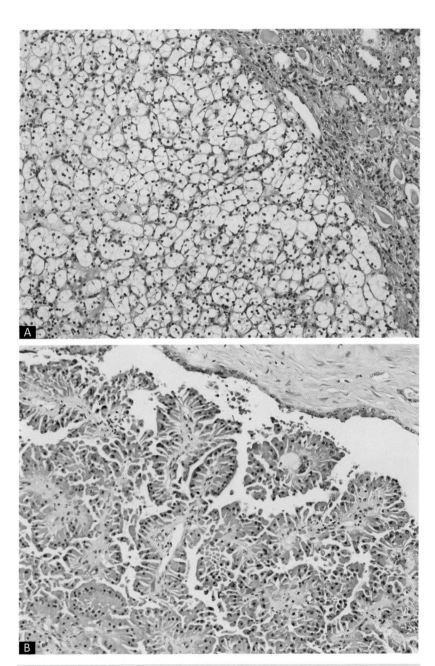

**Figs 7.20A and B:** Renal cell carcinoma

**A.** Clear cell carcinoma is composed of sheets of clear cells that have hyperchromatic nuclei. **B.** Papillary renal cell carcinoma is composed papillae lined by cuboidal cells which have eosinophilic cytoplasm.

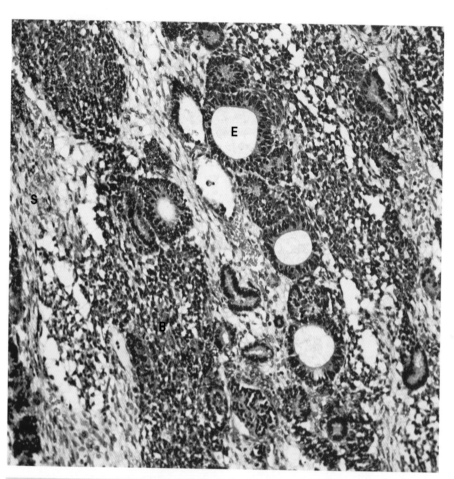

**Fig. 7.21:** Wilms' tumor

The tumor is composed of immature cells forming tubules and called epithelial cell (E), forming dense aggregates of hyperchromatic cells, called blastema cell (B), and loosely arranged cells called stromal cells (S).

THE URINARY SYSTEM

CHAPTER

7

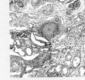

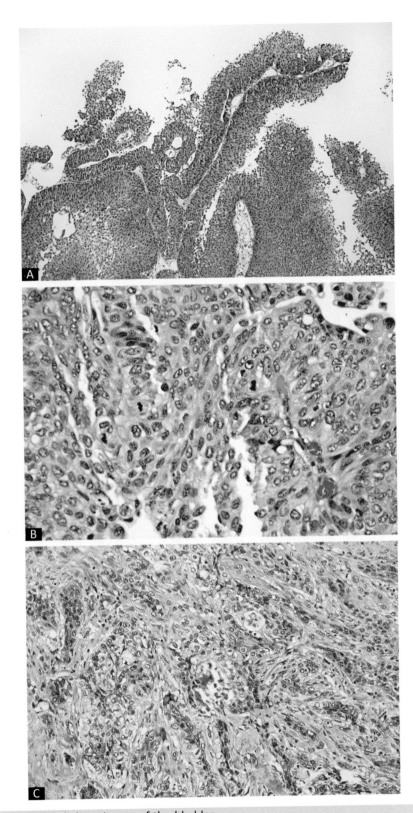

**Figs 7.22A to C:** Urothelial carcinoma of the bladder

**A.** Papillary carcinoma of low grade malignancy forms papillae by relatively uniform cells. **B.** Papillary carcinoma of high grade malignancy forms papillae lined by cells that show much more pleomorphism and mitotic activity. **C.** Invasive urothelial carcinoma is formed of cells that invade the muscle layer of the bladder.

# 8 The Male Genital System

*Ivan Damjanov*

## Introduction

*The male reproductive system consists of testes, excretory ducts, such as the epididymis, vas deferens, parts of the lower urinary tract, such as the urethra, adnexal genital glands, such as seminal vesicles and prostate, and the penis. In this chapter we will deal primarily with the pathologic changes of the testis, prostate and penis.*

## Testis

The testis is the male gonad, whose principal functions are to produce sperm and synthesize male sexual hormones. Spermatogenesis takes place within the seminiferous tubules, membrane bound hollow tubes containing germ cells in various stages of maturation and Sertoli cells (Fig. 8.1). The peritubular interstitial spaces contain Leydig cells, the primary source of testosterone.

*The most important diseases of the testis are:*

- Developmental disorders
- Infections
- Neoplasms.

### Developmental Disorders

The normal development of the testis begins with the formation of genital fold on the posterior side of the fetal abdominal (coelomic) cavity. Once formed, the testes slowly descend through the inguinal canal into the scrotum, which they reach during the last stages of pregnancy. Incomplete descent of the testes into their normal scrotal position is called cryptorchidism. Bilateral cryptorchidism may cause infertility. Cryptorchidism is also a risk factor for germ cell tumors.

*Cryptorchid testes* surgically positioned into the scrotum during early childhood develop normally and usually do not differ from normal testes. If the cryptorchid testes are left in the abnormal position, they will show variable signs of atrophy of seminal epithelium and incomplete or arrested spermatogenesis. The basement membranes of the seminiferous tubules become thickened and there is interstitial fibrosis (Figs 8.2A and B).

*Sertoli-only syndrome* is a term used to describe a group of infertile patients who have genetic azoospermia. Testicular biopsy will typically reveal a lack of germ cells in the seminiferous tubules, which are lined by Sertoli cells (Fig. 8.3). The interstitial spaces contain hyperplastic Leydig cells.

### Infections

The infection of the testis is called *orchitis,* whereas the infection of epididymis is called *epididymitis.* In many cases both organs are involved and the disease is therefore called *epididymo-orchitis.*

*Epididymitis* is typically a consequence of bacterial infection ascending through the vas deferens from the lower urinary tract. Clinically, it typically presents as suppurative inflammation (Fig.

8.3). In younger men, such infections are caused by *N. gonorrhoeae* and other sexually transmitted pathogens. In elderly men, epididymo-orchitis is caused by *E. coli* and other uropathogens. Acute infection may evolve into a chronic infection dominated by fibrosis.

*Orchitis* may be caused by viruses, such as mumps virus, or bacteria, such as *Treponema pallidum,* the cause of syphilis. Mumps orchitis, a prototype of viral infection of the testis is characterized by interstitial infiltrates of lymphocytes, macrophages and plasma cells invading and destroying the seminiferous tubules **(Figs 8.4A and B)**. Atrophy and hyalinization of seminiferous tubules may be the final outcome. Bilateral infections may cause infertility.

*Testicular atrophy* due to hyalinization of the seminiferous tubules is the final outcome of chronic orchitis (Fig. 8.5). It may, however, also be the end result of many other testicular diseases, including ischemia due to atherosclerosis, chronic disease, chemotherapy or radiation.

### Neoplasms

Primary testicular tumors are of germ cell origin in over 90% of all cases. The tumors of sex cord cells, i.e. the Sertoli and Leydig cell tumors are less common.

*Germ cell tumors* are almost all malignant and found predominantly in men in the age group of 25–45 years. They can be subdivided into two major groups: seminomas and nonseminomatous germ cell tumors (NSGCT). Almost all germ cell tumors originate from a preinvasive form of cancer called intratubular germ cell neoplasia (ITGN) **(Figs 8.6A and B)**.

*Seminoma* is the most common testicular neoplasm, accounting for 40% of all testicular tumors. It is composed of a single population of cells resembling spermatogonia **(Figs 8.7A and B)**. These cells are arranged into compact groups surrounded by fibrous strands infiltrated with lymphocytes.

*Nonseminomatous germ cell tumor (NSGCT)* is a term used to group all other germ cell tumors and separate them from seminoma. In contrast of seminomas, which are composed of a single cell type, NSGCT are composed of many cell types. The malignant stem cells of NSGCT are called *embryonal carcinoma cells*. Embryonal carcinoma cells can differentiate into somatic and nonsomatic (extraembryonic) tissues. Somatic tissues include derivatives of all three embryonic germ layers (ectoderm, mesoderm and endoderm), such as ski, cartilage, neural tissue, etc. Extraembryonic nonsomatic tissues include cells that resemble chorionic epithelium of the placenta and the yolk sac.

*Embryonal carcinoma* is a tumor composed of undifferentiated embryonic cells (Fig. 8.8). Embryonal carcinomas account for about 10% of all NSGCT. These tumors secrete no serologic markers.

*Teratocarcinoma or Malignant NSGCT, not otherwise specified*, is the most common NSGCT. It contains embryonal carcinoma as its stem cells and various somatic and extraembryonic (nonsomatic) elements **(Figs 8.9A to D)**. The most important extraembryonic elements are *choriocarcinoma* and *yolk sac carcinoma*, resembling the cells of the placental chorionic epithelium or the fetal yolk sac respectively. Choriocarcinoma cells secrete human chorionic gonadotropin (hCG) and the yolk sac carcinoma cells secrete α-fetoprotein (AFP), which serve as serologic tumor markers and are important for the diagnosis of these tumors.

*Choriocarcinoma* may occur in a pure form, but such tumors are very rare. Microscopically it is composed of mononuclear cytotrophoblastic and multinucleated syncytiotrophoblastic cells that secrete hCG (Fig. 8.10).

*Yolk sac tumor* is an early childhood tumor composed of yolk sac elements known to secrete AFP. Microscopically the tumor cells grow in a variety of patterns, such as reticular or papillary, glandular, just to mention a few. Cell form structures resembling endodermal sinuses in the rodent placenta and glomeruloid structures are called Schiller-Duval bodies **(Fig. 8.11)**.

*Sex cord cell tumors* are uncommon, usually benign tumors accounting for only 5% of testicular neoplasms. Exceptionally these tumors may be malignant. They are hormonally active or inactive and can occur at any age.

*Sertoli cell tumors* are uncommon benign tumors composed of cells that resemble normal sertoli cells (Fig. 8.12). These cells may form tubules resembling those of the testis or cords and nests surrounded by fibrous strands. Like their normal counterpart Sertoli cell tumors secrete inhibin, but many tumors are hormonally inactive.

*Leydig cell tumors* are composed of endocrine cells resembling normal Leydig cells (Fig. 8.13). Like the normal Leydig cells they have an eosinophilic cytoplasm with scattered small lipid droplets. The cytoplasm of these cells may also contain Reinke crystals. Leydig cell tumors may secrete testosterone, or less commonly estrogen, but some tumors are hormonally inactive.

## Prostate

*The prostate* is an exocrine gland attached to the urethra. It is composed of epithelial acinar glands and tubules embedded in a fibromuscular stroma (Fig. 8.14). The secretions of the prostate are excreted in seminal fluid.

The most important diseases of the prostate are:
- Benign prostatic hyperplasia
- Carcinoma of the prostate.

### Benign Prostatic Hyperplasia

*Benign prostatic hyperplasia* (BPH) is an age-related nodular enlargement of the periurethral portion of the prostate found in most, if not all, elderly men (Fig. 8.15). Microscopically the nodules are composed of hyperplastic glands and fibromuscular stroma (Figs 8.16A and B). It has been proposed that the increased number of glandular cells is related to their defective apoptosis; the proliferation of fibromuscular stroma results from dihydrotestosterone-induced growth factors. BPH may obstruct urinary outflow from the bladder. The subsequent retention of urine is associated with an increased incidence of urinary stones, recurrent cystitis, ascending urinary tract infections and even the infection of the prostate itself.

### Neoplasms

*Adenocarcinoma* is the most common prostatic neoplasm and also the most common malignant tumor in males. It occurs mostly in the posterior and lateral peripheral portion of the prostate (Fig. 8.15). It is a tumor of elderly men and is rarely found under the age of 40 years. Benign tumors and other forms of malignancy are rare and of limited clinical significance.

Adenocarcinoma develops from a preinvasive form of malignancy called *prostatic intraepithelial neoplasia* (PIN) (Fig. 8.17). The *invasive prostatic adenocarcinoma* is composed of small glands lined by a single layer of cuboidal cells (Figs 8.18A and B). In contrast to normal glands which are surrounded by an outer basal layer, the neoplastic glands are directly surrounded by the desmoplastic fibrous stroma. Neoplastic cells invade the periprostatic tissue, nerves and metastasize to lymph nodes and distant organs. The bones of the pelvis and vertebrae are the most common sites for these metastases.

The degree of differentiation of prostatic adenocarcinoma varies and the tumors could thus be classified as well differentiated, moderately differentiated or poorly differentiated. Tumors can be graded on a scale from 1 to 5 according to the system devised by Gleason (Figs 8.19A and B). Gleason's grade is assigned to the most prevalent pattern and the second most common pattern and the two grades are then combined into a final Gleason score (e.g. Gleason grade 3+4 = Gleason score 7). Gleason's score, usually combined with staging data, is used for predicting the clinical course of the disease.

## Penis

The penis is the main copulatory male organ. On its external surface it is covered with skin and squamous mucosa. In the central part of the penis there is the urethra, which serves as conduit for both the ejaculated seminal fluid and the urine. The urethra is surrounded by corpora cavernosa composed of vascular spaces that may expand due to congestion, leading to erection of the penis.

### Neoplasms

*Condyloma acuminatum* is the most common benign tumor of the penis. It presents as a wart-like papule or polyp, most often located in the coronal sulcus. Microscopically it is lined by thickened squamous epithelium showing koilocytic clearing of the cytoplasm human papillomavirus infection (Figs 8.20A and B).

*Squamous cell carcinoma* is the most common malignant tumor of the penis. On the shaft it may be preceded by preinvasive carcinoma called Bowen disease. Most carcinomas, however, occur on the glans and coronal sulcus or the inner surface of the prepuce. Microscopically it resembles squamous cell carcinoma in other sites (Fig. 8.21).

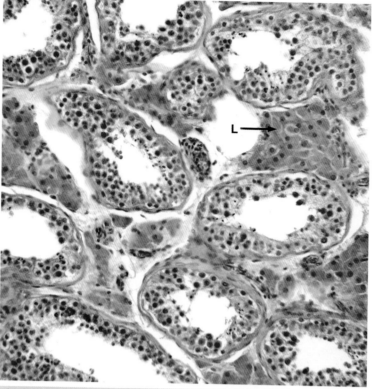

**Fig. 8.1:** Normal testis

The main components of the testis are the seminiferous tubules lined sperm-producing germinal epithelium and Sertoli cells and interstitial cells of Leydig (L). The seminiferous tubules are delimited from the interstitial spaces by a basement membrane.

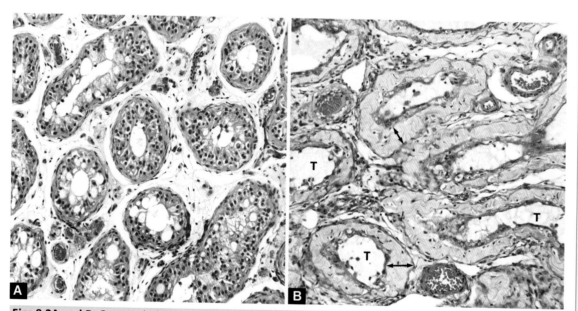

**Figs 8.2A and B:** Cryptorchid testis

**A.** The testis shows signs of atrophy. The seminiferous tubules show no signs of spermatogenesis and are lined by Sertoli cells. There basement membranes are thickened and the interstitial spaces contain increased amounts of fibrous tissue. **B.** Atrophy is the testis associated with partial hyalinization of tubules (T), which have markedly thickened basement membranes (arrows).

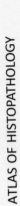

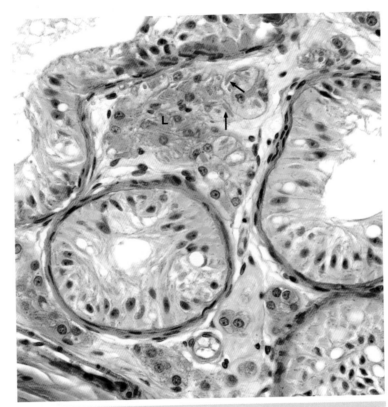

**Fig. 8.3:** Sertoli-only syndrome

The seminiferous tubules are lined by Sertoli cells and contain no germ cells or any evidence of spermatogenesis. Arrows point to Reinke crystals in Leydig cells (L).

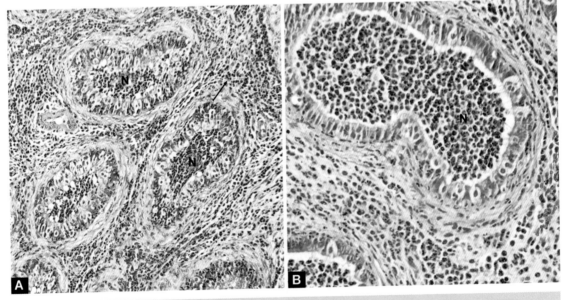

**Figs 8.4A and B:** Acute bacterial epididymitis

The epididymal duct contains neutrophils (N), which may also be seen in the periductal connective tissue (arrow).

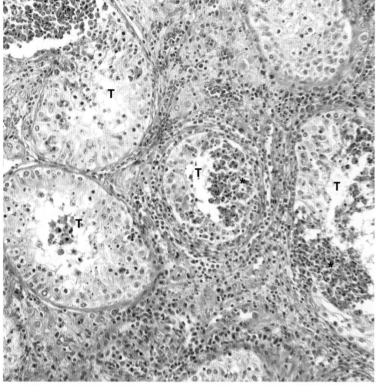

**Fig. 8.5:** Viral orchitis

The interstitial spaces are infiltrated with mononuclear cells, which also impinge upon the seminiferous tubules (T). Some tubules contain inflammatory cells (asterisk). There is no spermatogenesis.

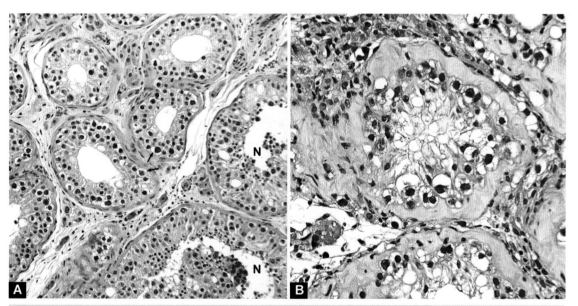

**Figs 8.6A and B:** Intratubular germ cell neoplasia

The seminiferous tubules, which have a thickened basement membrane, contain prominent neoplastic cells (arrows). Adjacent normal seminiferous tubules (N) show signs of spermatogenesis. These cells have a large centrally located nucleus surrounded by clear cytoplasm that imparts them a "fried egg appearance".

THE MALE GENITAL SYSTEM

CHAPTER

**8**

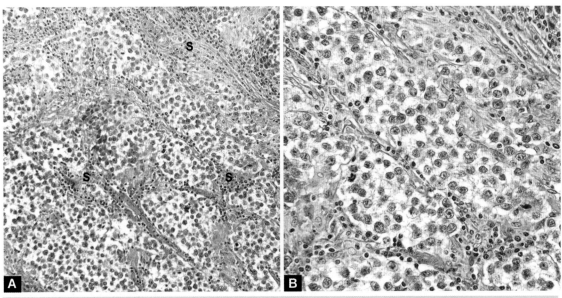

**Figs 8.7A and B:** Seminoma

**A.** The tumor is composed of clear cells arranged in groups surrounded by fibrous septa (S) infiltrated with lymphocytes. **B.** At higher magnification the tumor cells have centrally located vesicular nuclei surrounded by clear cytoplasm and distinct plasma membranes.

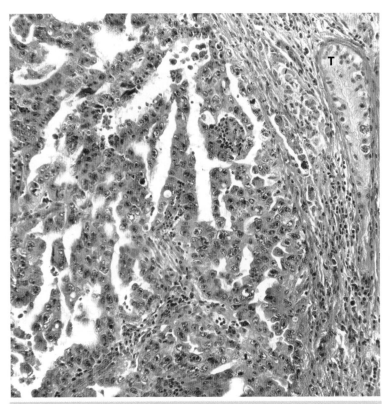

**Fig. 8.8:** Embryonal carcinoma

These tumor cells have large vesicular nuclei with prominent nucleoli and scant cytoplasm. The borders of individual cells are not clearly visible and their nuclei seem to be overlapping because there is not enough cytoplasm to separate them from one another. The adjacent seminiferous tubule (T) contains intratubular germ cell neoplasia.

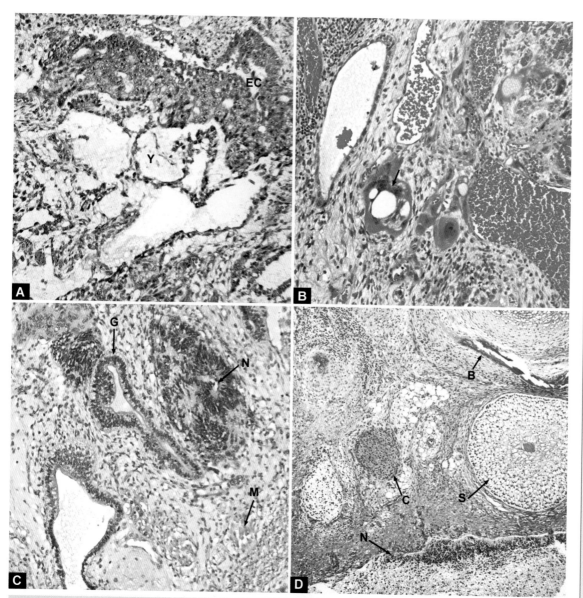

**Figs 8.9A to D:** Teratocarcinoma. The tumor consists of heterogeneous tissues.
**A.** Hyperchromatic embryonal carcinoma cells (EC), arranged in a group adjacent to loosely textured yolk sac carcinoma cells (Y). **B.** Multinucleated choriocarcinoma cells (arrow), some mononuclear cytotrophoblastic cells (C) are adjacent to pools of extravasated blood. **C.** Immature somatic cells include cells forming neural tubes (N), and fetal intestinal glands (G), and loosely structured fetal stroma that contains eosinophilic cells, most likely representing muscle cells (M). **D.** Somatic tissues include bone (B), cartilage (C), neural tissue (N), and nests of squamous epithelium composed of clear cells (S).

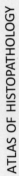

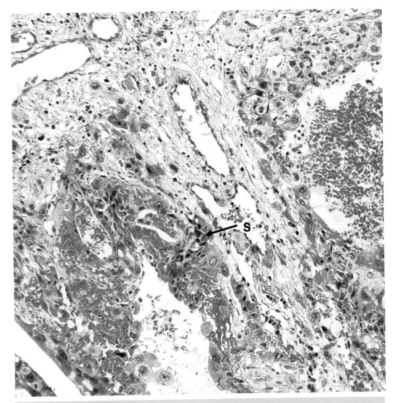

**Fig. 8.10:** Choriocarcinoma

The tumor is composed of multinucleated syncytiotrophoblastic cells (S) and mononuclear cytotrophoblastic cells surrounded by clotted blood.

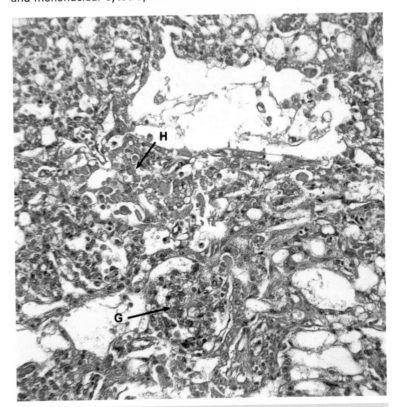

**Fig. 8.11:** Yolk sac tumor

The tumor is composed of loosely arranged cells forming strands, nests or glomeruloid structures (G) called Schiller-Duval bodies. There are also prominent round hyaline globules (H).

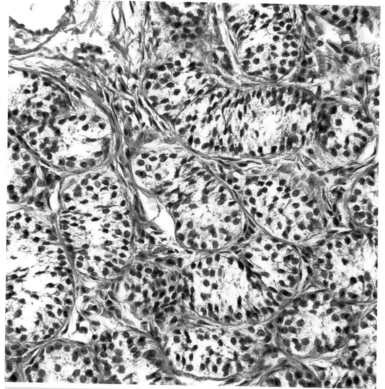

**Fig. 8.12:** Sertoli cell tumor

Tumor cells form tubules similar to those in the testis, but lined by Sertoli cells only and devoid of germ cells.

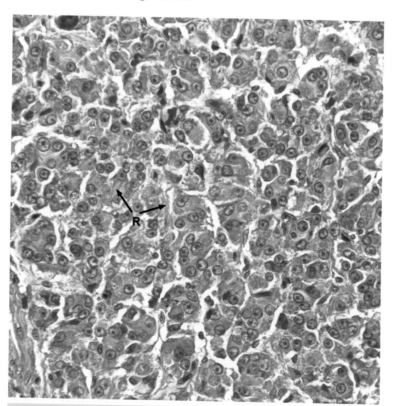

**Fig. 8.13:** Leydig cell tumor

The tumor is composed of a uniform population of cells which have round nuclei and abundant cytoplasm. Eosinophilic Reinke crystals are also seen (R arrows).

THE MALE GENITAL SYSTEM

CHAPTER

**8**

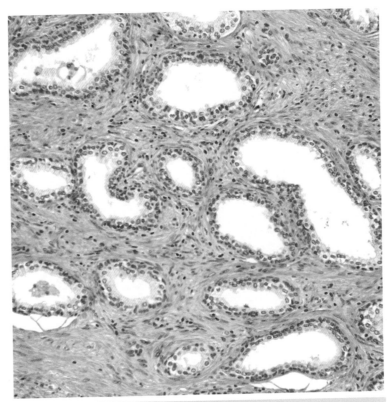

**Fig. 8.14:** Normal prostate

The prostate is formed of glands lined by two layers of cells: luminal cuboidal cells surrounded by a basal layer separating the glands from the fibromuscular stroma.

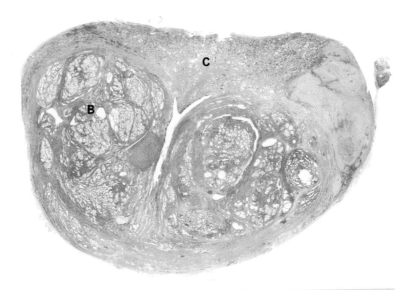

**Fig. 8.15:** Abnormal prostate

The prostate is nodular due to benign prostatic hyperplasia (B). Solid areas in the peripheral part correspond to carcinoma (C).

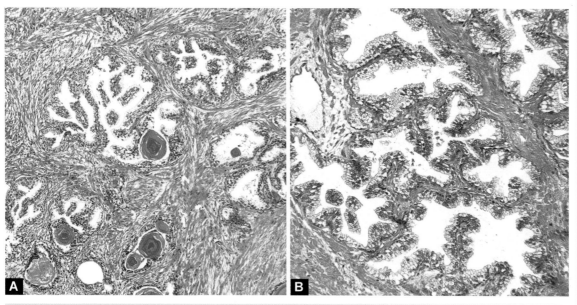

**Figs 8.16A and B:** Benign prostatic hyperplasia

**A.** The prostate contains hyperplastic glands enclosed by abundant fibromuscular stroma. **B.** Hyperplastic glands are lined by cells which have abundant clear cytoplasm and small, round, basally located nuclei.

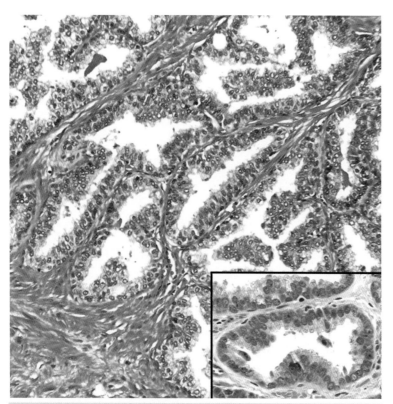

**Fig. 8.17:** Prostatic intraepithelial neoplasia

Normal glands with well-defined lumina are lined by atypical cells with enlarged nuclei, resembling those in invasive carcinoma. The inset shows at higher magnification the enlarged nuclei with prominent nucleoli in neoplastic cells.

THE MALE GENITAL SYSTEM

CHAPTER

**8**

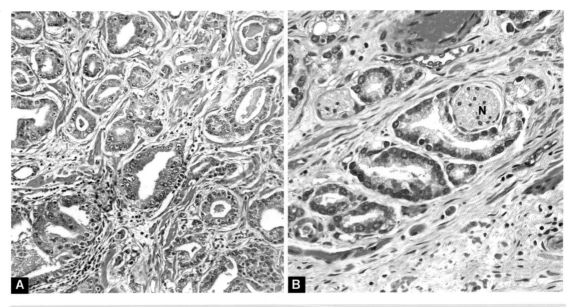

**Figs 8.18A and B:** Adenocarcinoma of the prostate

The neoplastic glands are composed of a single layer of cuboidal cells directly abutting on the fibrous stroma. Tumor cells have enlarged vesicular nuclei and prominent nucleoli. The basal layer is missing. Perineural invasion is seen as rapping of neoplastic glands around a nerve (N).

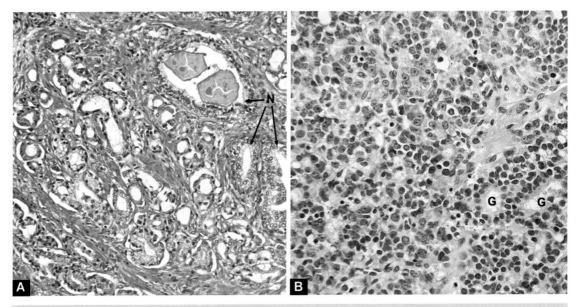

**Figs 8.19A and B:** Adenocarcinoma of the prostate

**A.** Gleason score 3 + 4 = 7 carcinoma consists in part of discrete glands separated one from another by strands of stroma and interlacing or fused glands. In the upper part of the figure there are three normal glands (N). **B.** Gleason score 5 + 5 = 10 carcinoma consists of solid sheets of cells and a few abortive glands (G).

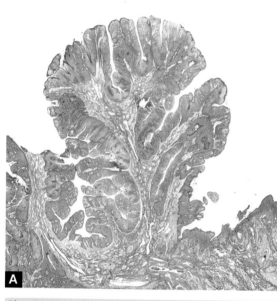
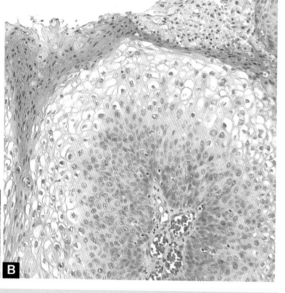

**Figs 8.20A and B:** Condyloma acuminatum

**A.** The lesion is lined by thickened epithelium showing clearing of the cytoplasm, corresponding to koilocytic changes induced by human papillomavirus. **B.** Higher power view of koilocytes, which have enlarged irregular nuclei and clear cytoplasm.

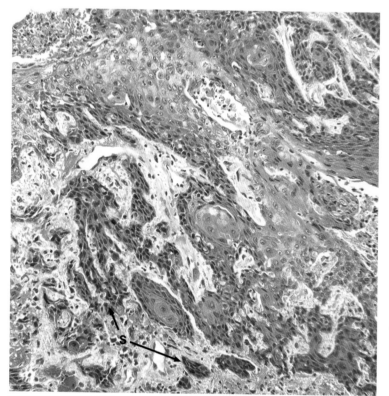

**Fig. 8.21:** Squamous cell carcinoma of the penis

The tumor is composed of squamous cells which form strands (S) invading the underlying stroma.

THE MALE GENITAL SYSTEM

# 9 Female Reproductive System

*Fang Fan*

## Introduction

*The female reproductive system consists of vulva, vagina, cervix, uterine corpus, ovary and fallopian tubes. Important diseases of these organ systems as well as some pregnancy related changes will be discussed in this chapter.*

## Vulva, Vagina and Cervix

The vulva is lined by keratinized squamous epithelium **(Fig. 9.1A)**. On the labia majora, the surface covering has all the features of the skin, and includes hair follicles and adnexal glands as well subcutaneous fat tissue. The labia minora are skin folds without hair follicles and adipose tissue but rich in blood vessels, elastic fibers and sebaceous glands. The vagina and the ectocervix are lined by non-keratinizing squamous epithelium; the endocervix is lined by glandular epithelium containing a single layer of columnar mucin-producing cells **(Fig. 9.1B)**.

The most important diseases of the vulva, vagina and cervix are:
- Non-neoplastic vulvar epithelial disorders
- Non-neoplastic lesions of the cervix
- Human papillomavirus-related squamous intraepithelial lesions
- Invasive squamous cell carcinoma
- Cervical adenocarcinoma
- Paget's disease of the vulva.

### Non-Neoplastic Epithelial Vulvar Disorders

This group of diseases of unknown etiology previously known as *vulvar dystrophy* presents clinically as whitish pruritic thickening, i.e. vulvar leukoplakia. It includes two entities: (a) lichen sclerosus and (b) squamous cell hyperplasia, which may coexist. These lesions are often biopsied because they may clinically resemble specific skin diseases such as psoriasis, lichen planus, and squamous vulvar intraepithelial neoplasia.

*Lichen sclerosus* most often occurs in postmenopausal women, but may affect young adults and, occasionally, occur even in children. The characteristic histopathologic features of lichen sclerosus include the following: an atrophic epithelium with hyperkeratosis and loss of rete pegs, an edematous acellular subepithelial zone composed of homogenized and hyalinized collagen, and scattered infiltrates of chronic inflammatory cells in the lower dermis **(Fig. 9.2)**.

*Squamous cell hyperplasia* is a reactive change most likely resulting from irritation and scratching. Microscopically, it is characterized by thickening of the epidermis (*acanthosis*), thickening of the granular cell layer (*hypergranulosis*) and prominent surface keratinization (*hyperkeratosis*) **(Fig. 9.3)**. Mild chronic inflammatory infiltrate may be present in the dermis. The absence of epithelial dysplasia and atypia are important findings distinguishing this lesion from intraepithelial vulvar neoplasia.

## Non-Neoplastic Lesions of Cervix

*Non-neoplastic lesions of the cervix* are very common and include a spectrum of inflammatory and reactive proliferative conditions. These lesions are often biopsied, and it is very important not to confuse them with neoplasia. Here we shall mention just a few most important non-neoplastic lesions of the cervix such as: (a) chronic cervicitis; (b) microglandular hyperplasia and (c) endocervical polyps.

*Chronic cervicitis* is a very common condition and it usually affects the squamocolumnar junction and the endocervix. Microscopically, it shows congestion, surface erosion and chronic inflammation. The etiology of this inflammation is variable but in most instances it is of limited clinical significance. Occasionally it may be associated with pelvic inflammatory disease (PID).

*Endocervical polyps* are benign lesions protruding from the mucosa of the cervix and occasionally bulging through the cervical os. Microscopically, they are composed of dilated endocervical glands in fibrovascular stroma **(Fig. 9.4)**. The surface of polyps is covered with glandular cuboidal cells similar to those of the endocervix, although often it may undergo squamous metaplasia.

*Microglandular hyperplasia* of the endocervix is characterized by proliferation of small glands in a crowded and complex pattern **(Fig. 9.5)**. It is most often seen in women using oral contraceptives. The closely apposed glands are lined by a layer of cuboidal or flattened epithelium with almost no atypia. The intervening stroma often contains acute and chronic inflammatory cells. Microglandular hyperplasia is a benign proliferation and should not be confused with endocervical adenocarcinoma.

## Human Papillomavirus-Related Squamous Intraepithelial Lesions

Human papillomavirus (HPV) is a sexually transmitted DNA virus that affects most sexually active young women. It is now known that HPV causes almost all cervical squamous cell carcinomas and most cervical adenocarcinomas. It is the persistence of the HPV infection together with other host and environmental factors that enhances the progression of cervical neoplasia. The HPV-induced carcinogenesis is mediated through the interactions of E6 and E7 (the products of two early genes), with the tumor suppressor proteins TP53 and pRb respectively. These interactions result in abrogation of apoptosis and uninhibited proliferation of cells. The HPV are divided into low-risk and high-risk groups referring to their level of association with squamous cell carcinoma. The "high-risk" types are primarily 16 and 18, but also include 31, 33, 35, 39, 45, 51, 52, 56, 58, 59, 68, 73 and 82. The "low-risk" types include 6, 11, 40, 42, 43, 44, 54, 61, 70, 72 and 81.

The HPV may cause "flat" lesions including squamous intraepithelial neoplasia in the vulva (VIN), vagina (VAIN) and cervix (CIN), and may cause exophytic condyloma acuminata. The squamous intraepithelial neoplasias are further divided into VIN I-III, VAIN I-III and CIN I-III respectively. They share similar morphologic features, and therefore the cervical intraepithelial neoplasia (CIN) only will be described here.

*Cervical intraepithelial neoplasia I (CIN I)* or mild squamous dysplasia is characterized by the presence of koilocytes in the upper two-thirds of the epithelium with adequate epithelial maturation. Mitosis is limited to the basal third of the epithelium. Koilocytes are due to the cytopathic effect of HPV virus on superficial or intermediate squamous cells. The cells have mildly enlarged hyperchromatic nuclei with irregular nuclear membrane (rasinoid nuclei), and a characteristic perinuclear halo rimmed by a condensed peripheral cell border **(Fig. 9.6A)**.

*Cervical intraepithelial neoplasia II (CIN II)* is characterized by moderate squamous dysplasia, which involves the lower two-thirds of the epithelium. The cells have high nuclear to cytoplasmic ratio and nuclear atypia. Mitotic figures can be found in the middle to lower two-thirds of the epithelium, and atypical forms may be seen **(Fig. 9.6B)**.

*Cervical intraepithelial neoplasia III (CIN III)* is characterized by severe squamous dysplasia or squamous cell carcinoma in situ, in which the epithelium shows no maturation. Nuclear atypia and mitoses are present throughout the thickness of the epithelium **(Fig. 9.6C)**. Abnormal mitotic figures are frequent.

*Condyloma acuminatum* is a polypoid exophytic lesion characterized by papillomatosis, acanthosis and koilocytosis **(Fig. 9.7)**. It is most strongly associated with infection by HPV types 6 and 11. Occasionally it may be caused by high-risk HPV (HPV 16); in such cases the condyloma will contain microscopic changes corresponding to CIN II or CIN III.

### Invasive Squamous Cell Carcinoma

*Invasive squamous cell carcinoma* is the most common malignant tumor of the cervix. It is characterized by neoplastic squamous cells invading into the stroma. In the World Health Organization Classification of Tumors, squamous cell carcinoma of the cervix is divided into several microscopic subtypes including keratinizing, non-keratinizing, basaloid, verrucous, warty, papillary, lymphoepithelioma-like and squamotransitional types **(Fig. 9.8)**. A simple three-tiered grading system may be used to grade squamous cell carcinomas and classify them as well differentiated, moderately differentiated or poorly differentiated.

*Microinvasive squamous cell carcinoma* or early invasive squamous cell carcinoma is defined as a stromal invasion that is no greater than 3.0 mm in depth and 7.0 mm in horizontal spread. The measurement should be taken from the epithelial-stromal junction of the adjacent most superficial epithelial papilla to the deepest point of invasion **(Fig. 9.9)**.

### Cervical Adenocarcinoma

*Cervical adenocarcinoma* is less common than squamous cell carcinoma of the cervix but the overall incidence of endocervical adenocarcinoma is on the rise as compared to the decreasing trend of cervical squamous cell carcinoma. Most cervical adenocarcinomas are associated with HPV infections, particularly HPV 16 and 18. These lesions may present as: (a) endocervical adenocarcinoma in situ or (b) invasive endocervical adenocarcinoma.

*Endocervical adenocarcinoma in situ (AIS)* is diagnosed when the normal mucinous epithelium is replaced by pseudostratified hyperchromatic nuclei showing mitoses and numerous apoptotic bodies **(Fig. 9.10)**. Cytoplasmic mucin is depleted.

*Invasive endocervical adenocarcinoma* most often presents as a mucinous adenocarcinoma **(Fig. 9.11)**. Approximately 70% of all cervical adenocarcinomas are of the mucinous type, and are composed of cells resembling those of the normal endocervix. The cells have basal nuclei and cytoplasmic mucin. The nuclei show considerable atypia, pleomorphism, prominent nucleoli and frequent mitoses. The infiltrating tumor cells usually form glands or cribriform structures. The remaining 30% of endocervical adenocarcinomas are classified as endometrioid, clear cell, and serous adenocarcinomas.

### Vulvar Paget Disease

Paget's disease is a malignant intraepithelial carcinoma characterized by intraepidermal spreading of singly dispersed or clustered large malignant epithelial cells with abundant pale cytoplasm, large nuclei and prominent nucleoli **(Fig. 9.12)**. It presents clinically as an eczematous lesion. The tumor may originate from epidermis or derive from an underlying skin adnexal adenocarcinoma or an adjacent anorectal or urothelial carcinoma.

## Uterine Corpus

The uterine corpus is a hollow organ; with a cavity lined by endometrium surrounded by a thick muscular layer (myometrium) and a serosal covering. The endometrium is composed of endometrial glands and stroma and is divided into a superficial *functional layer* and a deep *basal layer*.

*The normal endometrium* undergoes cyclic changes during child-bearing age. Microscopic features of the *proliferative phase endometrium* are distinct from those of the *secretory phase endometrium* and can be readily recognized in endometrial biopsies. The changes involve both the endometrial glands and the stroma **(Figs 9.13A and B)**.

*Pregnancy related changes* involve the stroma and the glands. During pregnancy the endometrial stroma undergoes decidual transformation, and the glands appear hypersecretory **(Figs 9.14A and B)**. In some instances the endometrial glands may show hobnail nuclei with marked enlargement and hyperchromasia. Mitoses, even atypical forms, may be present. This phenomenon is called *Arias-Stella reaction*.

The most important diseases of the uterine corpus are:
- Endometritis
- Endometrial hyperplasia
- Endometrial epithelial tumors
- Endometrial stromal tumors
- Smooth muscle tumors
- Carcinosarcomas.

## Endometritis

*Acute endometritis* is usually seen in post-abortion or postpartum endometrial curetting specimens. There are neutrophils in endometrial glands and focal accumulations of neutrophils forming microabscesses within the lumens **(Fig. 9.15)**.

*Chronic endometritis* is diagnosed when there are infiltrates of lymphocytes and plasma cells in the endometrial stroma **(Fig. 9.16)**. Identification of plasma cells is the most important criterion for the diagnosis of chronic endometritis. The suspicion for chronic endometritis should be raised when dating the cyclic pattern of the endometrium is difficult, the endometrial stromal cells show a spindle or stellate pattern around the glands or there are focal areas of necrosis or calcifications.

## Endometrial Hyperplasia

Endometrial hyperplasia represents a progressive spectrum of morphologic changes from benign hyperplasia as a result of an unopposed estrogenic stimulus to premalignant conditions with genetically altered monoclonal neoplastic glands. The World Health Organization classifies endometrial hyperplasia based on cytologic features into *typical* and *atypical hyperplasia*, and then further according to the degree of architectural complexity into *simple* and *complex hyperplasia* **(Figs 9.17A to D)**.

*Simple hyperplasia* is characterized by crowding of glands with an increased ratio of glands to stroma. The glands are mostly tubular with minimal intraluminal budding or tufting, and there is no fusion of glands.

*Complex hyperplasia* is characterized by crowding of glands which are tortuous with intraluminal epithelial budding and tufting. There is expansion of crowded glands with back-to-back glands fused together to form cribriform structures. The cytologic atypia is shown as stratification of the nuclei with loss of polarity, hyperchromasia and increased mitoses.

## Endometrial Epithelial Tumors

Tumors of the uterus may originate from the endometrium or the myometrium, and may be being or malignant. We shall describe the following tumors: (a) endometrial polyp, and (b) endometrial adenocarcinoma.

*Endometrial polyp* is a benign polypoid growth projecting into the endometrial cavity. Microscopically it consists of fibrotic stroma containing thick-walled blood vessels and benign endometrial glands **(Fig. 9.18)**. The glandular component may be similar to normal endometrial glands but also may be involved by hyperplasia or carcinoma.

*Endometrial carcinomas* are classified into two types according to different pathogenesis. Type 1 endometrial carcinoma is estrogen-dependent and accounts for 80–85% of endometrial carcinomas. Risk factors include early menarche, late menopause, nulliparous, obesity and diabetes. Tumors are usually low grade and of endometrioid type associated with endometrial hyperplasia. Type 2 endometrial carcinoma is non-estrogen dependent, occurs in older postmenopausal women and accounts for 10–15% of cases. Tumors are high grade, associated with atrophic endometrium and include serous and clear cell types.

*Endometrioid adenocarcinoma* is the most common type of endometrial carcinoma. The neoplastic glands are lined by stratified columnar cells resembling normal endometrial glands. Endometrioid adenocarcinomas can be graded on a scale from 1 to 3 according to the criteria developed by the International Federation of Gynecology and Obstetrics (FIGO) **(Figs 9.19A to C)**. In FIGO grade 1 tumors, more than 95% of the tumor forms glandular structures with back-to-back glands and complex folds and tufts. The squamous and morular components are excluded from the grading. In FIGO grade 2 tumors, 50–95% of the tumors show glandular differentiation; areas of solid tumor growth are increased. When less than 50% of the tumor shows glandular formation, it is FIGO grade 3. When there is marked nuclear atypia with bizarre nuclei, the FIGO grade should be raised by one.

*Variant forms of endometrioid adenocarcinoma* include the following: (a) endometrioid adenocarcinoma with squamous differentiation; (b) villoglandular adenocarcinoma (villous fronds with delicate central cores and lined by cells with low grade cytological atypia); (c) secretory variant; (d) ciliated cell variant, and (e) mucinous adenocarcinoma. The latter variant secretes mucin and must be distinguished from endocervical mucinous adenocarcinoma, with which it shares some common features.

*Serous adenocarcinoma* is the prototypical type 2 endometrial carcinoma. It is usually composed of papillary structures with broad fibrovascular cores, and is lined by tumor cells with high cellular atypia including hyperchromasia, high nuclear to cytoplasmic ratio, lack of polarity, frequent mitoses with atypical forms, and giant tumor cells **(Fig. 9.20)**. Serous carcinoma is considered by definition to be a high-grade malignancy.

*Clear cell adenocarcinoma* is another type 2 endometrial carcinoma. It is composed of clear, glycogen-filled tumor cells with distinct cell borders **(Fig. 9.21)**. Tumors may display several microscopic patterns classified as tubular, papillary or solid. The hobnail cells, the cells that have lost most of their cytoplasm and protrude into the gland lumen with hyperchromatic and pleomorphic nuclei, are readily recognized in tubular and papillary tumors but are not prominent in solid tumor nests.

## Endometrial Stromal Tumors

*Endometrial stromal tumors* are mesenchymal tumors of the uterus that resemble the endometrial stroma of proliferative phase endometrium. The category includes three entities: (a) endometrial stromal nodule; (b) low grade endometrial stromal sarcoma and (c) undifferentiated endometrial sarcoma.

*Endometrial stromal nodule* is a benign endometrial stromal tumor characterized by well-circumscribed expansile growth of bland and uniform oval to spindle cells resembling proliferative phase endometrial stromal cells **(Fig. 9.22)**. The tumor cells are closely packed and supported by rich small arterioles. They are strongly immunoreactive for CD10 and estrogen receptor.

*Low-grade endometrial stromal sarcoma* shows an infiltrative margin invading into the surrounding myometrium and/or vascular spaces **(Fig. 9.23)**. It is composed of cells resembling proliferative endometrial stromal cells. Marked atypia and pleomorphism are absent although focal high mitotic count (> 10/10 high power fields) may be seen. Low-grade endometrial stromal sarcoma has an indolent clinical course with a high late local recurrence rate.

*Undifferentiated endometrial sarcoma* is a high-grade sarcoma showing no specific differentiation or resemblance toward endometrial stroma. The tumor cells have marked pleomorphism with high mitotic activity. Differential diagnosis includes carcinosarcoma.

## Smooth Muscle Tumors

*Smooth muscle tumors* represent the most common mesenchymal tumors of uterus. They are classified by histologic features including cytologic atypia, mitotic activity and tumor necrosis into three groups:

(a) leiomyoma; (b) smooth muscle tumor of uncertain malignant potential (STUMP) and (c) leiomyosarcoma.

*Leiomyoma* is a very common benign neoplasm of uterus composed of proliferation of smooth muscle cells. Leiomyomata are usually multiple, firm spherical nodules and have submucosal, intramural or subserosal distributions. Microscopically, they are composed of uniform spindle cells in a fascicular arrangement. The cells have elongated nuclei with blunt ends, fine chromatin and small inconspicuous nucleoli **(Fig. 9.24)**. Mitoses are infrequent. Degenerative changes are common and include hyaline fibrosis, edema, hemorrhage and calcification. Necrosis is unusual in leiomyomas but may be observed during pregnancy or in relation to progestin treatment. Some histologic variants of leiomyomas are mitotically active leiomyoma, cellular leiomyoma, epithelioid leiomyoma and atypical (bizarre) leiomyoma.

*Smooth muscle tumor of uncertain malignant potential* has ambiguous and indeterminate histologic features, which preclude a clear-cut distinction between a benign leiomyoma on one the hand and malignant leiomyosarcoma on the other. For example, when the tumor shows moderate nuclear atypia and focally increased mitoses (> 15/10 high power fields), but the presence of necrosis is uncertain, this tumor is categorized as STUMP.

*Leiomyosarcoma*, the most common uterine sarcoma, is composed of malignant smooth muscle cells. It is usually located intramurally with a fleshy cut surface and poorly defined margins. Areas of hemorrhage and necrosis are common. Microscopically, these tumors are cellular and show moderate to severe nuclear atypia, high mitotic index (> 15/10 high power fields) and foci of coagulative tumor necrosis **(Fig. 9.25)**. Vascular invasion may be identified. The smooth muscle cell nature of the tumor can be confirmed by positive immunohistochemical stains for smooth muscle actin and desmin.

### Carcinosarcoma

*Carcinosarcoma or malignant mixed mullerian tumor (MMMT)* is a highly malignant uterine tumor which commonly occurs in elderly postmenopausal women. On gross examination it appears polypoid and bulky with prominent areas of hemorrhage and necrosis. Microscopically, it consists of malignant epithelial and mesenchymal components **(Fig. 9.26)**. The epithelial component may have features of endometrioid or serous carcinoma. The mesenchymal component may be homologous with features of endometrial stromal sarcoma, leiomyosarcoma or undifferentiated sarcoma, or it may be composed of heterologous stromal cells which do not have a normal counterpart in the uterus, and are microscopically classified as rhabdomyosarcoma or chondrosarcoma. Carcinosarcoma has a poor prognosis.

## Fallopian Tube

The fallopian tube is a tubular structure that runs between the uterine cornus and the ovary. It is divided into four portions: (1) intramural; (2) isthmus; (3) ampulla and (4) infundibulum (with an ending opening to the peritoneal cavity as fimbriae). The mucosa is lined by three cell types: (1) secretory; (2) ciliated and (3) intercalated. The muscular wall is composed of an inner circular and an outer longitudinal layer of smooth muscle bundles.

The most important diseases of the fallopian tube are:
- Acute and chronic salpingitis
- Tubal pregnancy
- Carcinoma

### Acute and Chronic Salpingitis

Acute and chronic salpingitis represents part of the PID. In acute salpingitis, the lumen is infiltrated and filled with acute inflammation and pus (*pyosalpinx*) **(Fig. 9.27)**. The inflammatory exudate may spread to the adjacent ovary and cause a *tubo-ovarian abscess*. When the inflammation enters into a chronic stage, the tubal wall becomes fibrotic and partially obstructed leading to *hydrosalpinx*. In chronic salpingitis the inflammatory infiltrate consists of lymphocytes and plasma cells. Chronic *granulomatous salpingitis* is a feature of tubal tuberculosis, but it may be seen in sarcoidosis and Crohn disease as well.

### Tubal Pregnancy

In tubal pregnancy, the fallopian tube is markedly dilated containing a gestational sac. Microscopically, chorionic villi are identified within the lumen and invading the tubal wall **(Fig. 9.28)**. Marked hemorrhage is usually seen distending the fallopian tube in the form of a *hematosalpinx*.

### Carcinoma

Primary fallopian tube carcinoma is rare, and the involvement of the adjacent ovary often makes it difficult to determine if the tumor represents a primary ovarian or fallopian tube tumor. Serous carcinoma is the most common carcinoma identified in the fallopian tube. The tumor resembles serous carcinoma of the ovary and shows a papillary growth pattern lined by tumor cells with high nuclear grade **(Fig. 9.29)**.

## Ovary

The ovaries are located on the bilateral sides of the uterus and are covered by a single layer of surface epithelium. The ovary has a cortical and medullary parts **(Fig. 9.30)**. The ovarian stroma is composed of spindle-shaped cells arranged in a storiform pattern. Embedded within the ovarian stroma are ovarian follicles including primordial, maturing and atretic follicles. The maturing follicle is composed of the oocyte, the granulosa layer and the two theca layers. The corpus luteum is made of luteinized granulosa cells and theca cells, and the corpus albicans represents the scarring of the corpus luteum. In corpora albicans the luteinized granulosa cells, and theca cells are replaced by hyalinized fibrous tissue.

The most important diseases of the ovary are:
- Non-neoplastic cysts
- Endometriosis
- Surface epithelial –stromal tumors
- Germ cell tumors
- Sex cord-stromal tumors
- Metastatic tumors.

### Non-Neoplastic Cysts

Non-neoplastic cysts are common findings in ovaries. The most common non-neoplastic cysts of the ovary are: (a) inclusion cysts; (b) follicular cysts and (c) corpus luteum cysts.

*Inclusion cysts* are lined by a flattened, cuboidal or columnar epithelium, and probably arise from invagination of the surface epithelium. Tubal metaplasia of the cyst lining is common.

*Follicular cysts* are formed from the distension of maturing or atretic follicles and are lined by granulosa cells **(Fig. 9.31)**.

*Corpus luteum cysts* develop in pregnancy or at the end of the menstrual cycle. The cyst wall is composed of luteinized granulosa cells and the cyst contents are often bloody.

### Endometriosis

The ovary is the most common location for endometriosis, defined as the presence of endometrial glands and stroma outside the uterus **(Fig. 9.32)**. Repeated hemorrhage may totally destroy the epithelial lining and replace it with hemosiderin-laden macrophages. The entire ovary may be replaced by a hemorrhagic cyst containing dark brown-red partially hemolyzed blood (chocolate cyst).

### Surface Epithelial-Stromal Tumors

*Surface epithelial-stromal tumors* derive from the ovarian surface epithelium and are the most common tumors of the ovary. These tumors are classified into several groups which include: (a) serous;

(b) mucinous; (c) endometrioid; (d) clear cell; (e) transitional and (f) undifferentiated tumors. Serous tumors account for most of neoplasms in this group.

*Serous cystadenomas* are typically unilocular or multilocular cysts with a smooth inner surface containing small papillary projections. Cysts are lined by a flattened layer of epithelium (resembling the surface epithelium) or ciliated tubal epithelium **(Fig. 9.33)**. Tumors containing a prominent fibrous stroma in the wall of the cyst are diagnosed as serous cystadenofibromas.

*Serous borderline tumors* are also cystic. The cysts are lined by serous cells forming papillae, and usually show prominent epithelial hyperplasia and stratification. Tufting of cells and micropapillae are yet other features, and there is mild to moderate cytologic atypia **(Fig. 9.34)**. Detached or floating cell clusters are characteristic findings. Serous borderline tumor is distinguished from serous carcinoma by lack of stromal invasion in serous borderline tumor.

*Serous adenocarcinoma* is a malignant tumor which is usually partially cystic but it may be largely solid. The cells grow in a papillary growth pattern, but they also form solid cords invading the stroma **(Fig. 9.35)**. Glandular and solid nests are also seen. Metastases to the omentum, peritoneal surfaces and abdominal wall (as well as other organs) are common.

*Mucinous tumors* are also similarly divided into *benign mucinous tumors, mucinous borderline tumors and mucinous adenocarcinomas* **(Figs 9.36A to C)**. Tumor cells contain mucin in the cytoplasm. These tumors may resemble metastatic mucinous adenocarcinomas of the gastrointestinal tract. Accordingly, before the diagnosis of a primary mucinous adenocarcinoma of the ovary is made, it is very important to exclude metastases from other sites, especially if both ovaries are involved and the tumors are more solid than cystic.

## Germ Cell Tumors

*Germ cell tumors* arise from oocytes or their precursors in the ovary. They account for 30% of primary ovarian tumors and 60% of primary ovarian tumors in women under the age of 21. These tumors are classified as: (a) mature teratoma; (b) immature teratoma; (c) dysgerminoma; (d) embryonal carcinoma; (e) yolk sac carcinoma; (f) choriocarcinoma and (g) mixed germ cell tumors.

Ovarian germ cell tumors correspond to germ cell tumors of the testis. Accordingly, to avoid repetition, here we shall illustrate only the teratomas, the most common germ cell tumor of the ovary. Teratomas account for more than 90% of all ovarian germ cell tumors.

*Mature teratomas* occur most frequently in young women. They are usually cystic and rarely solid tumors composed of mature adult-type tissue derived from two or three embryonic layers. The most common histological finding is a cystic structure lined by epidermis with skin appendages in the wall, the so-called "dermoid cyst" clinically **(Fig. 9.37)**. The cyst is often filled with keratin debris, sebaceous material and hair. Teeth or bone may be identified grossly.

*Immature teratoma* is composed of a variable amount of immature embryonal-type tissues, most commonly immature neuroectodermal tissue, admixed with mature tissue. The immature neuroectodermal component is characterized by small blue cells forming rosettes **(Fig. 9.38)**. Other less common immature components may include immature mesenchyme and immature endodermal tissues such as hepatic tissue and intestinal-type epithelial tissue. Immature teratoma is graded from 1 to 3 based on the quantity of the immature neuroepithelial component.

## Sex Cord-Stromal Tumors

*Sex cord-stromal tumors* are formed of cells that are normally found in the stroma of the ovary and are thus classified as: (a) fibroma; (b) thecoma; (c) granulosa cell tumor; (d) Sertoli-Leydig cell tumor and (e) steroid cell tumor.

*Fibromas* represent the most common hormonally inactive stromal tumors of the ovary. Microscopically they are composed of bland spindle cells in a collagenous stroma **(Fig. 9.39)**. Cytologic atypia is minimal and mitoses are rare. *Thecomas* are also composed of spindle cells resembling those seen in fibromas. Some tumor cells may have abundant pale and lipid-rich cytoplasm. The cytoplasmic lipid may be confirmed by Oil-Red-O stain, which is the best way of distinguishing them from fibromas.

*Granulosa cell tumor* is composed of neoplastic granulosa cells in a fibrothecomatous background. Neoplastic granulosa cells have round to oval nuclei, scant cytoplasm and characteristic longitudinal nuclear grooves. Tumor cells grow in various patterns, including a microfollicular pattern, characterized by the formation of Call-Exner bodies, trabecular pattern, insular pattern and gyriform pattern **(Figs 9.40A and B)**. Tumor cells are positive for alpha-inhibin and calretinin. The Sertoli-Leydig cell tumor and steroid cell tumor are discussed in the testicular tumor section.

### Metastatic Tumors

Metastases to the ovaries may occur from many primary tumors, but most often they originate from malignant tumors of the gastrointestinal system. Many mucinous cystadenocarcinomas, especially those that involve both ovaries, are actually metastases from a gastrointestinal primary tumor. Bilateral ovarian involvement, multinodular growth pattern and the presence of ovarian surface tumor implants favor a metastatic mucinous adenocarcinoma. Common primary tumor origins include colon, appendix, pancreas and stomach.

*Krukenberg tumor* refers to metastatic signet ring/mucinous adenocarcinoma of the ovaries which usually originates from the stomach or the colon **(Figs 9.41A and B)**.

## Pregnancy Related Changes

The normal placenta is composed of umbilical cord, fetal membrane, chorionic villi and maternal decidua tissue. The umbilical cord contains two arteries and one vein embedded in highly mucoid connective tissue (Wharton's jelly). Fetal membrane consists of amnion which lines the innermost surface of amniotic cavity, and chorion which carries the fetal vasculature. Chorionic villi are composed of villous structures lined by mononuclear cytotrophoblastic and multinuclear syncytiotrophoblastic cells **(Fig. 9.42)**. The intermediate trophoblasts are more numerous in the extravillous region and form the deepest component of the implantation site.

The most important pregnancy-related diseases are:
- Blighted ovum
- Hydatidiform mole
- Choriocarcinoma.

### Blighted Ovum

Blighted ovum or hydropic abortus occurs when there is failure of development or early demise of the embryo. The villi are distended by edema; however, they do not assume the large size as found in molar pregnancy **(Fig. 9.43)**. There is no trophoblastic hyperplasia.

### Hydatidiform Mole

Hydatidiform moles are placental abnormalities arising from abnormal conceptions. They are characterized by enlarged, swollen and vesicular chorionic villi accompanied by trophoblastic proliferation. On the basis of cytogenetic and clinicopathologic features, hydatidiform moles are classified as: (a) partial or (b) complete.

*Partial moles* result from fertilization of a normal egg by two sperms resulting in a triploid zygote. Histologically, partial moles are characterized by the presence and admixture of two populations of villi: one of normal size and the other enlarged and hydropic. The hydropic villi have irregular contour with minimal trophoblastic hyperplasia, and many trophoblastic inclusions **(Fig. 9.44)**. Evidence of fetal development is often present including nucleated fetal red blood cells.

*Complete moles* result from fertilization of an empty egg by a haploid sperm which then replicates its own chromosomes. Most complete moles have a 46, XX karyotype. Histologically, all villi are abnormally enlarged with marked villous edema, central cistern formation and circumferential trophoblastic hyperplasia with cytologic atypia **(Fig. 9.45)**. Fetal tissue is not found.

## Choriocarcinoma

Gestational choriocarcinoma may occur subsequent to molar pregnancy, abortion, normal pregnancy or ectopic pregnancy. It is composed of sheets of syncytiotrophoblast, cytotrophoblast and intermediate trophoblast with marked cytologic atypia. Hemorrhage, necrosis and vascular invasion are always present **(Fig. 9.46)**. Structures resembling chorionic villi are usually not found.

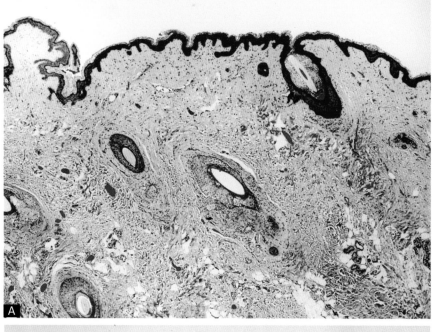

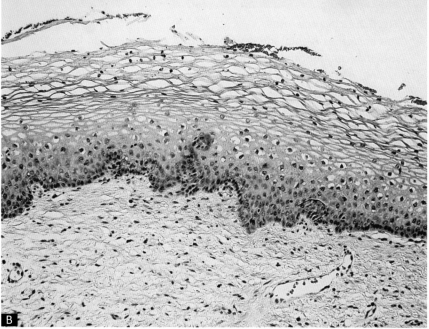

**Figs 9.1A and B:** Normal histology of the lower part of the female reproductive system.

**A.** Vulva (labium major) is covered with normal skin. **B.** Cervix is covered with non-keratinizing squamous epithelium.

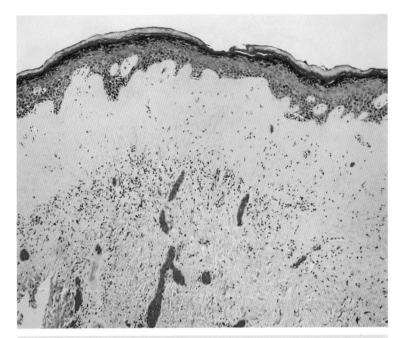

**Fig. 9.2:** Lichen sclerosus

The epidermis is thin and covered with a surface keratin layer. The subepidermal dermis is composed of acellular homogenized and hyalinized collagen. The lower dermis contains scattered infiltrates of chronic inflammatory cells.

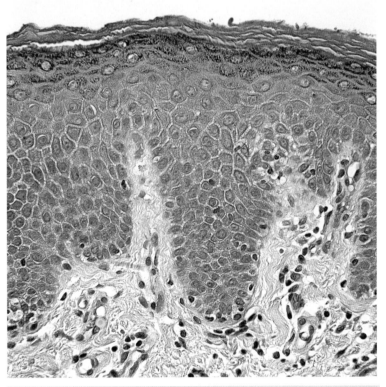

**Fig. 9.3:** Squamous cell hyperplasia

There is acanthosis, hypergranulosis and hyperkeratosis of the epidermis. The dermis contains scattered chronic inflammatory cells.

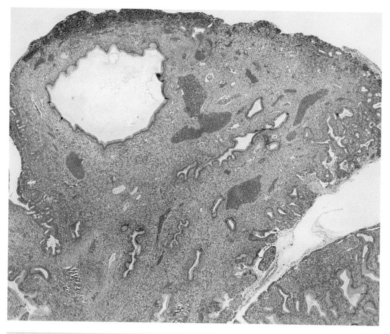

**Fig. 9.4:** Endocervical polyp

It is a polypoid endocervical lesion composed of benign endocervical glands and fibrovascular stroma tissue.

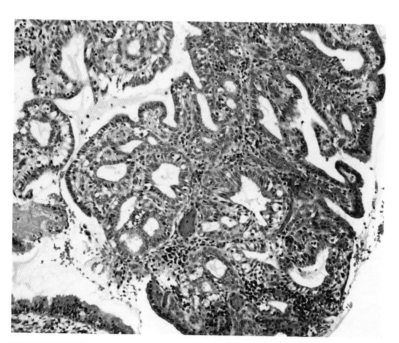

**Fig. 9.5:** Microglandular hyperplasia

The lesion is composed of small closely apposed glands lined by cuboidal epithelium. The intervening stroma shows signs of chronic inflammation.

FEMALE REPRODUCTIVE SYSTEM

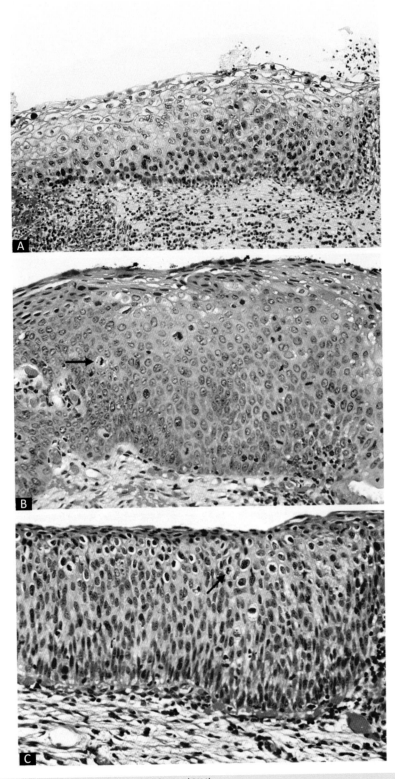

**Figs 9.6A to C:** Cervical intraepithelial neoplasia (CIN)

**A.** CIN I is characterized by the presence of koilocytes in the upper layers of the epithelium. **B.** CIN II is characterized by dysplastic changes involving the lower two-thirds of the epithelium. A mitosis is identified in the middle third of the epithelium (arrow). **C.** CIN III is characterized by severe dysplasia involving the entire epithelium, which shows no evidence of surface maturation. A mitosis is identified in the upper third of the epithelium (arrow).

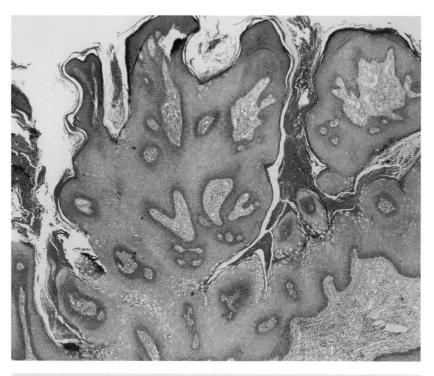

**Fig. 9.7:** Condyloma acuminatum
This exophytic lesion shows papillomatosis, acanthosis and koilocytosis.

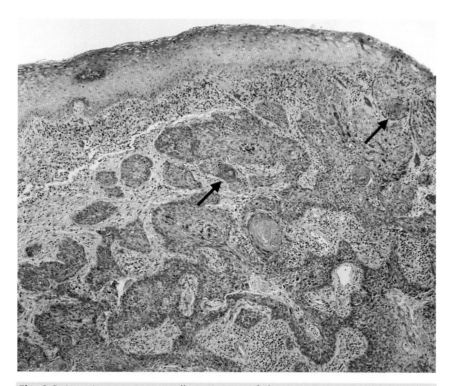

**Fig. 9.8:** Invasive squamous cell carcinoma of the cervix
The tumor is composed of squamous cells forming strands which invade into the connective tissue stroma. Foci of keratin pearl formation are seen (arrows).

FEMALE REPRODUCTIVE SYSTEM

CHAPTER
**9**

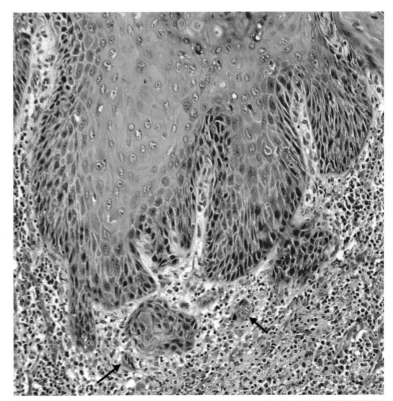

**Fig. 9.9:** Microinvasive squamous cell carcinoma of the cervix
In addition to the intraepithelial carcinoma in situ there are short strands of neoplastic cells invading into the underlying stroma (arrows).

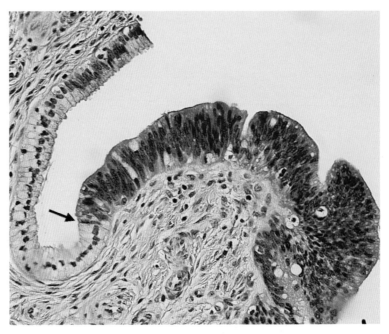

**Fig. 9.10:** Endocervical adenocarcinoma in situ
The neoplastic cells with pseudostratified hyperchromatic nuclei are seen replacing the normal mucinous epithelium (arrow).

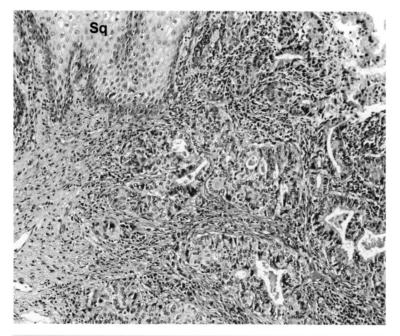

**Fig. 9.11:** Invasive endocervical adenocarcinoma
Malignant tumor cells form glands and invade into the stroma under the normal squamous epithelium (Sq).

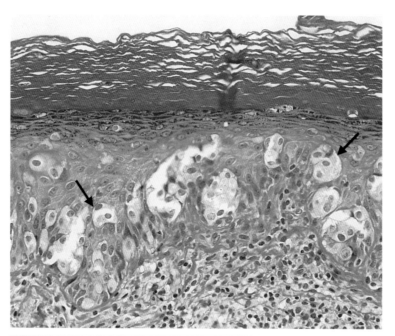

**Fig. 9.12:** Vulvar Paget disease
Neoplastic cells with abundant pale cytoplasm, large nuclei and prominent nucleoli are seen intermixed with the normal cells of the epidermis (arrows).

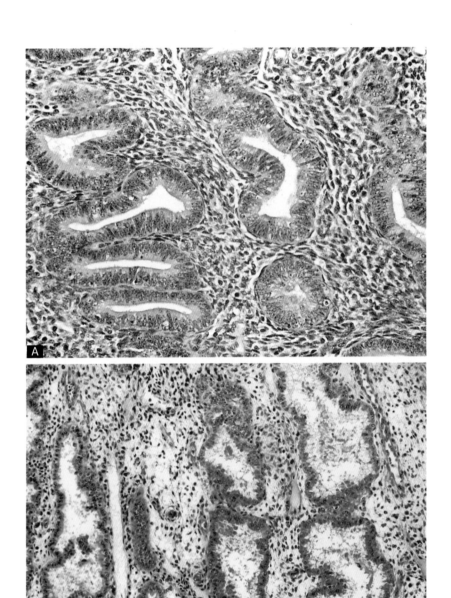

**Figs 9.13A and B:** Normal endometrium

**A.** Proliferative phase endometrium is composed of dense stroma and straight and narrow glands, lined by cells that have elongated pseudostratified nuclei. **B.** Secretory phase endometrium consists of loosely structured stroma and dilated glands lined by cells showing signs of secretion.

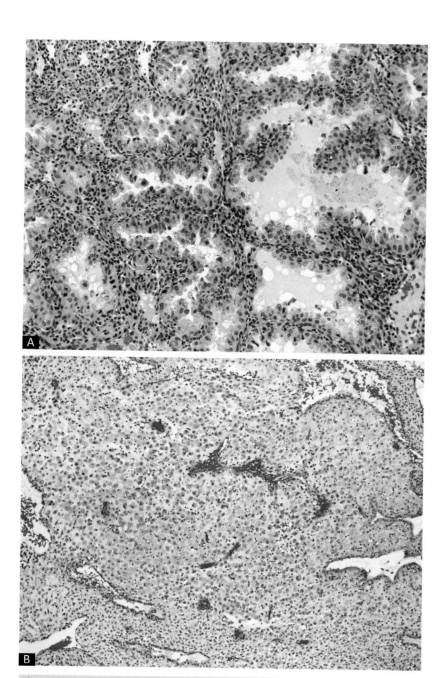

**Figs 9.14A and B:** Gestational endometrium

**A.** The glands are dilated and contain secretary material. The glandular epithelial cells have abundant clear cytoplasm. **B.** The endometrial stroma shows diffuse decidual changes. The decidual cells have uniform, round to oval nuclei, abundant eosinophilic cytoplasm and distinct cell borders.

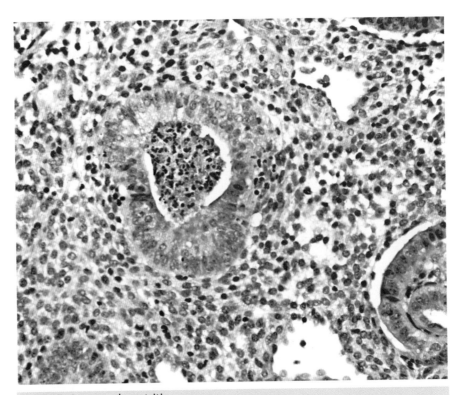

**Fig. 9.15:** Acute endometritis
The endometrium shows an endometrial gland filled with neutrophils.

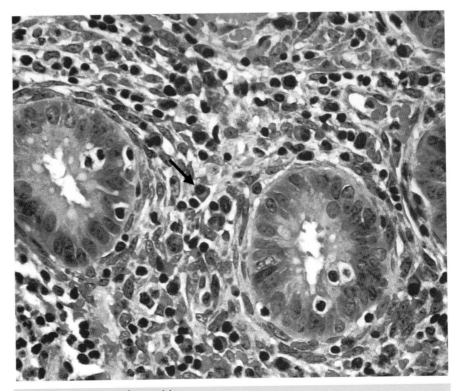

**Fig. 9.16:** Chronic endometritis
The stroma of the endometrium is infiltrated with lymphocytes and plasma cells (arrow).

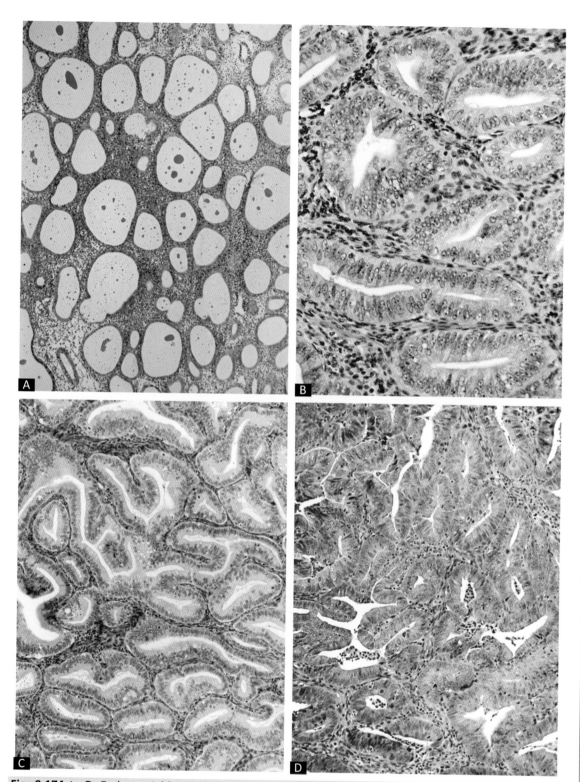

**Figs 9.17A to D:** Endometrial hyperplasia

**A.** Simple hyperplasia without atypia. There are more glands than stroma. Glands are in simple dilated cystic structures without complex architectural patterns. Cells do not show significant cytologic atypia. **B.** Simple hyperplasia with atypia. Cells lining the simple proliferating glands show enlarged nuclei with vesicular chromatin and prominent nucleoli. **C.** Complex hyperplasia without atypia. Proliferating glands show crowded growth pattern and irregular branching with back-to-back glands and little intervening stroma. Significant cytologic atypia is absent. **D.** Complex hyperplasia with atypia. Proliferating glands show complex architectural pattern and cells with hyperchromasia and frequent mitoses.

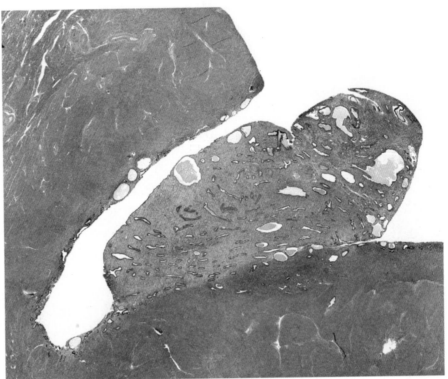

**Fig. 9.18:** Endometrial polyp

The picture shows a polypoid lesion arising from endometrium. It is composed of dilated benign endometrial glands and stroma.

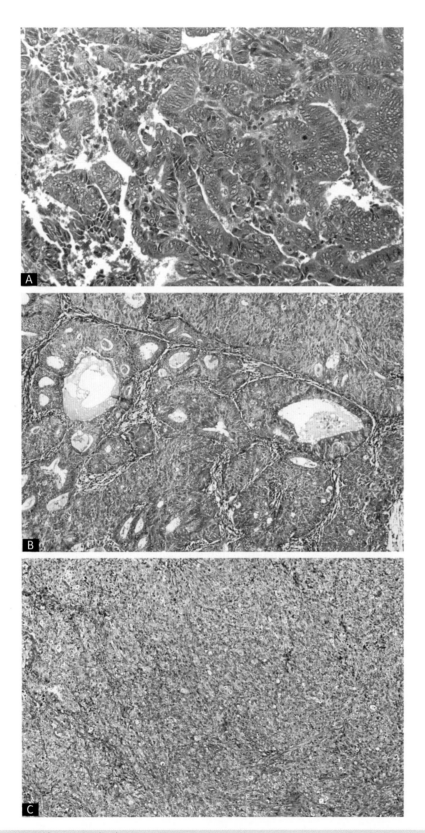

**Figs 9.19A to C:** Endometrioid adenocarcinoma
**A.** FIGO grade 1 tumors are composed of well-formed glands, which form 95% or more of the entire tumor.
**B.** FIGO grade 2 tumors are composed of solid and glandular areas. The glandular areas account for 50–95% of the entire tumor. **C.** FIGO grade 3 tumors consist predominantly of solid areas, and less than 50% of the entire tumor shows glandular differentiation.

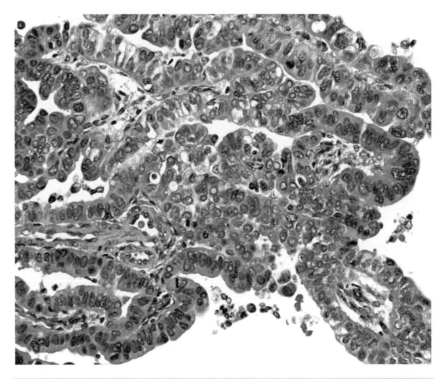

**Fig. 9.20:** Serous adenocarcinoma of endometrium
The tumor is composed of papillary structures lined by cells with hyperchromatic nuclei and frequent mitoses.

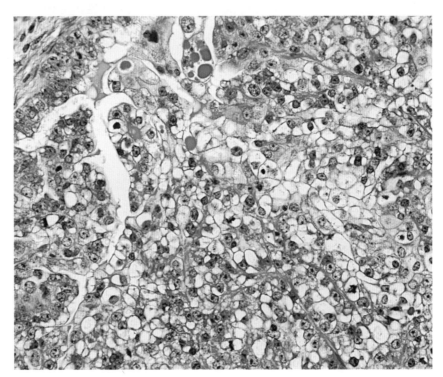

**Fig. 9.21:** Clear cell adenocarcinoma of endometrium
The tumor is composed of clear, glycogen-filled cells with distinct cell borders.

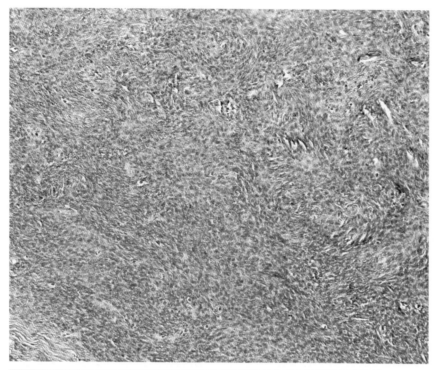

**Fig. 9.22:** Endometrial stromal nodule

The nodule is composed of densely packed spindle cells resembling normal endometrial stromal cells.

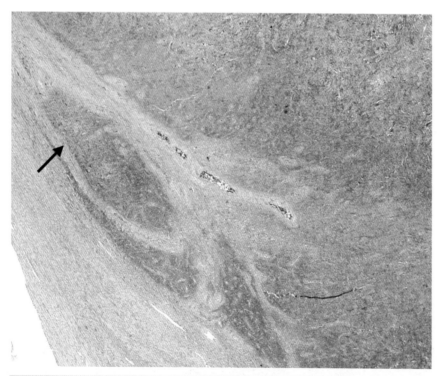

**Fig. 9.23:** Low-grade endometrial stromal sarcoma

In contrast to the endometrial stromal nodule which is well-circumscribed, low-grade endometrial stroma sarcoma is composed of spindle cells that form strands invading the surrounding myometrium (arrow).

FEMALE REPRODUCTIVE SYSTEM

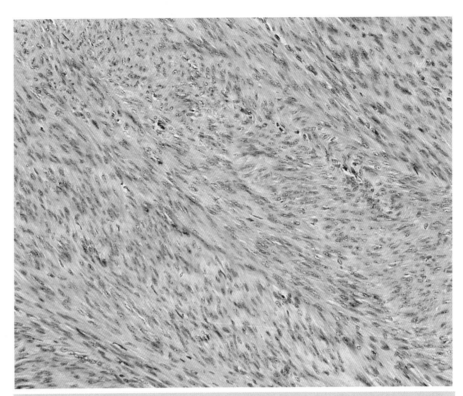

**Fig. 9.24:** Leiomyoma

The tumor is composed of elongated cells which have uniform cigar-shaped nuclei and well developed eosinophilic cytoplasm, similar to the cells of the normal myometrium.

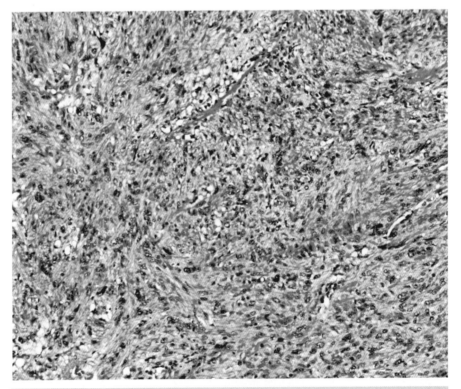

**Fig. 9.25:** Leiomyosarcoma

The tumor is composed of cells showing nuclear hyperchromasia, pleomorphism and increased number of mitoses.

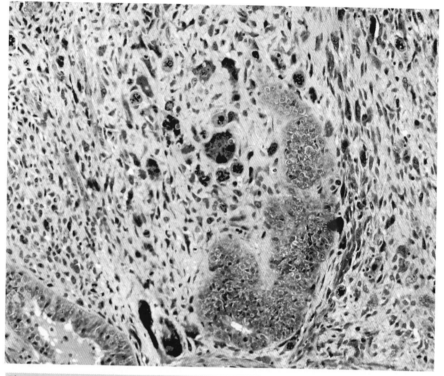

**Fig. 9.26:** Carcinosarcoma

The tumor is composed of malignant glands (epithelial component) and malignant stroma.

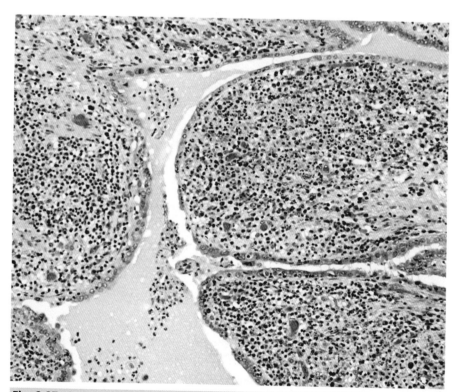

**Fig. 9.27:** Acute salpingitis

The fallopian tube mucosa is widened and filled with abundant neutrophils and lymphocytes. Neutrophils are also present in the lumen.

FEMALE REPRODUCTIVE SYSTEM

CHAPTER

**9**

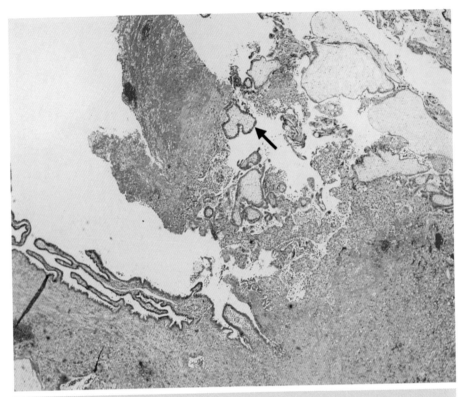

**Fig. 9.28:** Tubal pregnancy
The fallopian tube contains hemorrhagic decidua and chorionic villi (arrow).

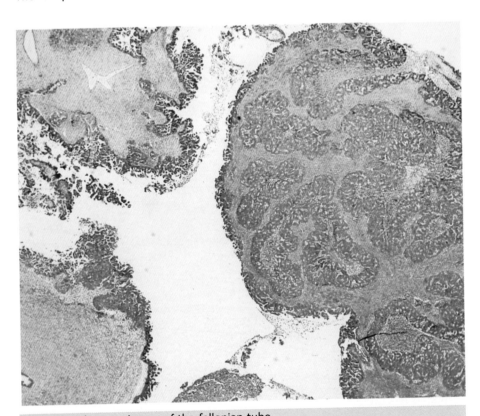

**Fig. 9.29:** Adenocarcinoma of the fallopian tube
The tumor arises from the tubal epithelium and invades into the underlying stroma. Serous carcinoma as shown here is the most common type of fallopian tube carcinoma.

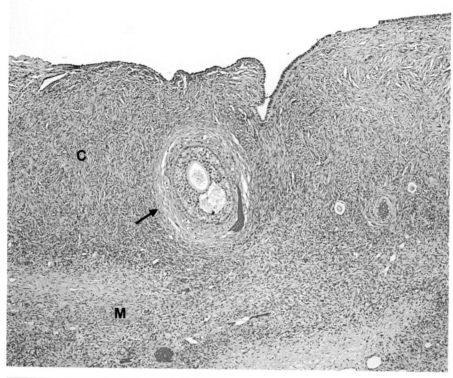

**Fig. 9.30:** Normal ovary

The ovary has a cortical (C) and medullary part (M). The cortical stroma is composed of spindle-shaped cells arranged in a storiform pattern. Embedded within the ovarian stroma are ovarian follicles including primordial and maturing follicles (arrow).

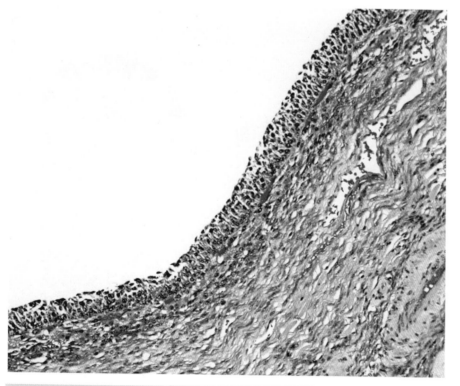

**Fig. 9.31:** Follicular cyst

The cyst is lined by granulosa cells resembling those that form the normal follicle.

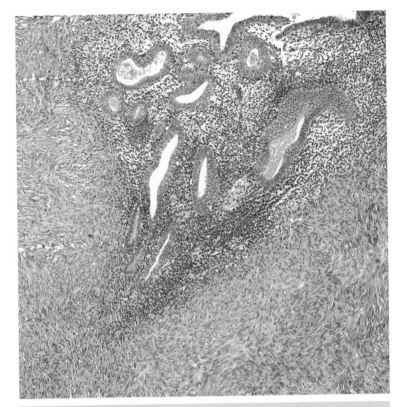

**Fig. 9.32:** Endometriosis

The lesion consists of endometrial glands and stroma, with some extravasated blood.

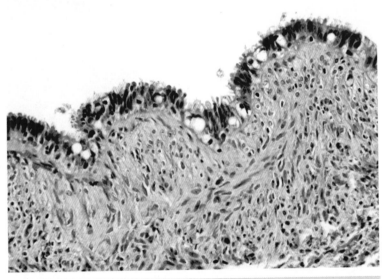

**Fig. 9.33:** Serous cystadenoma

The cyst is lined by an epithelium resembling that of the fallopian tube with cilia. Complex epithelial growth patterns including papillary projections, tufting, cribriform and micropapillary arrangements are absent.

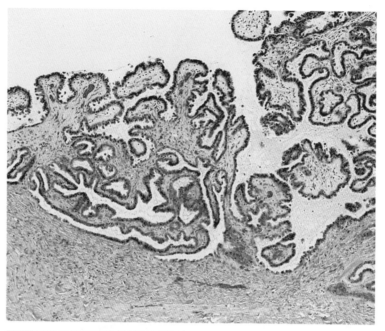

**Fig. 9.34:** Serous borderline tumor

This figure shows a typical pattern of serous borderline tumor. Hyperplastic epithelial cells form papillary structures with complex branching. Stromal invasion is not present.

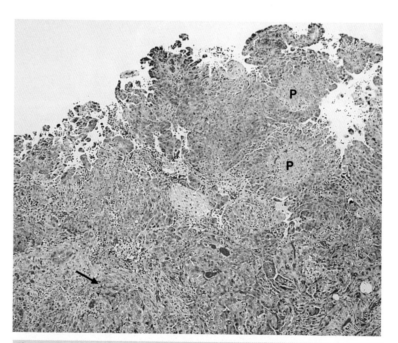

**Fig. 9.35:** Serous adenocarcinoma

The tumor shows a papillary (P) and solid growth pattern with invasion into the underlying stroma (arrow).

FEMALE REPRODUCTIVE SYSTEM

ATLAS OF HISTOPATHOLOGY

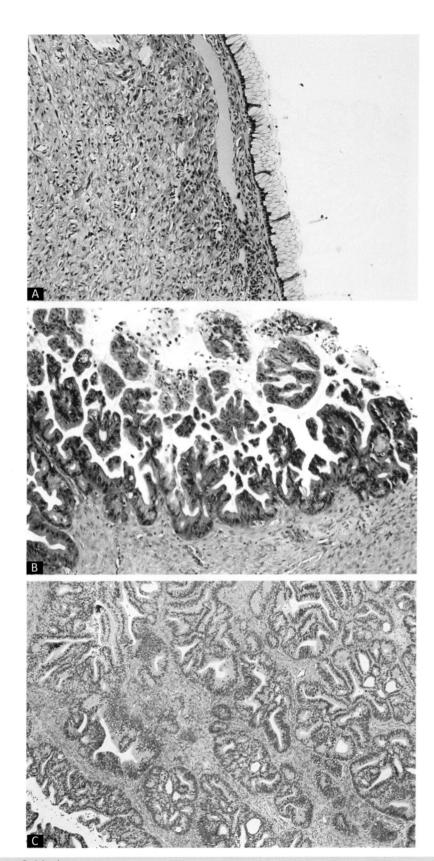

**Figs 9.36A to C:** Mucinous tumors

**A.** Mucinous cystadenoma: The cyst is lined by a single layer of mucinous epithelium. Marked nuclear stratification and atypia is absent. **B.** Mucinous borderline tumor: Nuclear stratification, hyperchromasia and papillary projections are evident. There is no stromal invasion. **C.** Mucinous adenocarcinoma: The tumor is composed of invasive infiltrating mucinous glands.

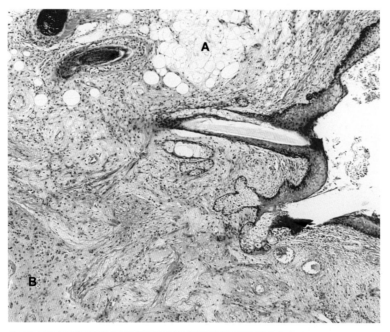

**Fig. 9.37:** Mature teratoma

The tumor is composed predominantly of skin-like structures, including hair shaft/follicles and sebaceous glands. Mature adipose tissue (A) and brain tissue (B) are also present.

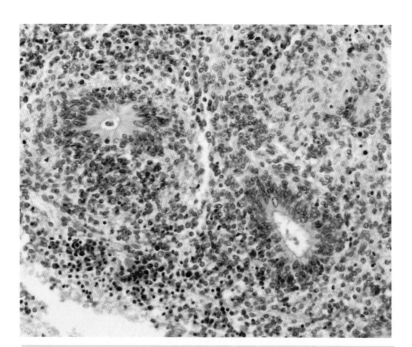

**Fig. 9.38:** Immature teratoma

The tumor contains immature neuroectodermal tissue in the form of neuroectodermal rosettes.

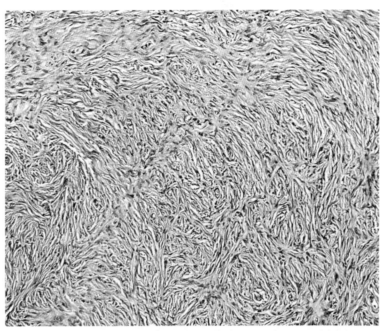

**Fig. 9.39:** Fibroma
The tumor is composed of densely packed elongated cells which have uniform spindle cell nuclei.

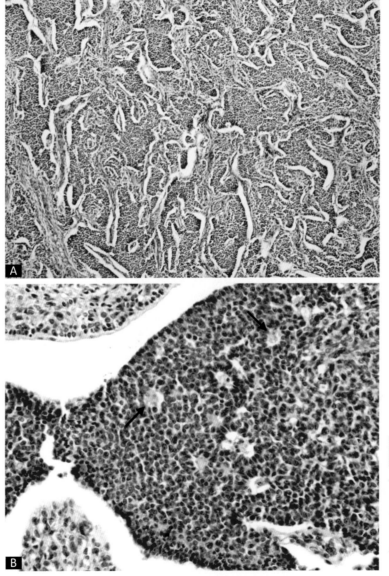

**Figs 9.40A and B:** Adult granulosa cell tumor
**A.** The tumor is composed of neoplastic granulosa cells arranged in a trabecular pattern.
**B.** An aggregate of neoplastic granulosa cells contain Call-Exner bodies (arrow).

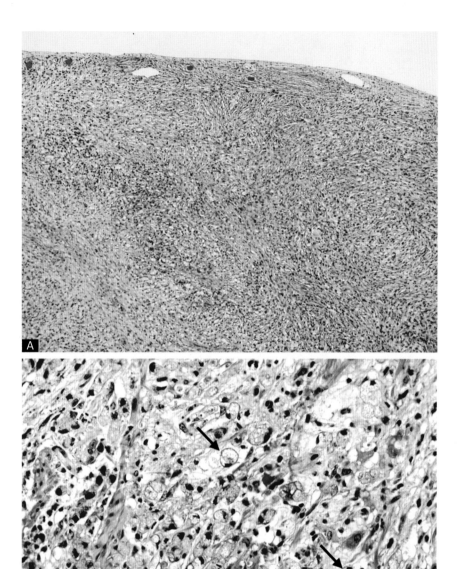

**Figs 9.41A and B:** Krukenberg tumor

**A.** The ovarian parenchyma is almost completely replaced by solid sheets of tumor. **B.** High magnification shows that the tumor is composed of signet ring cells (arrows) invading the ovarian stroma.

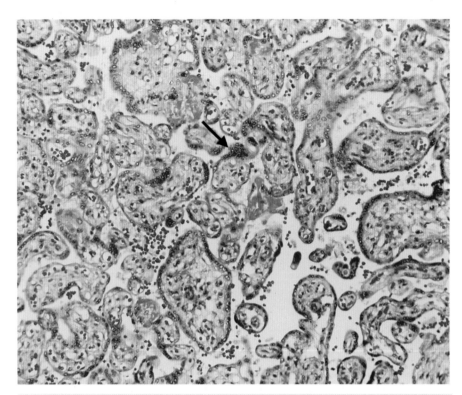

**Fig. 9.42:** Normal chorionic villi of a term placenta

The villi are variable and small in size and lined by syncytiotrophoblasts. The cytotrophoblastic layer is not evident and focally incomplete. The nuclei of syncytiotrophoblasts are piled up focally forming syncytial knots (arrow).

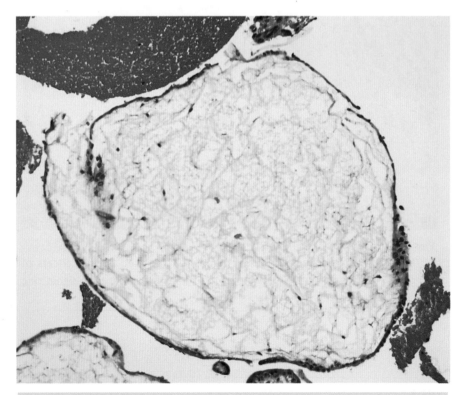

**Fig. 9.43:** Blighted ovum

The chorionic villus is round with marked edema.

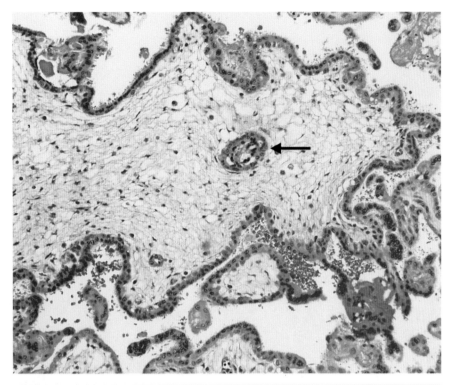

**Fig. 9.44:** Partial hydatidiform mole

It consists of a mixture of large edematous villi and small fibrotic villi. The markedly enlarged villus at the left has an irregular contour, focal trophoblastic hyperplasia and trophoblastic inclusion (arrow) formed by invagination of the surface.

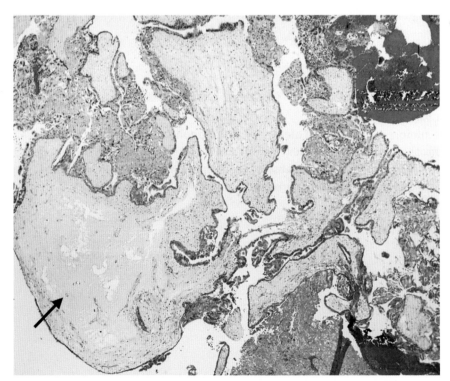

**Fig. 9.45:** Complete hydatidiform mole

It consists of abnormally enlarged villi showing marked edema, central cistern formation (arrow) and haphazard trophoblastic hyperplasia along the surface of the villi.

FEMALE REPRODUCTIVE SYSTEM

CHAPTER

**9**

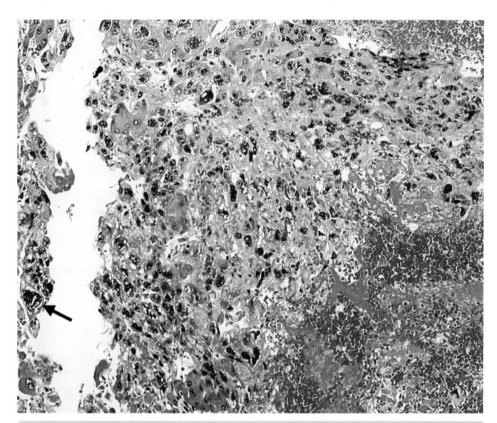

**Fig. 9.46:** Choriocarcinoma

The tumor is composed of malignant mononuclear cells corresponding to cytotrophoblastic cells, and multinucleated cells corresponding to syncytiotrophoblastic cells (arrow). Chorionic villi are absent. Choriocarcinoma tends to invade normal tissues and typically associated with marked hemorrhage (right lower corner).

# 10 Breast

*Fang Fan*

## Introduction

*The adult female breast is composed of successively branching ducts and ductules that originate from the nipple and end as terminal ductal lobular units (TDLUs). It is only after pregnancy and lactation that the breast fulfills its physiologic function. Breast milk provides complete nourishment and protection against infection and allergies for the baby.*
   *The most important diseases of the breast are:*
* *Reactive and inflammatory lesions*
* *Nonproliferative fibrocystic changes*
* *Adenosis*
* *Intraductal proliferative lesions*
* *Lobular neoplasia*
* *Fibroepithelial lesions*
* *Papillary lesions*
* *Invasive breast carcinoma*
* *Male breast lesions*

## Normal Breast

The TDLU is the functional secretory unit of the breast. It contains a variable number of blind-ending ductules or acini (Fig. 10.1A). The lobular acini are surrounded by loose, delicate and myxomatous intralobular stroma containing a few lymphocytes, plasma cells, macrophages or mast cells. The ductules and acini are lined by an inner ductal epithelium and an outer myoepithelial layer invested by a basal lamina composed of type IV collagen (Fig. 10.1B). The interlobular stroma consists of fibroconnective tissue admixed to adipose tissue. The TDLU exhibits morphologic changes through the menstrual cycle: the lobules are quiescent in the follicular phase; after ovulation, the number of acini per lobule increase, there is vacuolization of epithelial cells and marked intralobular stromal edema.

During pregnancy, the lobules are increased in number and size. The marked expansion of lobules may result in coalescence of adjacent lobules. True secretory glands form in the lobules with epithelial cells showing secretory lipid vacuoles in the cytoplasm (Fig. 10.2).

The lactating breast shows further distension of TDLUs by prominent epithelial cell vacuolization and abundant secretory material. The epithelial cells during pregnancy and lactation may appear atypical with enlarged nuclei, prominent nucleoli and vacuolated cytoplasm; however, these lobular changes should not be mistaken for malignancy. After cessation of lactation, the lobules regress.

The breast in a postmenopausal woman shows atrophy of acini and ducts with shrinkage of intralobular and interlobular stroma. The dense interlobular stroma is gradually replaced by adipose tissue (Fig. 10.3). The lobular acini may totally disappear.

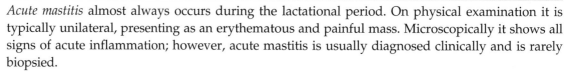

## Reactive and Inflammatory Lesions

*Acute mastitis* almost always occurs during the lactational period. On physical examination it is typically unilateral, presenting as an erythematous and painful mass. Microscopically it shows all signs of acute inflammation; however, acute mastitis is usually diagnosed clinically and is rarely biopsied.

*Subareolar abscess (periductal mastitis)* is not associated with lactation but has a strong association with cigarette smoking. Clinically it presents as a painful erythematous subareolar mass. This lesion is associated with squamous metaplasia of lactiferous ducts, subsequent formations of keratin plugs, and rupture of the ducts accompanied by an inflammatory response.

*Mammary duct ectasia* occurs in older women and is not associated with smoking. The inspissation of breast secretions leads to dilatation and rupture of the ducts and strong inflammatory response (Fig. 10.4). Clinically it presents as a poorly defined periareolar mass and thick-cheesy, "toothpaste-like" nipple discharge.

*Fat necrosis* of the breast follows a prior history of trauma or surgery and may present as a palpable mass or mammographic calcifications. Histologically, it shows necrotic fat cells surrounded by foamy macrophages (Fig. 10.5).

## Nonproliferative Fibrocystic Change

Fibrocystic change represents the most common finding in the breast biopsies of women in the age group of 20–40 years, clinically recognized as "lumpy bumpy" breasts. However, this change should not be classified as a disease and it does not confer any increased risk for developing breast carcinoma. Histologically, the involved breast tissue contains cysts with distorted TDLUs, fibrosis and apocrine metaplasia (Figs 10.6A and B).

## Adenosis

Adenosis refers to an increased number of lobular units (acini) per TDLU. The most common type is sclerosing adenosis in which there is proliferation of glands and tubules accompanied by dense stromal proliferation causing compression and distortion of acini. The compression and distortion of glands is most prominent in the center of the lesion, which may consist of fibrous tissue intermixed with epithelial strands and cords with barely visible lumens (Fig. 10.7). The glands and tubules are more dilated toward the periphery of the lesion and are obviously lined by an inner epithelial layer surrounded by a myoepithelial layer. The diagnosis is best made under low power, where sclerosing adenosis presents as a circumscribed, lobulocentric lesion, commonly associated with calcifications. Immunohistochemical stain for myoepithelial markers will highlight the myoepithelial cells around glands and confirm the diagnosis.

## Intraductal Proliferative Lesions

Intraductal proliferative lesions are characterized by an increased number of cells in the ductal epithelium of TDLU. This group of disorders includes: (a) usual ductal hyperplasia (UDH); (b) atypical ductal hyperplasia (ADH) and (c) ductal carcinoma in situ (DCIS). They are associated with an increased risk of developing breast cancer, but the magnitude of the risk varies from one lesion to another.

*Usual ductal hyperplasia (UDH)* is characterized by proliferation of ductal epithelial cells without architectural and cytological atypia. The internal lining of ducts usually has more than four cell layers. Two architectural patterns are recognized: a solid pattern in which the cells fill the entire lumen and a cribriform (sieve-like) pattern with fenestrations. The secondary lumens are variable in size and shape, irregular and often slit-like (Fig. 10.8). The cells are heterogenous with variable size and shape. Cell borders are poorly defined with areas of nuclear overlapping. Cellular bridges are stretched and thinned; cells in these bridges are usually attenuated with nuclei oriented in the same direction as the bridges. Cells also show swirling and streaming. Usual ductal hyperplasia may be associated with microcalcifications, which are usually detectable by mammography.

Usual ductal hyperplasia is associated with a 1.5- to 2-fold increased risk for breast cancer in both breasts.

*Atypical ductal hyperplasia (ADH)* is characterized by proliferation of the ductal epithelium showing cytologic and architectural atypia. The nuclei of these cells are small, round, monotonous and evenly spaced. However, the cytologic atypia is neither qualitatively nor quantitatively sufficient to make the diagnosis of ductal carcinoma in situ. For example, only parts of the duct may be involved by atypical cells whereas other parts contain cells resembling those of usual ductal hyperplasia (Fig. 10.9A). The architectural features of atypia include secondary lumens which are more round with polarization of cells around them. Bridges and arcades are more uniform in thickness and appear rigid (Fig. 10.9B). Micropapillae are bulbous, i.e. club shaped and wider at their tips than at their bases. These atypical architectures only involve portions of the duct. Differentiation of atypical ductal hyperplasia from low-grade ductal carcinoma in situ may be difficult or subjective. The size or extent of the lesion may be used as a criterion in equivocal lesions; in these instances a diagnosis of low grade ductal carcinoma in situ is favored over atypical ductal hyperplasia in lesions that measure greater than 2 mm.

Atypical ductal hyperplasia is associated with a 4–5 fold increased risk in developing breast cancer in both breasts.

*Ductal carcinoma in situ (DCIS)* is a preinvasive form of breast carcinoma composed of neoplastic epithelial cells which are confined to the inside of the ducts and do not invade through the basement membrane. The neoplastic cells fill and distend ducts and lobules in the terminal ductal lobular units. Ductal carcinoma in situ is graded according to cytologic features and presence/absence of necrosis as detailed below. It is associated with an 8–10 fold increased risk of breast cancer in the same breast at the same site.

*Low-grade ductal carcinoma in situ* is composed of monotonous round cells with small nuclei (1–1.5 red blood cells in diameter), evenly distributed chromatin and inconspicuous nucleoli. The secondary lumens are smooth and round (Fig. 10.10A); cells polarize around the lumens. Bridges and arcades are rigid and uniform in thickness. Comedo-type necrosis is usually not present.

*Intermediate-grade ductal carcinoma in situ* shows cells with mild to moderate pleomorphism, nuclei (1–2 red blood cells in diameter) contain coarse chromatin and occasional nucleoli. Comedo-type necrosis is usually present (Fig. 10.10B).

*High-grade ductal carcinoma in situ* is characterized by large pleomorphic cells with vesicular or coarse chromatin and prominent nucleoli. Mitoses are frequent and may be atypical. Central, comedo-type necrosis is often present (Fig. 10.10C). The architecture patterns may be solid, cribriform, micropapillary or flat.

*Paget's disease of the nipple* represents extension of high-grade DCIS to the skin of the nipple. Malignant cells apparently travel within and along the ducts to involve the large nipple ducts and extend to the nipple skin and areola. Clinically, Paget's disease presents as erythema and erosion of the nipple skin. Histologically, it shows large tumor cells with vesicular nuclei and prominent nucleoli involving the epidermis (Fig. 10.11).

## Lobular Neoplasia

*Atypical lobular hyperplasia (ALH) and lobular carcinoma in situ (LCIS)* are sometimes grouped under the name of "lobular neoplasia". Both lesions are characterized by filling and distending acini in the terminal ductal lobular units by small and loosely cohesive cells. The cells have small and uniform nuclei and inconspicuous nucleoli. There is no definitive sharp dividing line between LCIS and ALH and the difference is more or less quantitative. In general, LCIS is defined as at least one half of the spaces in a given lobule filled with and distended by tumor cells. Cases with lesser degree of involvement or cases in which all acini are involved but not distended are called atypical lobular hyperplasia (Figs 10.12A and B). LCIS and ALH can both involve and spread through ducts. A loss of E-cadherin, best seen by immunohistochemistry is a characteristic feature for the neoplastic cell in LCIS and ALH. This feature helps distinguish LCIS/ALH from DCIS.

LCIS and ALH also differ in the magnitude of associated breast cancer risk. LCIS is associated with a 7–10 fold increase in breast cancer risk bilaterally while ALH is associated with a lower risk (3–5 fold), also bilateral.

## Fibroepithelial Lesions

Fibroepithelial lesions, as the name implies, are lesions composed of both epithelial and stromal growth. They usually present as discrete masses clinically. The most important fibroepithelial lesions are: (a) fibroadenoma and (b) phyllodes tumor.

*Fibroadenoma* is the most common benign tumor of the female breast. It most often occurs in young women 20–30 years of age. Grossly it forms a well-circumscribed firm nodule, which can be shelled out from the adjacent parenchyma as a "marble". The cut surface is bosselated with slit-like spaces. Microscopically, it is composed of elongated and distorted ducts compressed by the surrounding proliferating myxoid stroma (intracanalicular pattern, Fig. 10.13); or ducts with open lumina surrounded by stroma (pericanalicular pattern). The epithelial component may be involved by any of the intraductal proliferative lesions discussed above, including UDH, ADH and DCIS; the stromal component may show prominent myxoid degeneration or hyalinization and calcification.

*Phyllodes tumor* is an uncommon tumor that usually occurs in older women. The cut surface is tan fleshy with clefts and cystic spaces. Microscopically, phyllodes tumor is characterized by stromal hypercellularity and projections of epithelial-lined stroma into clefts and spaces (leaf-like appearance) (Fig. 10.14). The stroma is often more condensed under the epithelium.

Phyllodes tumor is classified as benign, borderline or as malignant based on the degree of stromal cellularity, cellular pleomorphism, mitoses, margins and the stromal growth pattern. Malignant phyllodes tumor shows marked stromal cellularity and atypia with numerous stromal mitoses (> 10/10 high-power fields). The margins are typically invasive. Areas of stromal overgrowth are also seen. Phyllodes tumors, regardless of their classification, are treated by wide local excision to prevent local recurrence. Distant metastases are uncommon.

## Papillary Lesions

Papillary lesions of the breast are a heterogenous group of lesions characterized by papillary architecture (fibrovascular cores covered by epithelium).

*Intraductal papilloma* is a benign tumor characterized by the intraductal growth of papillary fronds with fibrovascular cores covered by epithelial and myoepithelial cells (Fig. 10.15). Two types are recognized: *central papillomas,* which are usually solitary and located within major lactiferous ducts; and *peripheral papillomas,* which involve the terminal ductal lobular units and are usually multiple. Intraductal papillomas may show marked stromal fibrosis (sclerosing papilloma) or involved by adenosis.

## Invasive Breast Carcinoma

The histopathologic classification of invasive breast carcinomas is based upon the cytologic features and growth pattern of the tumor. Most invasive breast carcinomas arise in the terminal ductal lobular units regardless of the histologic subtypes. Several microscopic subtypes are recognized such as: (a) Invasive ductal carcinoma, no special type; (b) invasive lobular carcinoma; (c) tubular carcinoma; (d) mucinous carcinoma and (e) medullary carcinoma.

*Invasive ductal carcinoma, no special type* is the most common type of invasive breast cancer, accounting for 70–75% of all breast cancers. Grossly, it presents as a firm, gritty, stellate mass with irregular borders. Microscopically, it is composed of infiltrating tubules, cords and nests of tumor cells with variable cytologic features and mitotic activity. The background is often composed of a desmoplastic stroma. The grading of invasive ductal carcinomas, according to the widely used *Nottingham grading system*, is based on nuclear grade, the extent of tubule formation and mitotic count (Figs 10.16A to C).

*Invasive lobular carcinoma* is the second most common type of invasive breast carcinomas. It is characterized by a unique pattern of tumor growth and distinctive cytologic features. Tumor cells are often small and uniform and invade the stroma in a single-file pattern. Tumor cells may also show characteristic concentric encircling of benign ducts (Fig. 10.17). The nuclei are bland with little pleomorphism; mitosis is rare. There may be intracytoplasmic lumina which contain eosinophilic globules. There is loss of E-cadherin in the tumor cells of invasive lobular carcinoma.

*Tubular carcinoma* is composed of well-formed glands growing in a haphazard fashion in a desmoplastic stroma. The glands are ovoid in shape with pointed ends. The tumor cells have small and relatively uniform nuclei which lack hyperchromasia. On the luminal side the tumor cells usually form apical snouts (Fig. 10.18). The diagnosis of tubular carcinoma should only be made when more than 90% of the tumor shows the above characteristic features. Tubular carcinomas are associated with excellent prognosis.

*Mucinous carcinoma* is characterized by clusters of tumor cells dispersed within pools of extracellular mucin, accounting for at least 90% of the tumor (Fig. 10.19). Tumor cells usually have low to intermediate nuclear grade. Mucinous carcinoma is another special type of invasive breast cancer that has a favorable prognosis.

*Medullary carcinoma* is a rare subtype of invasive breast carcinoma and is associated with a more favorable prognosis if strict diagnostic criteria are followed. The WHO criteria for the diagnosis of medullary carcinoma include: > 75% syncytial growth pattern; absence of glandular structures; diffuse moderate to marked lymphoplasmacytic infiltrate; moderate to marked nuclear pleomorphism and complete histologic circumscription (Fig. 10.20). Tumors that have some but not all of the above features are called "atypical medullary" carcinoma by some authors, but should be categorized under invasive ductal carcinoma. Breast carcinomas arising in *BRCA1* carriers often show a subset of medullary features.

## Male Breast Lesions

Male breast tissue is composed of branching ducts and terminal ductules embedded in a fibrous stroma without terminal ductal lobular units (Fig. 10.21).

*Gynecomastia* is the most common lesion of the male breast. In the early or florid stage, it shows increased number of ducts surrounded by a loose myxoid periductal stroma (Fig. 10.22). Ductal epithelium shows hyperplasia with tapering tufts, or even cribriform, solid and papillary patterns. In the late stage, the ductal epithelium becomes atrophic; the periductal stroma shows fibrosis and hyalinization.

*Male breast carcinomas* are rare and usually present at higher stages. The histology is similar to that of female breast cancer with invasive ductal carcinoma being the most common type. When matched with stage, male breast cancers have similar prognosis as female breast cancers.

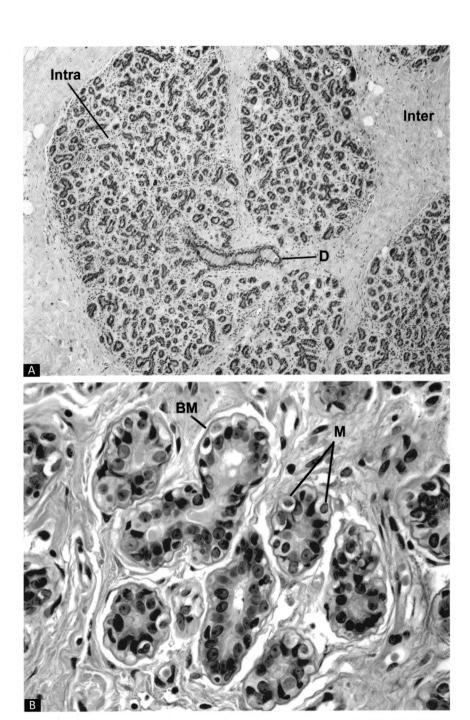

**Figs 10.1A and B:** Histology of normal female breast tissue

**A.** Normal terminal ductal lobular unit (TDLU) is composed of a duct (D) and a variable number of blind-ending ductules or acini with a smooth contour. Within TDLU is loose, delicate and myxomatous intralobular stroma (Intra). The interlobular stroma is composed of fibroconnective tissue admixed with adipose tissue (Inter). **B.** The acini are lined by an inner layer of epithelial cells and an outer layer of myoepithelial cells (M) invested by basement membrane (BM).

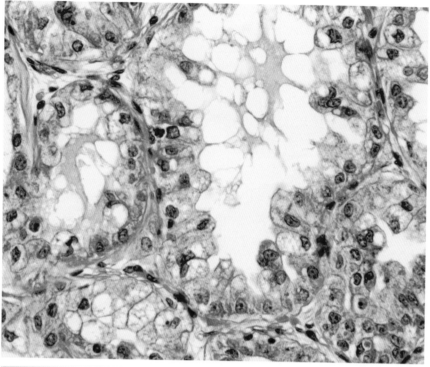

**Fig. 10.2:** Pregnancy/lactational changes

The epithelial cells are enlarged with abundant vacuolated cytoplasm containing lipoproteinaceous material. Scant secretions may appear in the lumen.

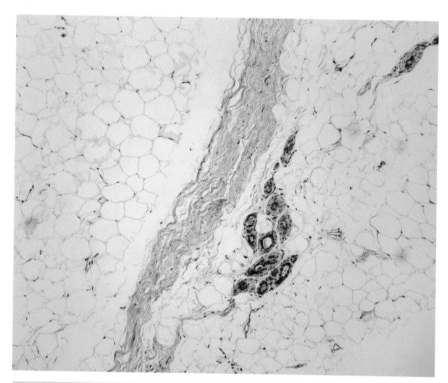

**Fig. 10.3:** Atrophy

After menopause, the terminal ductal lobular units decrease in size and number. The intralobular stroma is diminished; the interlobular stroma is in part replaced by adipose tissue.

BREAST

CHAPTER

**10**

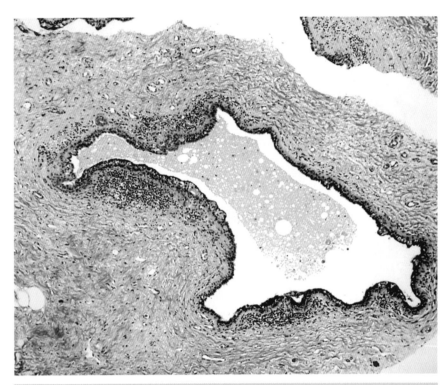

**Fig. 10.4:** Mammary duct ectasia

Mammary duct ectasia usually occurs in older women due to inspissation of secretions leading to dilatation of ducts. The ducts are filled with secretions and surrounded by chronic inflammatory cells.

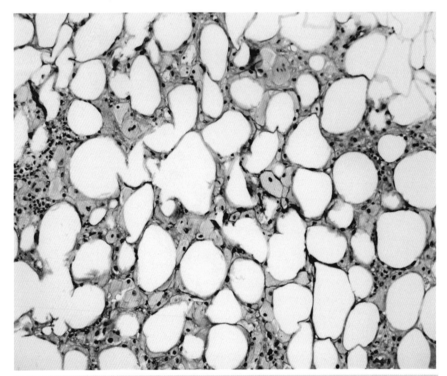

**Fig. 10.5:** Fat necrosis

Breast fat necrosis is commonly associated with a prior history of trauma or surgery and presents as a mass-like lesion or abnormal mammography. Histology shows necrotic fat cells devoid of nuclei surrounded by macrophages.

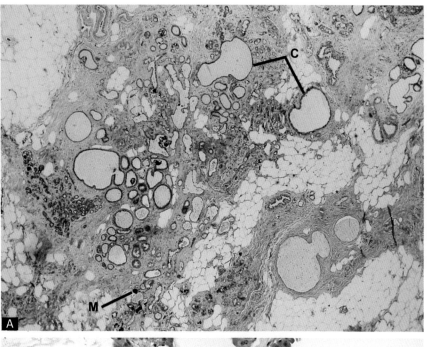

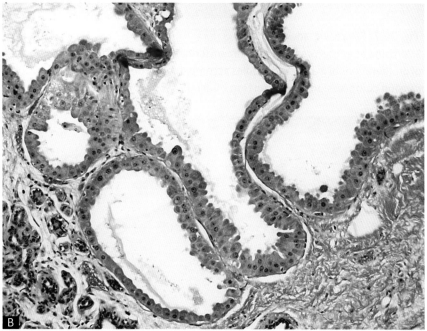

**Figs 10.6A and B:** Fibrocystic changes. Fibrocystic changes are very common findings in benign breasts and may be associated with abnormal mammography **A.** Characteristic microscopic features include distorted terminal ductal lobular units by dilated cysts (C) and fibrosis. Multiple foci of intraluminal micro-calcifications (M) are seen. **B.** Apocrine metaplasia is one of the histologic features of fibrocystic changes. It is characterized by epithelial cells with abundant eosinophilic and granular cytoplasm with apical snouting.

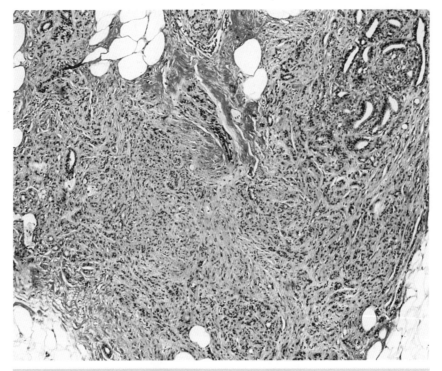

**Fig. 10.7:** Sclerosing adenosis

Sclerosing adenosis presents as a circumscribed, lobulocentric lesion composed of proliferations of glands and tubules accompanied by dense stromal proliferation causing compression and distortion of acini.

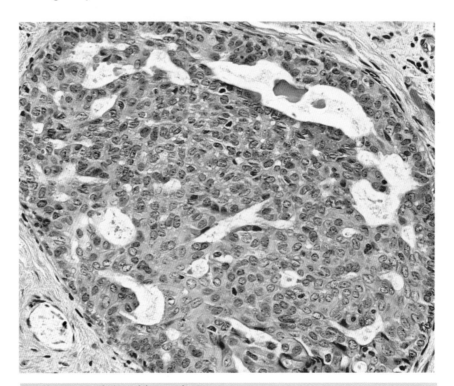

**Fig. 10.8:** Usual ductal hyperplasia

This benign intraductal proliferative lesion is composed of proliferating epithelial cells that vary in size and shape. The secondary lumens also vary in size and shape and are often slit-like.

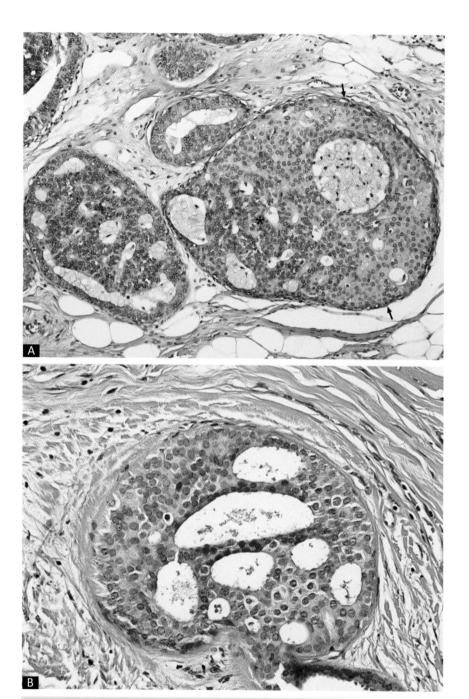

**Figs 10.9A and B:** Atypical ductal hyperplasia

**A.** A portion of the duct is filled with cells that are monotonous, small and uniform with rounded nuclei (arrows). The cells are evenly spaced with well-defined cell borders. The remaining population of the cells resembles cells in usual ductal hyperplasia (asterisk). **B.** The secondary lumens are more round and rigid.

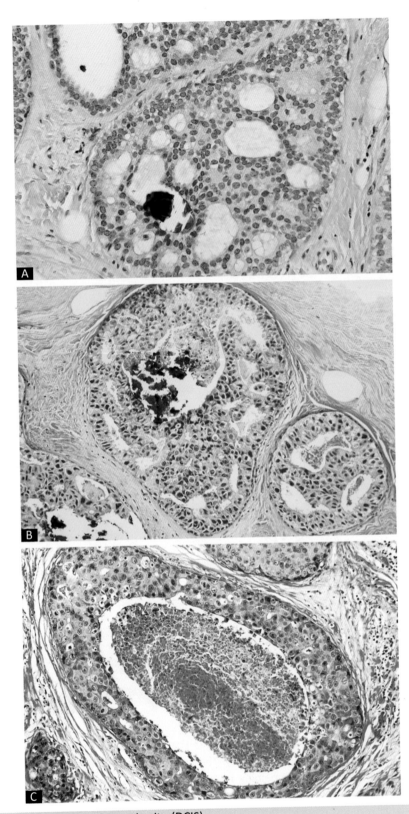

**Figs 10.10A to C:** Ductal carcinoma in situ (DCIS)

**A.** Low-grade DCIS is composed of small and monotonous cells filling the duct. The secondary lumen is smooth and round. An associated focus of microcalcification is present. **B.** Intermediate-grade DCIS is composed of cells with mild to moderate pleomorphism and nuclei (1–2 red blood cells in diameter) containing coarse chromatin and occasional nucleoli. Central luminal necrosis is usually present. **C.** High-grade DCIS is characterized by large pleomorphic cells with coarse chromatin and prominent nucleoli. Mitoses are frequent and may be atypical. There is central, comedo-type necrosis.

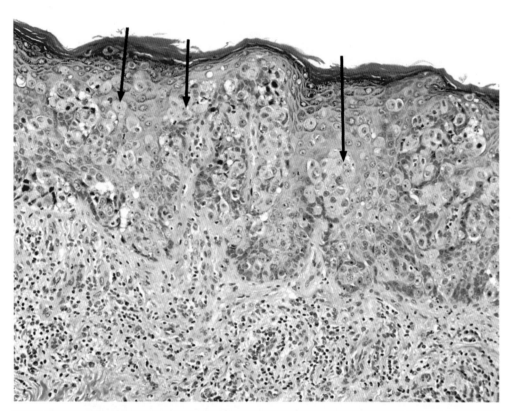

**Fig. 10.11:** Paget's disease of the nipple
The epidermis contains large tumor cells with abundant pale cytoplasm (arrows).

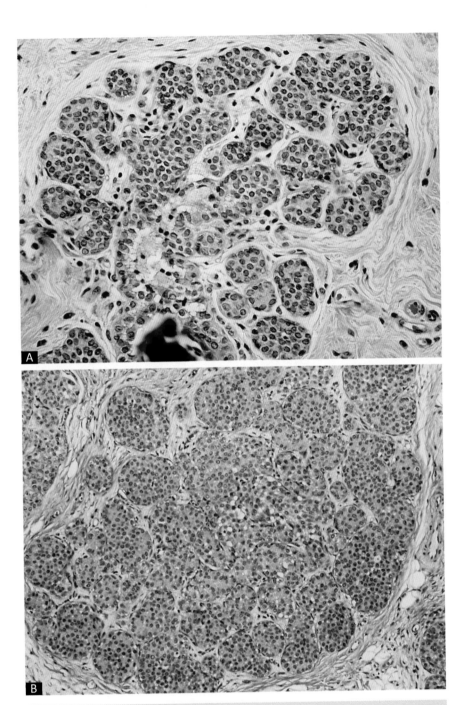

**Figs 10.12A and B:** Lobular neoplasia

**A.** Atypical lobular hyperplasia shows filling and mild expansion of the terminal ductal lobular system by small, monotonous and loosely cohesive cells. **B.** Lobular carcinoma in situ is characterized by further expansion and filling of the lobules by small and monotonous cells.

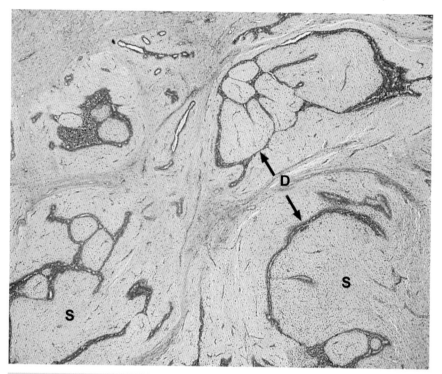

**Fig. 10.13:** Fibroadenoma

It is a benign biphasic neoplasm composed of elongated and distorted ducts (D) compressed by the surrounding proliferating intralobular myxoid stroma (S).

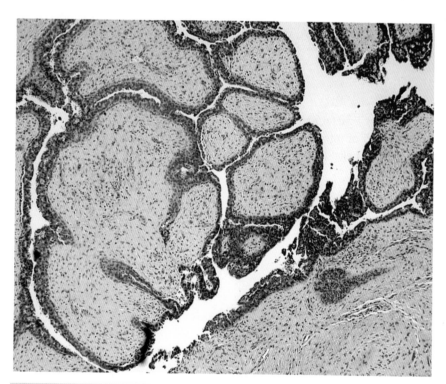

**Fig. 10.14:** Phyllodes tumor

It is characterized by leaf-like projections covered by epithelium and hypercellular stroma.

BREAST

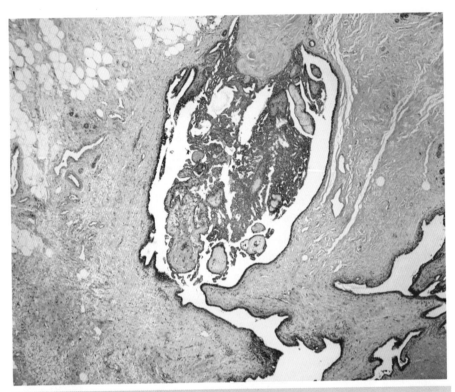

**Fig. 10.15:** Intraductal papilloma

It is composed of intraductal growth of papillary fronds. Fibrovascular cores are covered by epithelial and myoepithelial cells.

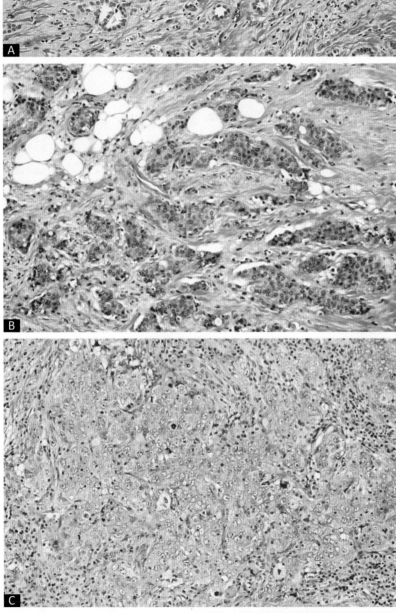

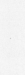

**Figs 10.16A to C:** Invasive ductal carcinomas

**A.** Invasive well-differentiated ductal carcinoma is composed of infiltrating ducts with open lumens lined by small bland cells. **B.** Invasive moderately differentiated ductal carcinoma shows less tubule formation with cells of moderate pleomorphism. **C.** Invasive poorly differentiated ductal carcinoma is composed of sheets of large pleomorphic cells with prominent nucleoli and frequent mitoses.

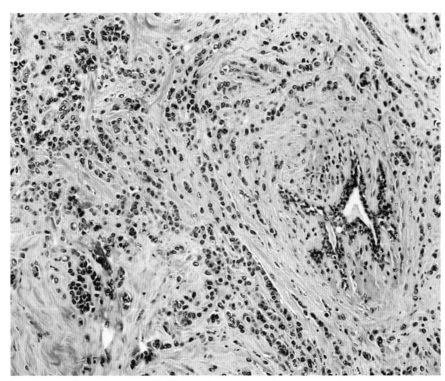

**Fig. 10.17:** Invasive lobular carcinoma
It shows a characteristic single-file and discohesive growth pattern. The cells are typically small and monotonous.

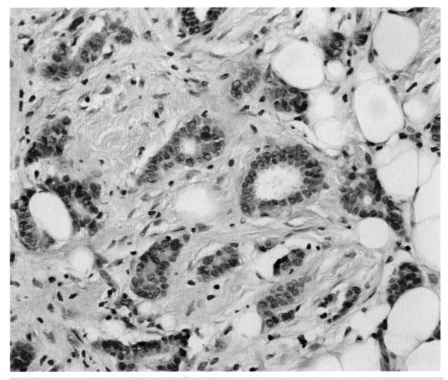

**Fig. 10.18:** Invasive tubular carcinoma
It is composed of tubules with open lumens lined by bland nuclei with apical snouting.

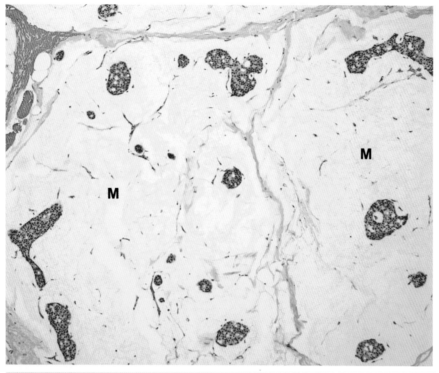

**Fig. 10.19:** Invasive mucinous carcinoma
The tumor cells are present in a background of mucin pools (M).

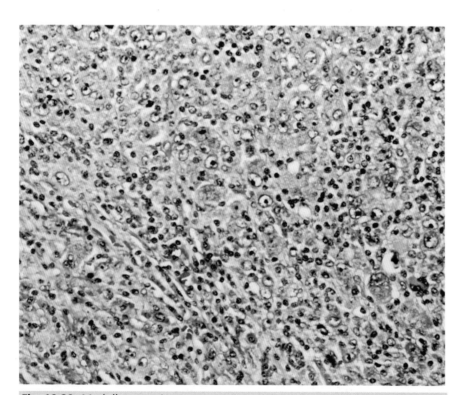

**Fig. 10.20:** Medullary carcinoma
These tumor cells are large and display a syncytial growth pattern. They have
vesicular nuclei and prominent nucleoli. The background contains lymphocytes
and plasma cells.

BREAST

CHAPTER
**10**

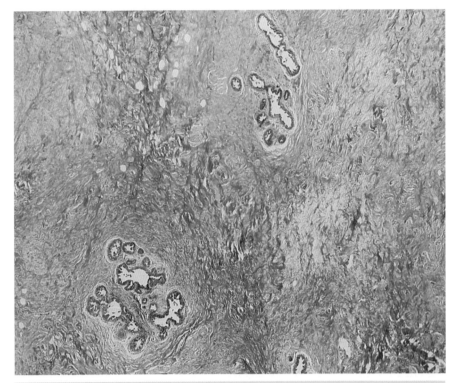

**Fig. 10.21:** Male breast tissue

It is composed of blind-ended ducts in a fibrous stroma. Terminal ductal lobular units are not formed.

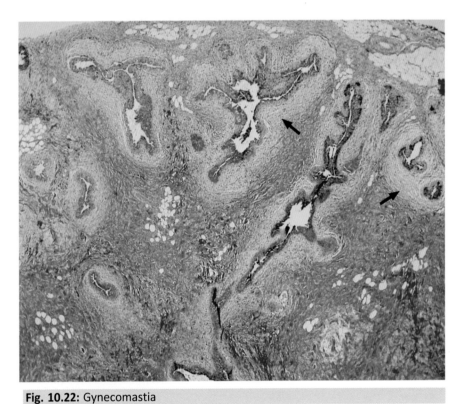

**Fig. 10.22:** Gynecomastia

Typically, there is prominent stromal edema (arrows) surrounding elongated/dilated ducts with mild epithelial hyperplasia.

# 11 The Endocrine System

*Paul St. Romain, Ivan Damjanov*

## Introduction

*The cells of the endocrine system form endocrine organs, parts of some organs or are dispersed throughout organ systems of the body. All of them are united by a common function: secretion of hormones into the bloodstream in order to maintain homeostasis. In this chapter we will discuss only the main endocrine organs (e.g. pituitary, thyroid, parathyroids and adrenals).*

## Pituitary

The pituitary gland is divided into two histologically distinct parts: (a) the anterior pituitary, derived from the pouch of Rathke (oral ectoderm) and (b) the posterior pituitary, derived from neuroectoderm, and linked to the hypothalamic nuclei by unmyelinated axons.

*The anterior pituitary* is composed of several cell types, i.e. cells that produce specific polypeptide hormones: thyrotropin (TSH), luteotropin (LH), follicle stimulating hormone (FSH), corticotropin (ACTH), growth hormone (GH) and prolactin (PRL) secreting cells. By light microscopy these cells can be classified either acidophilic, basophilic or chromophobic depending on their staining pattern. These cells are organized in nests and cords with intervening fenestrated sinusoidal capillaries (Fig. 11.1).

*The posterior pituitary* is composed of unmyelinated axons, which store antidiuretic hormone (ADH) and oxytocin, supported by modified glia cells called pituicytes. Pathologic changes in the posterior pituitary are usually secondary to those affecting the hypothalamus or the pituitary stalk and will not be discussed here.

Pituitary diseases may present in the following two forms:
- Hypopituitarism due to a deficiency of pituitary hormones.
- Hyperpituitarism due to an excess of pituitary hormones.

*Hypopituitarism* usually results from pituitary destruction, which may be caused by hemorrhage, infarction, infections, tumors or systemic diseases such as sarcoidosis or hemochromatosis. Nonfunctioning pituitary adenomas may compress the normal pituitary and cause hypopituitarism as well.

*Hyperpituitarism* typically results in clinical syndromes caused by the overproduction of one of the pituitary hormones. The best known examples are hyperprolactinemia due to an excess of PRL, Cushing syndrome due to an excess of ACTH and acromegaly and gigantism due to an excess of GH. Pituitary carcinomas may also occur but are extremely rare.

### Neoplasms

Pituitary adenomas are benign, usually hormonally active tumors composed of a single cell type. By light microscopy they can be classified as acidophilic, basophilic or chromophobe adenomas. This classification is of no clinical value, and accordingly most tumors are classified immunohistochemically by demonstrating the functional nature of the tumor cells. Approximately 25% of all primary pituitary tumors are hormonally inactive and are composed of either nonfunctioning stem cells or oncocytes.

*Prolactinomas* account for almost one-third of hyperfunctioning pituitary adenomas and are thus the most common hormonally active pituitary tumor. Prolactin provides negative feedback on GnRH, resulting in the clinical presentation of amenorrhea and galactorrhea in women or impotence in men. Most prolactinomas are composed of chromophobic cells, but the final diagnosis is always based on immunohistochemical demonstration of prolactin in the cytoplasm of tumor cells (Figs 11.2A and B).

## Thyroid

The thyroid is an endocrine organ composed of follicular and parafollicular cells (C cells) arranged into colloid-filled follicles (Figs 11.3A and B). *Follicular cells* produce triiodothyronine (T3) and tetraiodothyronine or thyroxine (T4) hormones that regulate basal metabolic rate and the intermediary metabolism of carbohydrates, lipids and proteins, thus affecting the growth, development and function of all major organs. *Parafollicular* or *C cells* secrete calcitonin, a hormone involved in the regulation of the homeostasis of calcium and phosphate.

The most important diseases of the thyroid are as follows:
• Goiter
• Thyroiditis
• Neoplasms.

### Goiter

Goiter is a term for enlargement of the thyroid gland, which may be diffuse or nodular. It develops due to disturbances of thyroid hormone production, which may be secondary to iodine deficiency, certain hereditary metabolic defects or metabolic disturbances related to drugs and toxins. In many instances the cause of goiter remains unknown, and the disease is then called *idiopathic* or *sporadic* goiter. Goiter developing in iodine-deficient parts of the world is called *endemic* goiter. *Hereditary* goiter is often referred to as *familial* goiter, and the goiter related to identifiable causes as *secondary food induced, toxin related* or *iatrogenic* goiter. All these forms of goiter present with the same pathologic changes.

*Nodular goiter* involving one or both thyroid lobes is the most common form of this disease. It results from impaired production of thyroid hormones in some thyroid follicles followed by compensatory changes in other follicles. Microscopically the goiter is composed of follicles that vary in size and shape (Fig. 11.4). Secondary changes caused by the expanded follicles compressing the normal thyroid include hemorrhage, extravasation of colloid with secondary inflammation, fibrosis and calcification. Some hyperplastic nodules may resemble follicular adenomas, and occasionally they may also be hormonally hyperactive.

### Thyroiditis

Thyroiditis is an inflammation of the thyroid that is in most instances immunologically mediated. Depending on the causes and the underlying pathology, thyroiditis may present as hyperthyroidism or hypothyroidism, or in some instances it may produce no hormonal changes. All forms of thyroiditis have a strong female preponderance. The most important forms of thyroiditis are: (a) granulomatous (de Quervain) thyroiditis; (b) Hashimoto thyroiditis; (c) Graves disease and (d) Riedel struma.

*Granulomatous (de Quervain) thyroiditis* usually has a sudden onset, and presents as a self-limited, painful enlargement of the thyroid thought to result from viral infection. Reactive cytotoxic T-lymphocytes damage the follicles, resulting in release of colloid. Colloid elicits a foreign body giant cell reaction, explaining the presence of granulomas (Fig. 11.5).

*Hashimoto thyroiditis* is an autoimmune disease of the thyroid resulting in hypothyroidism. It is most common in middle-aged women and has a strong genetic component. The etiology is probably related to a breakdown in regulation of cytotoxic T-cells, which subsequently infiltrate and damage the gland to release thyroid autoantigens. Antibodies to these autoantigens, including antithyroglobulin and antithyroid peroxidase, serve as disease markers but are probably not as important pathogenetically as the T-cell response. Lymphocytic infiltrates with germinal centers are found throughout the thyroid, destroying and replacing the normal follicles **(Figs 11.6A and B)**. In later stages of the disease fibrosis predominates. The remaining follicular cells undergo oncocytic transformation, evidenced as eosinophilic enlargement of the cytoplasm related to an excessive accumulation of mitochondria. Hashimoto thyroiditis is associated with an increased incidence of papillary carcinoma formation.

*Graves disease* is an autoimmune disease characterized by hyperthyroidism, ophthalmopathy and pretibial myxedema in the classical form. Incidence peaks at ages 20–40 years, and the disease has a strong female preponderance and a strong genetic component. Activating autoantibodies to the TSH receptor stimulate the gland to cause hyperthyroidism, and provoke an autoimmune attack on TSH-receptor-expressing preadipocyte fibroblasts in the orbit to cause ophthalmopathy. Histological hallmarks of Graves disease are follicles lined by hyperplastic tall columnar cells abutting with their apical portion on peripherally vacuolated or "scalloped" colloid **(Fig. 11.7)**. These changes imply hyperfunction of follicular cells, which are absorbing colloid at a rapid rate. Lymphocytic infiltrates may also be present, consistent with the autoimmune nature of this disease.

*Riedel struma* is a disease of unknown etiology characterized by progressive fibrosis of the thyroid. The disease is usually associated with other fibromatoses suggesting that it is a part of a multisystemic disorder, and is possibly immunologically mediated. The fibrous tissue also contains scattered lymphocytes which are usually most visible in the wall of small veins. Fibrous tissue replacing the thyroid follicles leads to hypothyroidism. The thyroid is rock-hard and firmly attached to the larynx **(Fig. 11.8)**.

## Neoplasms

Most thyroid tumors originate from follicular cells. The only exception is medullary carcinoma, which originates from C cells. Benign tumors (adenomas) are much more common than malignant tumors (carcinomas). Benign tumors are not considered to represent precursors of carcinomas. Primary tumors are more common than metastases, which are relatively rare. Most tumors are hormonally inactive and present as cold nodules characterized by low uptake of radioactive iodine. Nevertheless, some tumors may be hormonally active and take up radioactive iodine. Except for the anaplastic form of carcinoma and to some extent medullary carcinoma, most malignant thyroid tumors have a favorable prognosis.

The most important thyroid tumors are: (a) follicular adenoma; (b) follicular carcinoma; (c) papillary carcinoma; (d) medullary carcinoma and (e) anaplastic carcinoma.

*Follicular adenoma* is a benign neoplasm of the thyroid composed of follicular cells, enclosed usually by a capsule. Tumor cells may form small or large follicles, which may contain variable amounts of colloid. The tumor cell nuclei are usually uniformly round or oval and there are no mitoses **(Figs 11.9A and B)**.

*Follicular carcinoma* makes up 5–15% of thyroid cancers, although it is more common in areas where iodine deficiency is endemic. Well differentiated forms may resemble follicular adenomas, and the diagnosis of malignancy is made by demonstrating capsular or vascular invasion **(Figs 11.10A and B)**. Poorly differentiated forms grow in sheets of cells that are more obviously malignant.

*Papillary carcinoma* accounts for the majority (> 85%) of thyroid cancers. The strongest risk factor is exposure to ionizing radiation in the head and neck area. In typical cases the tumor cells line papillae projecting into small cavities **(Figs 11.11A and B)**. For the proper diagnosis it is important to recognize the diagnostic nuclear features which include optically clear nuclei (Orphan Annie eye nuclei), nuclear grooves and eosinophilic intranuclear inclusions. The tumor cells have scant cytoplasm, which contributes to the overlapping of elongated nuclei arranged parallel to one another. The fibrous stroma of the papillae often contains psammoma bodies.

In addition to the classical type of papillary carcinoma some tumors contain few if any papillae and their cells are arranged in follicles (*follicular subtype of papillary carcinoma*). There are also several other histologic subtypes, such as columnar cell and tall cell papillary carcinoma, but those are less common than the typical papillary carcinomas. All papillary carcinomas tend to metastasize to local neck lymph nodes, but overall most of them have an excellent prognosis.

*Medullary carcinoma* makes up 5% of all thyroid cancers. Unlike the other types of thyroid cancer, it arises from the parafollicular cells (C cells). Like other neuroendocrine tumors, it is composed of cells that have round or oval, relatively uniform nuclei. The cells form nests, cords or solid sheets which may be surrounded by fibrous tissue (**Figs 11.12A and B**). Typically tumor cells produce calcitonin, which contributes to the formation of amyloid often found in the fibrous septa. Immunohistochemical stains with antibodies to calcitonin give positive results and amyloid can be demonstrated with Congo red. Both of these stains are useful for the diagnosis of medullary carcinoma.

*Anaplastic carcinoma* is a rare aggressive form of thyroid cancer, accounting for less than 2% of all malignant tumors. It is more common in older patients and has an extremely unfavorable prognosis due to its rapid invasive growth and a tendency to metastasize. It is believed to arise from well-differentiated papillary or follicular carcinoma in most instances. As with many poorly differentiated tumors, its cells are pleomorphic and do not grow in any characteristic pattern (**Figs 11.13A and B**).

## Parathyroid

The four parathyroid glands are predominantly composed of chief cells, with an admixture of eosinophilic (oxyphilic) cells, and a variable amount of stromal fat that increases with age (**Fig. 11.14**). Chief cells produce parathyroid hormone (PTH) in response to hypocalcemia; PTH acts on the kidneys to increase calcium retention and vitamin D production, intestine to increase calcium absorption, and bone to increase calcium release.

Clinical disorders involving parathyroids may present as: (a) hypoparathyroidism or (b) hyperparathyroidism. Hypoparathyroidism may be congenital or acquired, e.g. after inadvertent surgical removal of parathyroids. Hyperparathyroidism is caused by tumors or parathyroid gland hyperplasia.

The most important diseases of the parathyroids associated with histopathologic changes are as follows:
- Hyperplasia
- Adenoma.

### Hyperplasia

Parathyroid hyperplasia may be *primary* or *secondary* to any disease that causes hypocalcemia and thus forces the gland to grow in order to produce more PTH and raise serum calcium. Classically all four parathyroid glands are enlarged due to the proliferation of normal parathyroid cells. Chief cells proliferate most prominently, but there are also groups of eosinophilic cells. These cells replace the normal stromal fat cells and accordingly the enlarged parathyroids contain fewer fat cells (**Fig. 11.15**). The hyperplastic glands are 5–10 times larger than normal parathyroids. Normal glands have a combined weight of 100–120 mg whereas the hyperplastic glands weigh 800–1000 mg.

### Adenoma

Parathyroid adenoma accounts for 85–95% of all cases of primary hyperparathyroidism. The histologic pattern is similar to that observed in hyperplasia, but the tumor is often quite distinct from the adjacent normal gland (**Figs 11.16A to C**). Most adenomas are solitary, involving only one of the four glands. They weigh 0.5–5.0 gm, while the remaining three glands tend to atrophy. Some parathyroid tumors are malignant and invade local tissue or metastasize; such parathyroid carcinomas are extremely rare.

## Adrenal

The adrenal glands can be divided into two embryologically and functionally distinct zones: (a) cortex, which is derived from mesenchyme and (b) medulla, derived from the neural crest (**Figs 11.17A and B**).

The adrenal cortex is divided into three layers: (a) zona glomerulosa, which secretes aldosterone; (b) zona fasciculata, which secretes corticosteroids and (c) zona reticularis, which secretes adrenal sex hormones.

The adrenal medulla is composed primarily of basophilic nests of chromaffin cells with large clear nuclei and basophilic cytoplasm. These cells secrete the catecholamines adrenaline and noradrenaline.

Adrenal cortical diseases present clinically as hormonal insufficiency or hyperfunction. *Adrenal cortical insufficiency* presents clinically as hypocorticism. It may develop acutely due to hemorrhagic destruction of the adrenals, or in a chronic form such as Addison disease. *Adrenal cortical hyperfunction* may result in hormonal syndromes, such as hyperaldosteronism (Conn syndrome), hypercorticosteroidism (Cushing syndrome) or an excess of adrenal androgen production (e.g. adrenogenital syndrome). *Hyperfunction of the adrenal medulla* results in arterial hypertension.

The most important adrenal diseases associated with histopathologic changes are as follows:
- Acute adrenal insufficiency
- Chronic adrenal insufficiency
- Adrenal cortical hyperplasia
- Adrenal cortical adenoma
- Adrenal cortical carcinoma
- Medullary neoplasms
- Pheochromocytoma
- Neuroblastoma.

### Acute Adrenal Insufficiency

Acute adrenal insufficiency may arise in the context of chronic insufficiency, atrophy or infarction. The latter, also termed Waterhouse-Friderichsen syndrome, is a life-threatening emergency that generally results from overwhelming bacterial sepsis, classically *Neisseria meningitidis*, which leads to disseminated intravascular coagulation. Histologically, the cortex appears hemorrhagic and few cortical cells are preserved (**Fig. 11.18**).

### Chronic Adrenal Insufficiency

The most common cause of chronic adrenal insufficiency (*Addison disease*) is autoimmune adrenalitis, which may occur in an isolated form or as a part of polyglandular autoimmune syndrome. Destruction of the adrenal glands may be found in systemic amyloidosis, hemochromatosis, infections by bacteria (*Mycobacterium tuberculosis*) or fungi (*Histoplasma capsulatum*), and metastatic carcinoma of the lungs and breast. The morphology reflects the underlying cause of destruction; for example, in amyloidosis there is deposition of amyloid in the sinusoids accompanied by a loss of cortical cells (**Fig. 11.19**).

### Adrenal Cortical Hyperplasia

Hyperplasia of the adrenal may be primary or secondary (due to increased ACTH). An important cause is the category of adrenogenital syndromes, in which various genetic mutations result in ineffectual cortisol synthesis and lack of negative feedback on ACTH. Hyperplasia may be diffuse or nodular, and it is characterized by thickening of one or more layers of cortex due to an increased number of normal-appearing cells (**Fig. 11.20**).

## Adrenal Cortical Adenoma

Adrenal cortical adenomas may produce aldosterone (Conn syndrome), cortisol (Cushing syndrome) or androgens, but most frequently they are nonfunctional and clinically silent. They are well circumscribed with a yellow cut surface due to the presence of lipid. The microscopic appearance is similar to that of normal adrenal cortex although some cellular pleomorphism, termed *endocrine atypia*, is permitted (Figs 11.21A and B).

## Adrenal Cortical Carcinoma

Adrenal cortical carcinoma is a rare malignant tumor that may occur in any age group. Microscopically, the tumors may resemble cortical adenomas, but the presence of prominent mitoses, necrosis, hemorrhage and nuclear atypia support the diagnosis of carcinoma (Fig. 11.22). However, in some well differentiated forms, the only definitive way to distinguish the two is by the presence of invasion and metastasis in the malignant form.

## Pheochromocytoma

Pheochromocytoma is a neoplasm of chromaffin cells, most frequently occurring in the adrenal medulla. This neoplasm generally produces norepinephrine and epinephrine and thus composes a cause of surgically curable hypertension. The classic microscopic pattern is that of nests (zellballen) of polygonal or spindle-shaped cells with a finely granular cytoplasm. These cytoplasmic granules contain catecholamines. Due to the neurosecretory nature of the tumor, the chromaffin cells stain immunochemically with antibodies to chromogranin, synaptophysin and CD56 (Figs 11.23A and B). Although 10% of pheochromocytomas are malignant, the diagnosis of malignancy cannot be reliably established microscopically. Similar tumors may arise from autonomic paraganglia, in which case they are termed paragangliomas.

## Neuroblastoma

Neuroblastoma is a malignant tumor of infancy and childhood that is derived from primordial neural crest cells destined to populate the adrenal medulla and autonomic ganglia. These primitive neural crest cells are small, round cells with dark nuclei and scant cytoplasm. Architecturally, they may be arranged in rosettes around a region of neuropil (Homer-Wright pseudorosettes) or may grow in solid sheets (Fig. 11.24).

Ganglioneuroblastoma is a tumor closely related to neuroblastoma. In this tumor there are groups of neuroblasts adjacent to ganglion cells, which can be recognized due to their larger size, more abundant cytoplasm and vesicular nuclei with prominent nucleoli. The cytoplasmic processes of mature Schwann cells and fibroblasts form eosinophilic neuropil. If these mature regions are the predominant histology, the term *ganglioneuroma* is applied (Fig. 11.25). Either of these more differentiated tumor forms has a more favorable prognosis than undifferentiated neuroblastoma.

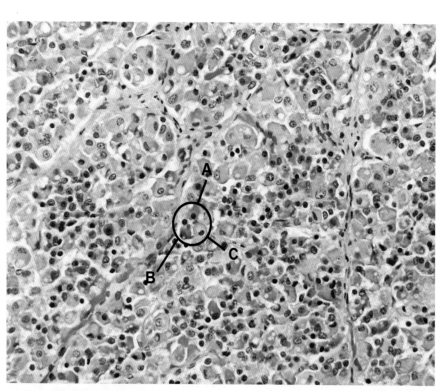

**Fig. 11.1:** Normal pituitary

In routine hematoxylin and eosin stained slides the anterior pituitary consists of acidophilic (A), basophilic (B) and chromophobe cells (C).

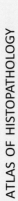

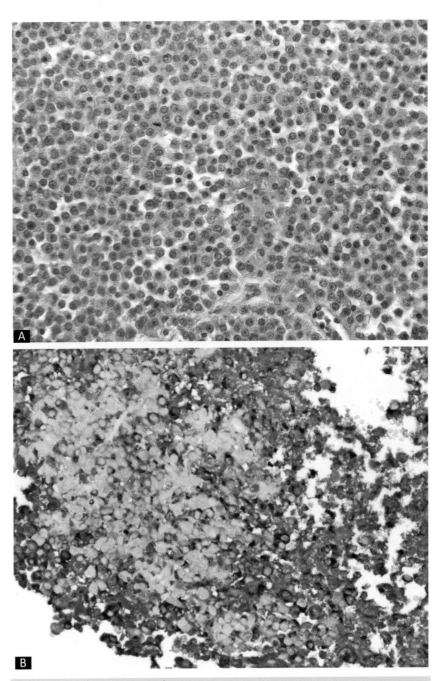

**Figs 11.2A and B:** Pituitary adenoma

**A.** The tumor is composed of a uniform population of small acidophilic cells. **B.** The exact nature of this adenoma could be determined only immunohisto-chemically using antibodies to one of the pituitary hormones. In this case the cells reacted with the antibodies to prolactin and thus the tumor was subclassified as a prolactinoma.

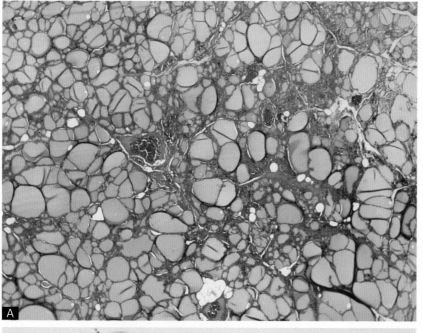

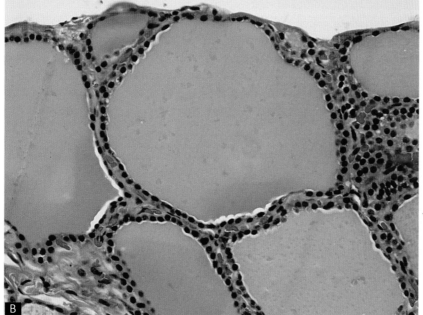

**Figs 11.3A and B:** Normal thyroid

**A.** The tissue is composed of follicles which vary slightly in size and shape. **B.** Each follicle is filled with homogenous pink colloid, a proteinaceous material composed primarily of thyroglobulin that has been produced by the follicular epithelial cells. The follicles are lined by a single layer of cuboidal cells. Parafollicular cells are generally not seen in H&E-stained sections of normal thyroid.

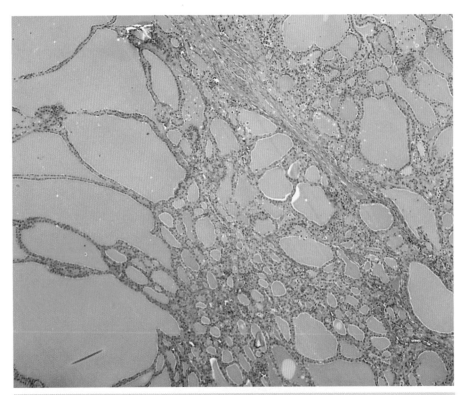

**Fig. 11.4:** Nodular goiter

Abnormally large follicles at left are located adjacent to much smaller follicles, shown at center of the photograph. Normal thyroid tissue is seen at upper right, separated from the nodular area by a fibrous band of connective tissue. This variation of follicular size is the most striking microscopic feature of nodular goiter.

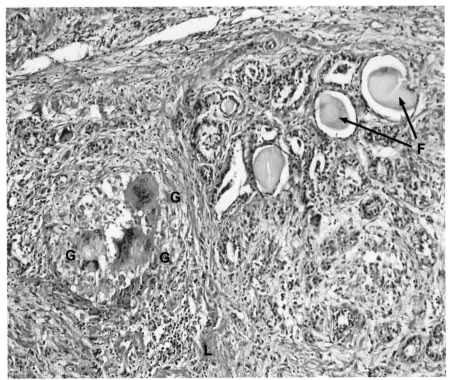

**Fig. 11.5:** Granulomatous (deQuervain) thyroiditis

Several multinucleated giant cells (G), the histologic hallmark of this disease, are seen near left-center. A prominent lymphocytic infiltrate (L) has destroyed much of the normal thyroid tissue even though several colloid-filled follicles (F) persist.

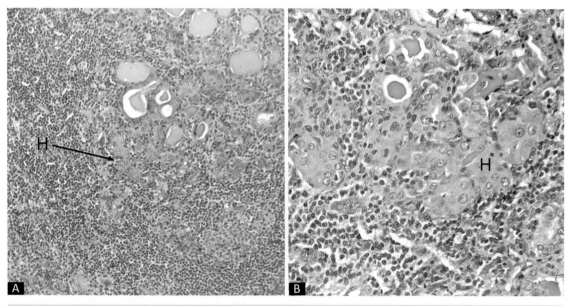

**Figs 11.6A and B:** Hashimoto thyroiditis

**A.** Dense lymphocytic infiltrates are seen replacing thyroid follicles. A few follicles and oncocytic follicular cells, called Hurthle cells (H), are visible. A germinal center is seen in the right lower corner. **B.** Hurthle cells (H) are epithelial follicular cells that have all the features of oncocytes, i.e. abundant eosinophilic cytoplasm and vesicular nuclei. These cells are surrounded by lymphocytes.

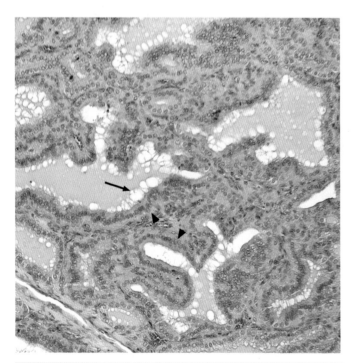

**Fig. 11.7:** Graves disease

Hyperplasia of the follicular epithelium in response to autoantibodies results in irregular projections and infoldings of the follicles. The epithelial cells appear columnar instead of cuboidal in some areas (arrowheads), and there are prominent vacuolated areas where the colloid abuts the follicular epithelium (scalloping) (arrow).

THE ENDOCRINE SYSTEM

CHAPTER

**11**

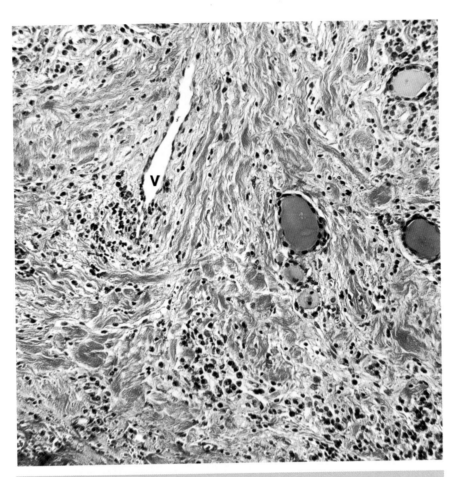

**Fig. 11.8:** Riedel thyroiditis

Dense bundles of pink collagen have replaced all normal tissue except for several atrophic follicles. The fibrotic tissue is rich in lymphocytes, reflecting the inflammatory etiology of the disease. Lymphocytes are also seen in the wall of an elongated vein (V).

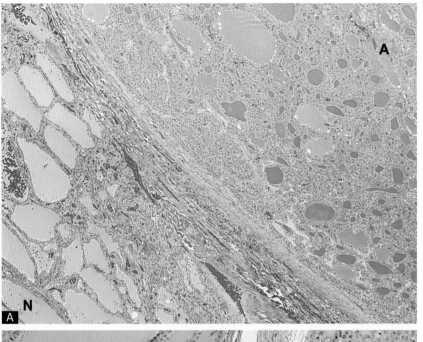

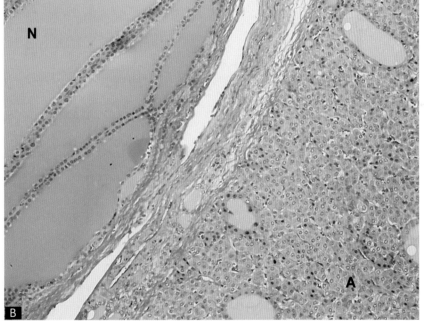

**Figs 11.9A and B:** Follicular adenoma

**A.** A dense, well-demarcated capsule separates normal thyroid tissue (N) from the adenoma (A). The tumor is not invading the capsule. The adenoma displays a solid and a microfollicular growth pattern distinct from the macrofollicular growth pattern of normal thyroid. **B.** A sharp border between normal thyroid (N) and adenoma (A), formed by a fibrous capsule, demonstrates the benign nature of the tumor.

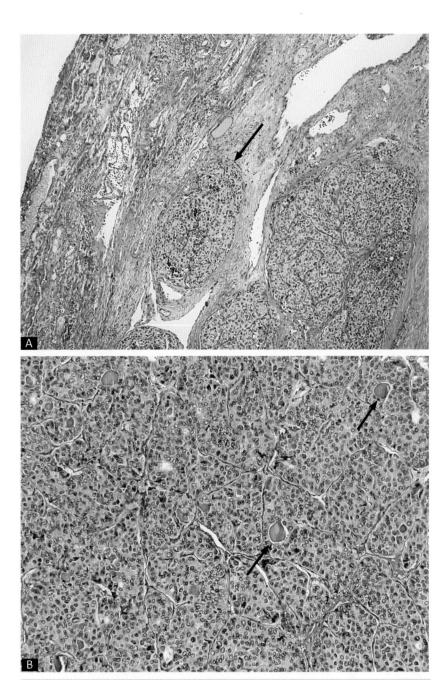

**Figs 11.10A and B:** Follicular carcinoma
**A.** The tumor resembles follicular adenoma but invades the fibrous capsule (arrow). **B.** Microfollicular growth pattern with occasional mild nuclear atypia are found but are not diagnostic, since similar histologic features can be seen in benign thyroid adenomas. Some follicles contain colloid (arrows).

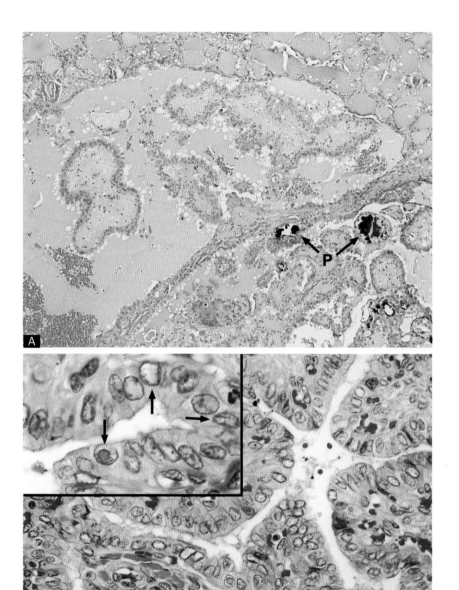

**Figs 11.11A and B:** Papillary carcinoma

**A.** Papillae lined by a single layer of cuboidal epithelium project into a serous fluid-containing cavity. Several psammoma bodies (P) are present. **B.** Nuclei are elongated and overlap one another. Optically clear nuclei, nuclear grooving and intranuclear inclusions (inset arrows) are diagnostic features of the tumor.

THE ENDOCRINE SYSTEM

CHAPTER

**11**

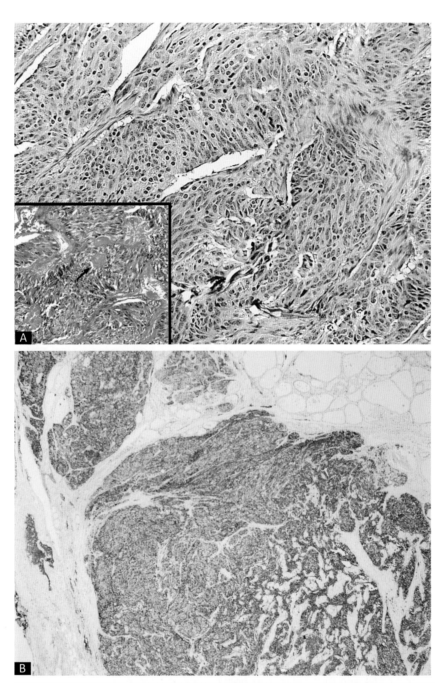

**Figs 11.12A and B:** Medullary carcinoma

**A.** Solid growth of spindle-shaped cells with regular round basophilic nuclei and finely stippled chromatin. Fibrils of amyloid appear pink, waxy and amorphous on H&E (arrow). **B.** An immunohistochemical stain for calcitonin (dark brown) is essential for the diagnosis of this tumor.

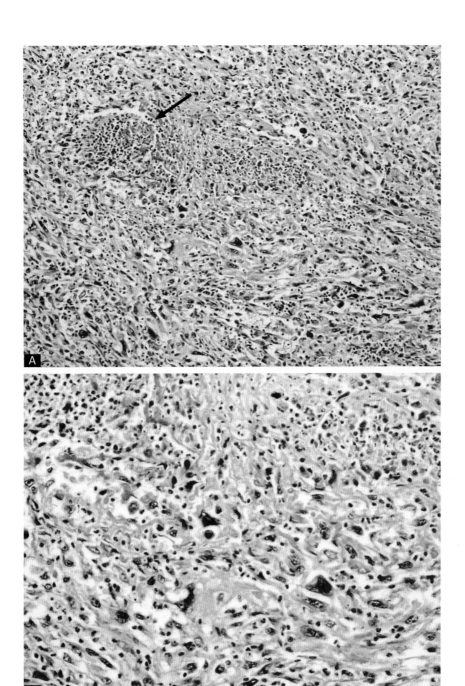

**Figs 11.13A and B:** Anaplastic carcinoma

**A.** Solid growth of tumor cells has obliterated the normal thyroid. Focal areas of necrosis are present (arrow). **B.** Cells show extreme variation in shape and size with high nuclear to cytoplasmic ratio and multiple prominent nucleoli. There is no resemblance to normal follicular epithelium.

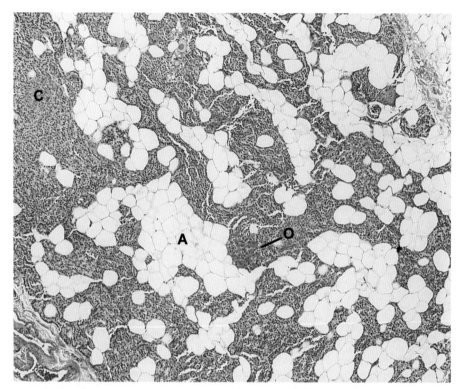

**Fig. 11.14:** Normal parathyroid
Chief cells (C), oxyphilic cells (O) and stromal adipose cells (A) are typical features of normal parathyroids.

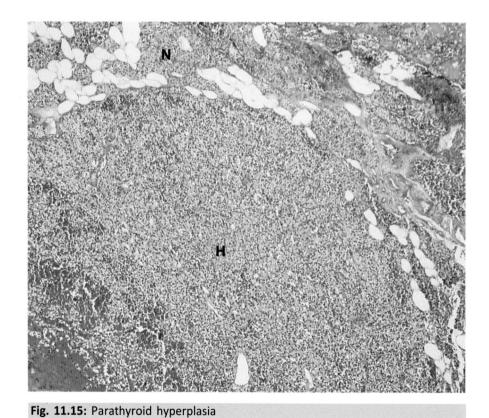

**Fig. 11.15:** Parathyroid hyperplasia
Chief cells in the center have grown to replace the stromal fat in the region of hyperplasia (H). Normal parathyroid tissue (N) surrounding the hyperplastic region contains fat cells.

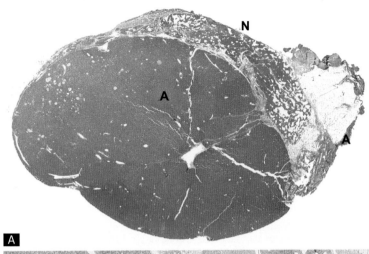

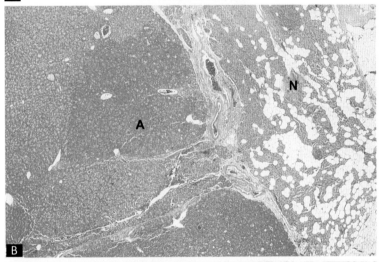

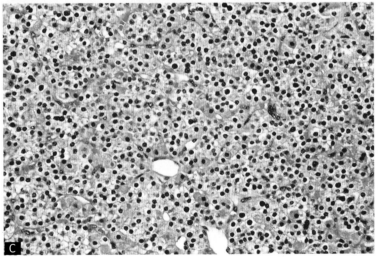

**Figs 11.16A to C:** Parathyroid adenoma

**A.** Adenoma (A) is distinctly separate from normal parathyroid (N) seen at low power. **B.** The adenoma (A) is separated from the normal tissue (N) by a fibrous capsule. **C.** Higher power view of chief cells within the adenoma shows that these cells have regular round nuclei and clear cytoplasm.

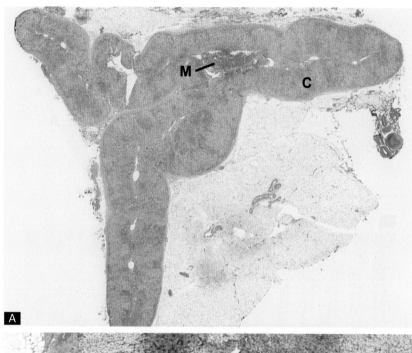

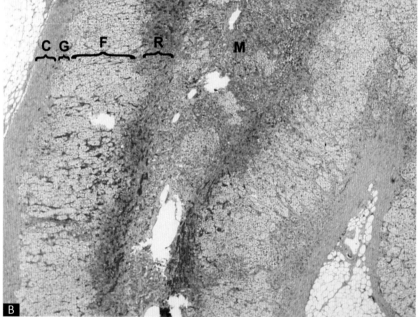

**Figs 11.17A and B:** Normal adrenal

**A.** The cortex (C) makes up most of the triangular adrenal gland and surrounds the medulla (M). **B.** Higher magnification demonstrating capsule (C), zona glomerulosa (G), zona fasciculata (F), zona reticularis (R) and medulla (M).

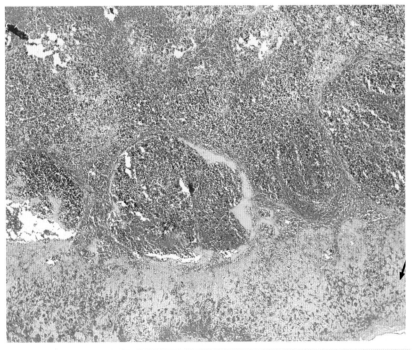

**Fig. 11.18:** Adrenal hemorrhage
Extensive hemorrhage obscures the normal features of the adrenal gland.
Some zona glomerulosa may be distinguished at bottom (arrow).

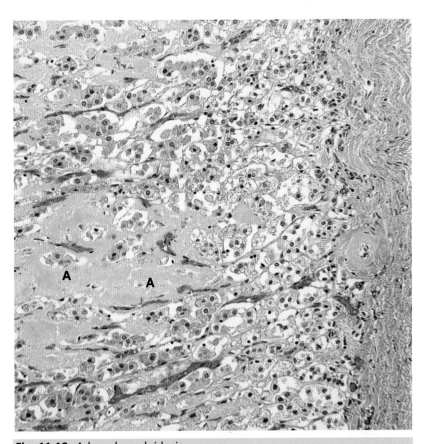

**Fig. 11.19:** Adrenal amyloidosis
Pink deposits of amyloid (A) infiltrating the adrenal gland are intermixed
with remaining cells of the zona glomerulosa.

THE ENDOCRINE SYSTEM

CHAPTER
**11**

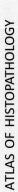

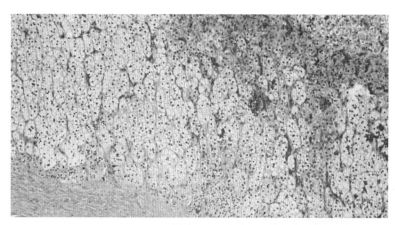

**Fig. 11.20:** Adrenal hyperplasia The zona glomerulosa is thick and prominent while other layers of the adrenal gland appear thinner in comparison.

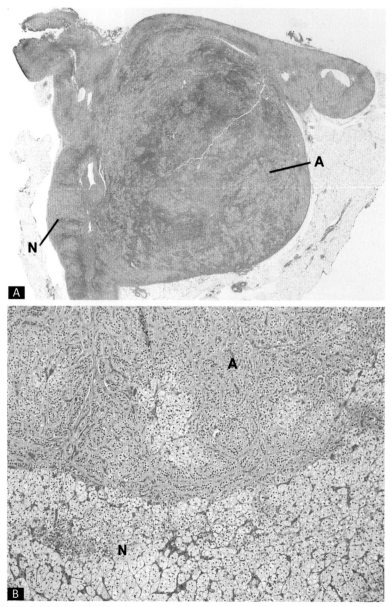

**Figs 11.21A and B:** Adrenal cortical adenoma
**A.** Low-power view of a cortical adenoma (A) protruding from the adrenal gland. Normal cortex (N) is present opposite to the adenoma. **B.** Higher magnification showing the clear demarcation between the normal adrenal (N) and the well-circumscribed adenoma (A). Adenoma cells have a bland, regular appearance.

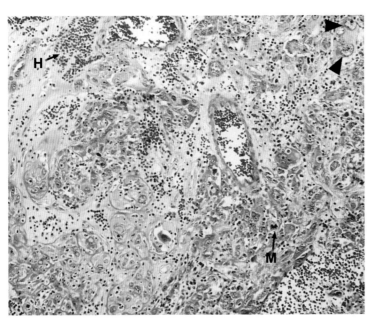

**Fig. 11.22:** Adrenal cortical carcinoma Areas of hemorrhage (H), mitosis (M) and nuclear pleomorphism (arrowheads) are indications of malignant tumor. Normal adrenal tissue is not seen.

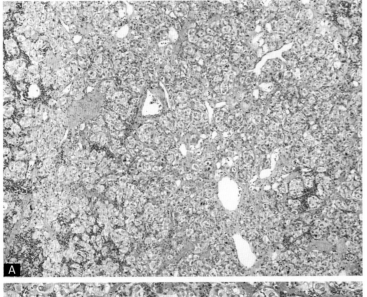

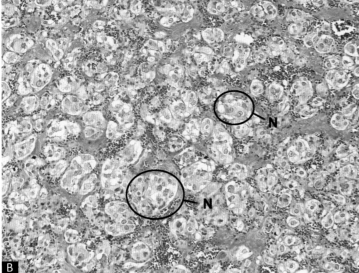

**Figs 11.23A and B:** Pheochromocytoma **A.** Tumor cells are arranged into groups surrounded by thin fibrous septa. **B.** Solid tumor nests (N), also known as "zellballen", are surrounded by vascular stroma.

CHAPTER
**11**

ATLAS OF HISTOPATHOLOGY

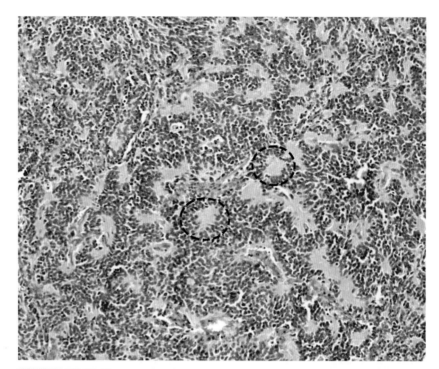

**Fig. 11.24:** Neuroblastoma

Neuroblasts are very dark blue on H&E with very little cytoplasm and display overlapping growth. Cells forming pseudorosettes are outlined with dotted lines.

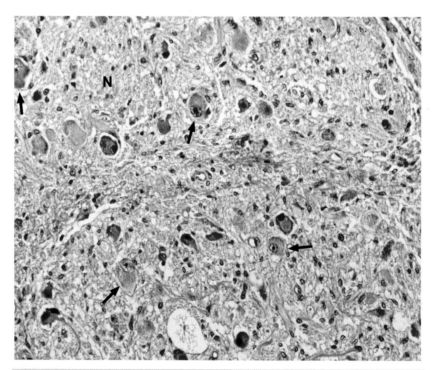

**Fig. 11.25:** Ganglioneuroma

The tumor is composed of ganglion cells (arrows) embedded in eosinophilic neuropil (N).

# 12 The Skin

*Garth Fraga*

## Introduction

*The skin forms the external surface of the body. It provides a protective barrier for the body, shielding it from physical trauma, infectious organisms and other environmental pathogens such as solar irradiation. The skin consists of the epidermis, dermis and subcutaneous tissue (Fig. 12.1). Skin diseases can be grouped into:*
- *Genodermatoses*
- *Inflammatory dermatoses*
- *Infections and infestations*
- *Neoplasms.*

## Genodermatoses

Skin changes in genodermatoses are mostly due to abnormal development of the epidermis.

*Ichthyosis vulgaris* is the most common genodermatosis with a prevalence of 1 in 250 (Fig. 12.2). It is associated with a deficiency in profilaggrin expression and produces dry skin with whitish scales located on the extensor surfaces of the arms and legs. The severity is quite variable, with many cases exhibiting relatively minor changes that are mistaken for common dry skin (*xerosis*).

## Inflammatory Dermatoses

Inflammatory dermatopathology can be challenging. The skin is reputed to suffer from over 2,000 separate inflammatory ailments, most of which have been given verbose Latin names, lack a known etiology, and produce overlapping gross and microscopic pathologies. In the interest of brevity, we will limit this discussion to the most common inflammatory dermatoses. The more common inflammatory dermatoses can be grouped into the following patterns:
- Spongiotic dermatitis
- Psoriasiform dermatitis
- Interface dermatitis
- Disorders of the hair follicle
- Perivascular dermatitis
- Granulomatous dermatitis
- Vesiculobullous/blistering dermatitis.

### Spongiotic Dermatitis

*Spongiotic dermatitis* is characterized by accumulation of fluid between cells of the epidermis. In its acute form, intraepidermal vesicles may form. Spongiotic dermatoses are typically pruritic, and, if the disease persists, the epidermis will thicken in response to the persistent itching and scratching. Although there are many different diseases in this category, they generally produce overlapping histopathologic changes and are usually best separated by clinical history and the configuration and distribution of lesions rather than by biopsy. Two common forms of spongiotic dermatitis are: (a) contact dermatitis and (b) atopic dermatitis.

*Contact dermatitis* is triggered by an exogenous allergenic or irritant substance (Fig. 12.3). Poison ivy dermatitis, nickel dermatitis to jewelry or occupational dermatitis to cleaners and solvents are common examples.

*Atopic dermatitis* usually presents prior to five years of age (Figs 12.4A and B). Patients have a genetic predisposition to allergy and often report a family history of atopic dermatitis, asthma, and respiratory and food allergies. Lesions in infants are often located on the face and extensor surfaces; whereas in childhood, they affect the flexor surfaces and hands. In adults, the head and neck, extremities and hands are often involved.

### Psoriasiform Dermatitis

*Psoriasis* is the stereotypic form of psoriasiform dermatitis and produces well-demarcated scaly plaques with a symmetric distribution and a predilection for the scalp, elbows, knees, palms/soles, gluteal cleft, genitalia and lower back (Figs 12.5A and B). *Seborrheic dermatitis* and chronic forms of spongiotic dermatitis can produce similar histopathologic findings, but can usually be separated from psoriasis by clinical and histopathological criteria.

### Interface Dermatitis

*Interface dermatitis* is defined by signs of T-cell mediated damage to the epidermis such as vacuolization of basilar keratinocytes, necrosis of keratinocytes and papillary melanophages. It is sometimes separated into lichenoid variants such as lichen planus in which a dense infiltrate of T-cells hugs the dermoepidermal junction, and vacuolar variants such as lupus erythematosus in which there is less inflammation at the dermoepidermal junction.

*Lichen planus* is an immunologically mediated disease that manifests with intensely pruritic papules of the wrists, genitalia and lower extremities. Microscopically it presents with dense lymphocytic infiltrates along the dermoepidermal junction (Fig. 12.6).

*Lupus erythematosus* is an autoimmune disease affecting the skin. It is the prototype of vacuolar interface dermatitis and sometimes produces systemic disease (Fig. 12.7). There are three primary subtypes of lupus erythematosus in the skin. *Discoid lupus erythematosus* produces hypopigmented plaques with scarring on the head and neck area, and is not usually associated with systemic disease. *Subacute lupus erythematosus* produces nonscarring annular erythematous plaques in the V-region of the neck and upper back. Approximately 50% of individuals with the subacute subtype have systemic disease, and it is often associated with antibodies to Ro and La. *Systemic lupus erythematosus* usually produces malar erythema, and 95% of individuals have a positive ANA.

### Disorders of the Hair Follicle

The four most common diseases involving the hair follicles are: (a) acne vulgaris; (b) rosacea; (c) infectious folliculitis and (d) alopecia.

*Acne vulgaris* is due to impaired desquamation of follicular corneocytes at the opening of the hair follicle, with subsequent occlusion, impaction of sebaceous debris and keratin, and overgrowth of *Propionibacterium acnes* (Fig. 12.8).

*Rosacea* may be mistaken for acne vulgaris (Figs 12.9A and B). It occurs at an older age (3rd and 4th decade) and does not produce comedones.

*Infectious folliculitis* is most commonly associated with *Staphylococcus*, dermatophytes, herpesviruses and *Pityrosporum* yeast (Fig. 12.10).

*Androgenetic alopecia* is the most common alopecia in both men and women. In men, there is frontal recession and thinning at the vertex. In women, androgenetic alopecia produces thinning at the top of the scalp with a widened part line and preservation of frontal scalp hair. Androgenetic alopecia is due to miniaturization of hair follicles by circulating androgens; since the follicles are preserved despite being abnormally small, it is considered a nonscarring alopecia.

## Perivascular Dermatitis

*Leukocytoclastic vasculitis* is perivascular dermatitis with signs of vascular injury such as extravasation of erythrocytes, fibrin and neutrophil fragment deposition in the vessel walls, endothelial cell swelling, a perivascular infiltrate of neutrophils and fragmentation of neutrophils (Fig. 12.11). Most cases of vasculitis in the skin affect superficial small venules. Leukocytoclastic vasculitis produces purpura, usually of the lower extremities and is due to vascular deposition of circulating immune complexes (type III hypersensitivity reaction).

*Perivascular dermatitis without vascular injury* is seen in: (a) pigmented purpuric dermatitis; (b) urticaria (Figs 12.12A and B); (c) viral exanthems and (d) drug reactions (Fig. 12.13).

*Pigmented purpuric dermatitis* is an idiopathic disorder that produces cayenne pepper-like dots on yellowish macules, usually on the lower legs. The yellowish background corresponds to dermal siderophages that have engulfed extravasated erythrocytes.

*Urticaria* produces pruritic, transient annular plaques. Urticaria is caused by a type I hypersensitivity reaction in which IgE binds to mast cells causing degranulation of histamine and other molecules that trigger vasodilation and exudation of serum into the dermis.

*Drug reaction* may present with skin changes resembling *viral exanthems*. Both drug reactions and viral exanthems often begin on the trunk and produce extensive macular erythema that may become confluent.

## Granulomatous Dermatitis

*Granulomatous dermatitis* may be a feature of: (a) sarcoidosis; (b) granuloma annulare; (c) foreign body reaction or (d) infections.

*Sarcoidosis* is a systemic disease that may involve the skin in one-third of individuals (Fig. 12.14). It produces red-brown plaques of the head, neck and extremities. Ninety percent of patients have lung disease. It is due to an abnormal T-cell mediated response to an unknown antigen that stimulates granuloma formation.

*Granuloma annulare* produces annular plaques, usually on the distal extremities in young adults and children (Figs 12.15A and B). The granulomas seen in granuloma annulare are remarkable for exhibiting central collagenolysis (so called "necrobiosis").

*Foreign bodies* inserted into the skin can produce a granulomatous reaction. Nevertheless, the most common foreign body giant cell reaction of the skin represents a response to keratin extruded from ruptured hair follicles and cysts (Fig. 12.16).

*Infectious granulomas* often contain collections of neutrophils at their centers (Fig. 12.17). Neutrophils in granulomas should prompt consideration of atypical mycobacteria and sporotrichosis.

## Vesiculobullous/Blistering Dermatitis

This group of vesiculobullous/blistering diseases includes several immunologically mediated diseases. The most important of which are: (a) bullous pemphigoid; (b) pemphigus vulgaris and (c) dermatitis herpetiformis.

*Bullous pemphigoid* is primarily seen in elderly individuals and manifests with tense blisters that usually spare mucous membrane (Fig. 12.18). The split occurs at the dermoepidermal junction resulting in a blister roof consisting of the full thickness of the epidermis. It is usually associated with copious eosinophils and direct immunofluorescence reveals linear deposition of IgG and C3

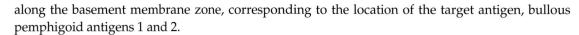

along the basement membrane zone, corresponding to the location of the target antigen, bullous pemphigoid antigens 1 and 2.

*Pemphigus vulgaris* is seen mostly in the 5th and 6th decade and produces painful flaccid blisters that form within the epidermis directly above the basal layer (Fig. 12.19). A positive Nikolsky sign can be produced by lifting the roof of the blister with extension of the blister into flanking intact skin. The oropharyngeal mucosa is often involved and direct immunofluorescence reveals a net-like pattern of IgG and C3 deposition on the exterior of keratinocytes corresponding to the target antigen, desmoglein 3.

*Dermatitis herpetiformis* produces extraordinarily pruritic papules in groups, particularly on the buttocks, elbows, knees and dorsal forearms. Direct immunofluorescence reveals granular deposits of IgA at the tips of the dermal papillae (Fig. 12.20).

## Infections and Infestations

Skin infections can be caused by any living pathogen, but most of them are caused by: (a) bacteria; (b) viruses; (c) fungi and (d) arthropods.

### Bacterial Infections

*Impetigo* is the most common bacterial infection of the skin and is due to *Staphylococcus aureus*. It is mostly seen in children and produces honey-colored crusts, usually of the face and extremities.

### Viral Infections

*Herpes simplex 1, herpes simplex 2 and varicella-zoster virus* produce painful vesicular eruptions (Figs 12.21A and B). They are histopathologically identical and are separated primarily by their anatomic distribution. The HSV1 affects the oral mucosa and lip, HSV2 affects the genitalia and VZV affects the face, trunk and extremities upon initial infection (chicken pox) and then may recur in a dermatomal distribution, usually on the trunk (shingles).

*Molluscum contagiosum (MC)* is seen in children and young adults and produces umbilicated papules (Figs 12.22A and B). It is transmitted by direct contact and caused by the MC virus. The virus accumulates in the cytoplasms of keratinocytes and forms eosinophilic molluscum bodies visible on a direct smear prepared from a papule.

*Verrucae/warts* are caused by human papillomavirus. More than 80 genotypes of HPV are recognized and associated with specific types of verrucae. *Verruca vulgaris*, or common warts, may be seen anywhere, but are common on the hands and other sites of trauma (Figs 12.23A and B). They produce firm hyperkeratotic elevated papules with loss of the skin markings (dermatoglyphs) and are caused by HPV types 1, 2 and 4. Keratinocytes with haloed hyperchromatic nuclei called koilocytes are often seen. *Verruca plantaris* or *palmoplantar* warts are caused by HPV types 1, 2, 4, 60, 63 and 65, and produce painful papules often situated at pressure points (Figs 12.24A and B).

### Fungal Infections

*Tinea* (ringworm) is caused by dermatophytes, filamentous fungi that include the genera *Trichophyton*, *Epidermophyton*, and *Microsporum* (Figs 12.25A and B). Dermatophytes colonize the cornified layer of the skin and produce expanding erythematous (red-pink) plaques studded with pustules and a raised annular border.

*Tinea versicolor* is caused by species of *Malassezia* and produces multiple flat, minimally scaly tan patches on the trunk (Fig. 12.26).

### Arthropods

*Scabies* is due to infestation of the skin by *Sarcoptes scabiei* (Fig. 12.27). It affects the genitalia, finger web spaces, belt area, buttocks, umbilicus, postauricular area and feet, and produces intractable pruritus that is worse at night. Only 10–15 mites are usually present at a time, so it is difficult to capture a mite in a biopsy, but signs of infestation, such as eosinophils, excoriations, egg casings and scybala (bug poop), can point to the right diagnosis.

*Arthropod bites* can be caused by a plethora of insects including mosquitoes, fleas, bedbugs and chiggers **(Figs 12.28A and B)**. They produce pruritic excoriated erythematous papules, usually on the extremities and usually in groups. Biopsies of arthropod bites are often centered on adnexa and contain eosinophils with deposition of fibrin on reticular collagen bundles.

## Neoplasms

Skin neoplasms may develop from: (a) epidermal cells; (b) melanocytes; (c) mesenchymal cells and (d) hematolymphoid cells. Epidermal cell tumors account for the vast majority of all skin neoplasms.

### Epidermal Neoplasms

*Seborrheic keratoses* are hyperpigmented raised tumors seen in adults and the elderly people. They have a stuck-on appearance and are limited to hair-bearing skin with a predilection for the upper back and extremities **(Fig. 12.29)**. Careful inspection with a hand lens will reveal white dots corresponding to the openings of the infundibular tunnels that produce the horn cysts seen in slide preparations. Seborrheic keratoses are benign.

*Basal cell carcinomas* are the most common malignant neoplasms of the skin **(Figs 12.30A and B)**. They have a predilection for the face, especially the nose. Most basal cells carcinomas have mutated *PTCH* and/or *p53* gene mutations that are due to solar UV damage. Although commonly thought of as epidermal tumors, basal cell carcinomas differentiate toward various parts of the hair follicle and are thought by some to be adnexal tumors. Several histological subtypes of basal cell carcinoma have been described. Nodular and superficial basal cell carcinomas are relatively indolent subtypes that form raised pearly nodules with telangiectasias and erythematous dermatitis-like plaques respectively. Infiltrating, sclerosing/morpheaform and micronodular subtypes of basal cell carcinoma form scar-like plaques and are more locally aggressive. Although basal cell carcinomas can produce extensive damage to the surrounding tissue, they almost never metastasize.

*Actinic keratoses* are scaly erythematous plaques of sun-damaged skin that are often felt more easily than seen **(Fig. 12.31)**. They are caused by mutation of the tumor suppressor gene *p53* by solar irradiation; hence its alternate term is "solar keratosis". Actinic keratoses are precursors to squamous cell carcinoma.

*Squamous cell carcinoma* is the second most common malignant neoplasm of the skin and produces keratotic or ulcerated nodules that have more substance than actinic keratoses **(Fig. 12.32)**. They rarely metastasize (significantly less than 1% in the author's experience), but squamous cell carcinomas of the lip, ear, sun-protected skin, within pre-existing scars or immunosuppressed individuals are at a higher risk.

### Melanocytic Neoplasms

Melanocytic neoplasms may be benign or malignant. The most important lesions are: (a) lentigines; (b) nevi and (c) melanoma.

*Lentigines* produce nonpalpable hyperpigmented macules and are due to hyperpigmentation of elongated rete ridges with a slight increase in individual melanocytes.

*Nevi* are nested proliferations of melanocytes that may be limited to the epidermis (junctional nevus), dermis (intradermal nevus) or both epidermis and dermis (compound nevus) **(Figs 12.33A and B)**. Congenital nevi are often present at birth, although many smaller nevi may exhibit a histologic congenital pattern despite the absence of a congenital history. Acquired nevi accumulate progressively in number over the first three decades and then steadily regress. The "dysplastic" or "atypical" nevus has produced more controversy than any other topic in dermatopathology. Most experts accept

| Table 12.1: Criteria for distinguishing nevus from melanoma ||
| Nevus | Melanoma |
| --- | --- |
| Small surface diameter | Large surface diameter |
| No evidence of sun damage | Signs of sun damage (solar elastosis) |
| Equal number of melanocytes in either half | More melanocytes on one side |
| Epidermal changes symmetric in either half | Epidermis different in two halves |
| Edges of lesion similar | Edges of lesion dissimilar |
| Pigmentation equal in either half | Pigmentation asymmetric |
| Melanocytes become smaller at base | Melanocytes are atypical at base |
| Small, uniform melanocytes | Large, pleomorphic melanocytes |
| Inconspicuous nucleoli | Large prominent nucleoli |
| Fine nuclear membranes | Thick nuclear membranes |
| Dermal mitoses rare/absent | Dermal mitoses present |
| Brown granular melanin pigment | Fine gray melanin pigment |

its existence as a distinct type of nevus, but it is not a precursor to melanoma, and its clinical significance lies primarily in distinguishing it from melanoma **(Table 12.1)**.

*Melanoma* is the most feared malignant neoplasm of the skin **(Figs 12.34A and B)**. The incidence has tripled in the past three decades, although some of the increase is likely due to increased recognition of early melanomas. Risk factors for melanoma include fair skin, signs of sun damage, a history of childhood sunburns, family or personal history of melanoma and more than 50 nevi or more than five atypical nevi. Melanomas are traditionally identified by the *ABCD criteria* of Asymmetry, irregular Borders, variation in Color and enlarging Diameter. Unfortunately, many benign nevi will exhibit these characteristics and many melanomas will lack them. The "ugly duckling" technique of examination takes advantage of the fact that most individuals have fairly uniform-appearing nevi. Any nevi that significantly differ from the patient's background population of nevi are usually sampled to exclude melanoma. Prognosis in melanoma is dependant on the Breslow thickness, which is the measurement from the granular layer to the point of deepest invasion. Melanomas that measure less than 1 mm in thickness are considered "thin melanomas" and are unlikely to metastasize.

Three basic subtypes of melanoma exist, which are thought to be derived from different populations of melanocytic stem cells. These subtypes are known as: (a) lentigo maligna; (b) superficial spreading melanoma and (c) nodular melanoma.

*Lentigo maligna* is the most common and most indolent form of melanoma. It is probably derived from melanocytic stem cells of the hair follicle and is seen in sun-damaged skin of the face and neck of elderly individuals.

*Superficial spreading melanoma* is probably derived from epidermal melanocytic stem cells, associated with solar irradiation, seen in middle-aged adults, with a predilection for the trunk in men and the legs in women, and associated with an intermediate prognosis.

*Nodular melanomas* are hypothesized to arise from dermal melanocytic stem cells, are less closely associated with solar irradiation and are the most aggressive subtype.

### Mesenchymal Neoplasms

There are numerous mesenchymal skin tumors, but we will discuss only a few examples.

*Dermatofibromas* are benign tumors derived from collagen-forming dermal dendrocytes **(Fig. 12.35)**. They are often located on the lower extremities. Squeezing the skin overlying a dermatofibroma may cause downward displacement of the lesion, the so-called "dimple sign". The pathogenesis of dermatofibromas is unknown, although some have postulated an unusual fibrosing reaction to the bite of an arthropod. Dermatofibromas-induced hyperpigmentation of the overlying epidermis is sometimes biopsied to rule out melanoma.

*Neurofibromas* are benign proliferations of nerve elements including Schwann cells, fibrocytes, mast cells and perineural cells **(Figs 12.36A and B)**. They are mostly sporadic, although multiple cutaneous neurofibromas are seen in neurofibromatosis. Neurofibromas are skin-colored nodules with a soft consistency.

*Pyogenic granulomas* are red nodules comprised of a lobular proliferation of capillaries and myxoid stroma. They often bleed copiously and are mostly seen on the gingiva, lip and fingers of children and young adults **(Fig. 12.37)**.

*Skin tags* (acrochordon and soft fibroma) are common polypoid excrescences seen on the eyelids, axillae, groins, neck and trunk. They increase in number with age and are due to localized overgrowth of dermal connective tissue.

## Hematolymphoid Neoplasms

*Hematolymphoid neoplasms* originate from mobile blood derived cells residing in the skin. Three most salient examples of tumors belonging to this group are discussed here.

*Juvenile xanthogranuloma* is the most common histiocytic proliferation and is mostly seen in infants and children **(Fig. 12.38)**. It produces a yellowish nodule due to a circumscribed, nonencapsulated proliferation of histiocytes in the dermis. Touton giant cells with peripherally xanthomatized cytoplasms are characteristic. Juvenile xanthogranulomas spontaneously involute over 3–6 years.

*Mastocytosis* can produce a solitary brown nodule (mastocytoma, mostly found in the children), multiple brown plaques (urticaria pigmentosa, mostly found in the children) or widely disseminated hyperpigmented papules with telangiectasias (telangiectasia macularis eruptiva, mostly found in the adults) **(Figs 12.39A to C)**. Rubbing a lesion of mastocytosis may cause it to urticate, the Darier sign. Mastocytosis in children is usually self-limited with spontaneous resolution, but in adults it may be persistent and associated with systemic disease.

*Mycosis fungoides* is a T-cell lymphoma of the skin **(Fig. 12.40)**. It produces erythematous patches and scaly atrophic plaques with a predilection for sun-protected skin, particularly the "double-covered" sites such as the buttocks. It is an indolent lymphoma with a characteristic waxing and waning course. Most cases have been present for many years prior to diagnosis.

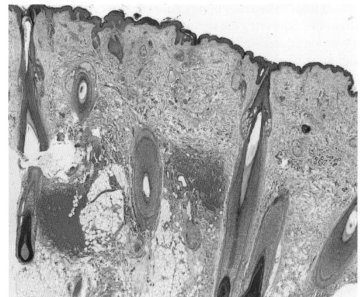

**Fig 12.1:** Normal skin

The integument consists of the *epidermis* which is comprised of keratinocytes, the *dermis* which comprised mostly of collagenic fibers and contains small (vellus) hair follicles, sebaceous glands, and blood vessels, and the *subcutaneum* which is comprised of lipocytes and contains large (terminal) hair follicles and the secretory segment of sweat glands.

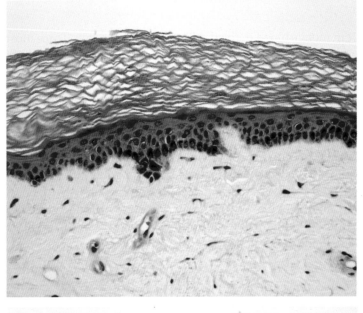

**Fig. 12.2:** Ichthyosis vulgaris

This disease is easily mistaken for normal skin. The absence of the granular layer is a useful clue to the diagnosis.

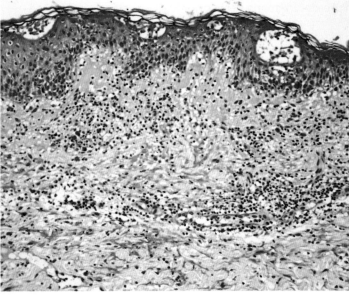

**Fig. 12.3:** Allergic contact dermatitis

The skin exhibits extreme spongiosis leading to formation of intraepidermal vesicles containing lymphocytes, Langerhans cells and eosinophils.

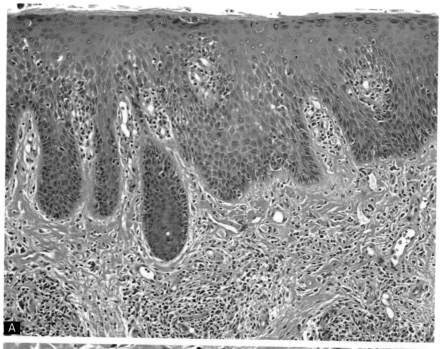

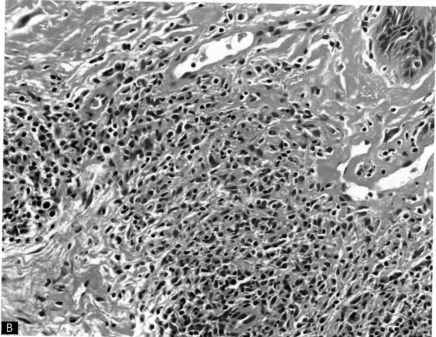

**Figs 12.4A and B:** Atopic dermatitis
**A.** Spongiosis is less obvious in this chronic spongiotic dermatitis characterized by uneven thickening of the epidermis, a fairly dense superficial infiltrate of lymphocytes and eosinophils, and coarsening of papillary collagen. **B.** The eosinophils and fibrovascular thickening of the dermis are a response to chronic rubbing.

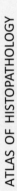

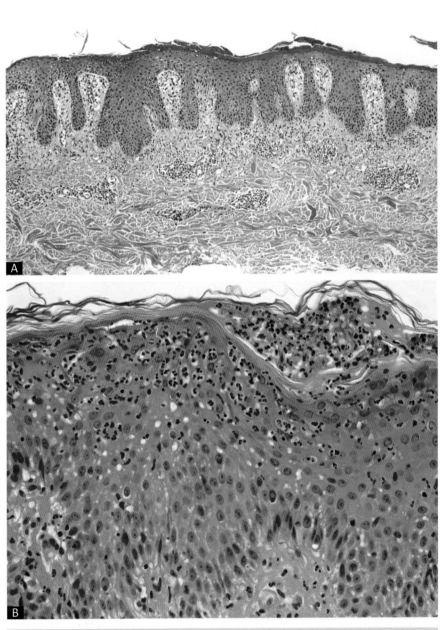

**Figs 12.5A and B:** Psoriasis

**A.** The rete ridges are evenly elongated, squared off and fused at the tips. The dermal papillae are edematous and contain dilated venules with stacks of erythrocytes. There is loss of space between the papillary venules and the base of the overlying epidermal arc. Neutrophils migrate into the epidermis and scale, where they accumulate atop scales in *Munro collections* and between necrotic keratinocytes in *Kogoj collections.* Eosinophils are scarce or absent. **B.** A Kogoj collection consists of neutrophils interspersed between superficial necrotic keratinocytes.

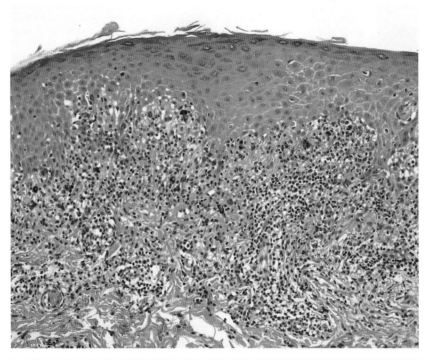

**Fig. 12.6:** Lichen planus

A dense infiltrate of lymphocytes hugs the dermoepidermal junction. The epidermis exhibits sawtooth-pattern acanthosis, wedge-shaped hypergranulosis and dense eosinophilic cytoplasmic keratin (so-called "squamatization"). The eosinophils in this example are unusual and should prompt consideration of a lichenoid drug eruption.

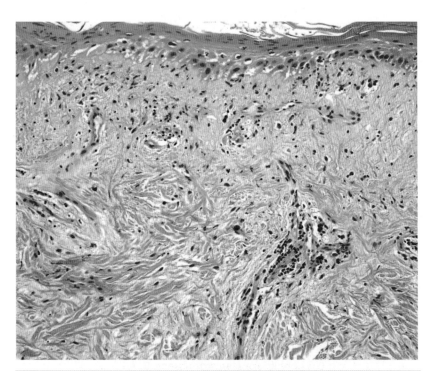

**Fig. 12.7:** Lupus erythematosus

This is a *vacuolar interface dermatitis* in which damage to the basal layer occurs without a band-like infiltrate of inflammatory cells. The pale blue mucin in the interstitial space is a useful clue to lupus erythematosus.

THE SKIN

CHAPTER

**12**

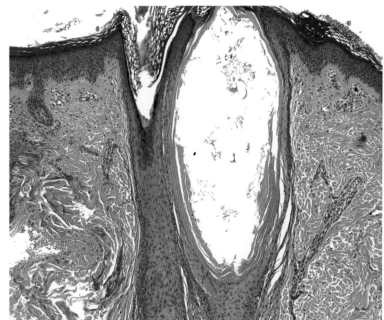

**Fig. 12.8:** Acne vulgaris
The initial event in acne vulgaris is the formation of a *comedone*— a dilated hair follicle with retained keratin and sebaceous debris.

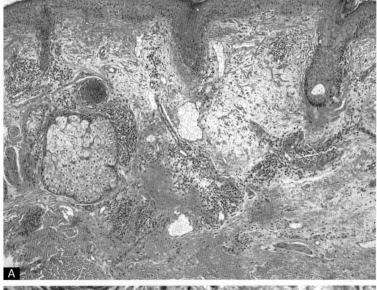

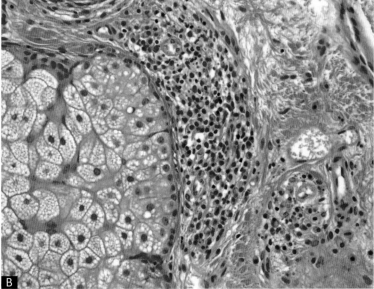

**Figs 12.9A and B:** Acne rosacea
**A**. Unlike acne vulgaris, comedones are not seen in rosacea. Instead there is perifollicular and peri-sebaceous lymphoplasmacytic dermatitis with telangiectasias and dermal edema. **B.** Note the frequent plasma cells in the inflammatory infiltrate.

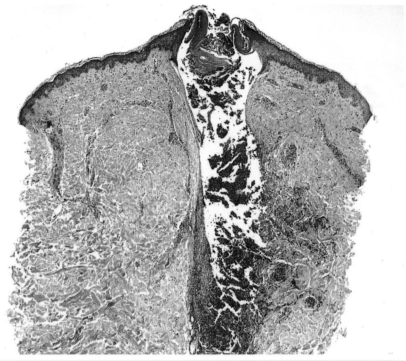

**Fig. 12.10:** Infectious folliculitis

A hair follicle is massively distended by neutrophils, leading to rupture at its edge and formation of a perifollicular abscess. *Staphylococcus aureus* was the culprit in this case, although similar changes are seen in infectious folliculitis due to *Pseudomonas* and *Pityrosporum*, and in the sterile folliculitis seen in some drug reactions.

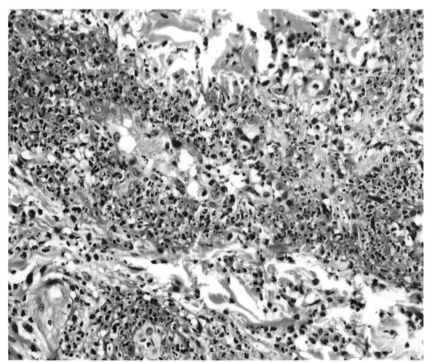

**Fig. 12.11:** Leukocytoclastic vasculitis

Signs of small vessel/leukocytoclastic vasculitis include a neutrophil-predominant infiltrate with perivascular hemorrhage, fragmentation of neutrophils (*leukocytoclasis*), swelling of endothelial cells, neutrophil fragments within vessel walls and fibrin deposition within vessel walls.

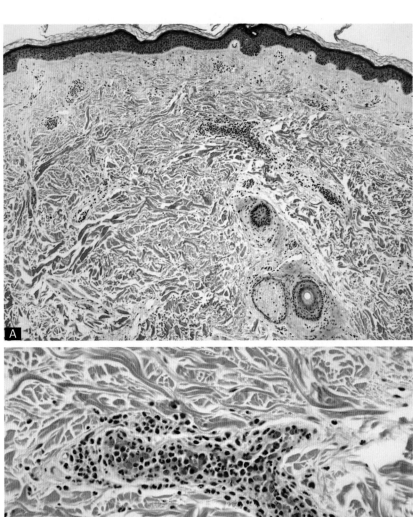

**Figs 12.12A and B:** Urticaria

**A.** The changes in urticaria can be deceptively subtle. Most of the clinical changes are due to tissue edema, which is not well demonstrated in histologic preparations. **B.** The vessels in urticaria are often abnormally dilated and house increased numbers of neutrophils and eosinophils. However, signs of vascular injury, such as perivascular hemorrhage or fibrin deposition in the vessel wall, are not present.

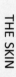

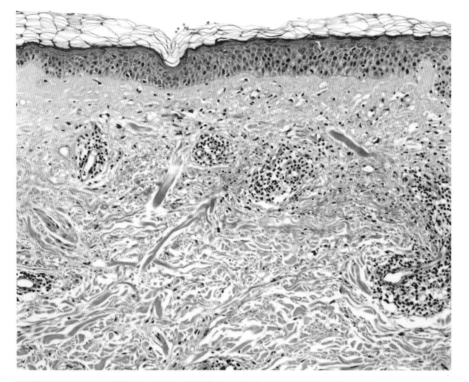

**Fig. 12.13:** Morbilliform drug reaction

Drug reactions are often subtle and may be mistaken for normal skin. A superficial infiltrate, particularly one associated with vacuolization of basal keratinocytes, eosinophils or extravasation of erythrocytes, is a clue to a drug reaction. The differential diagnosis includes a viral exanthem.

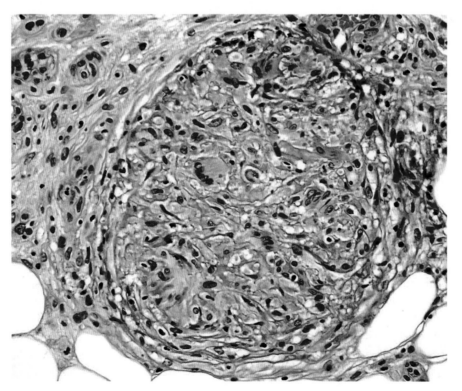

**Fig. 12.14:** Sarcoidosis

The "naked" granulomas of sarcoidosis are comprised predominantly of histiocytic uninucleate and multinucleate cells without a peripheral ring of lymphocytes.

THE SKIN

CHAPTER
**12**

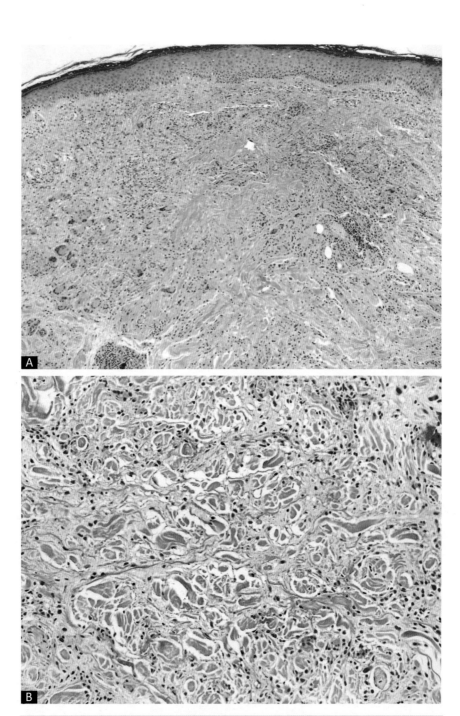

**Figs 12.15A and B:** Granuloma annulare

**A.** Although the epidermis is normal, the dermis is expanded by a nodular infiltrate of histiocytes that encircle degenerating collagenic fibers. This is colloquially called "necrobiosis". **B.** The granulomas are grouped around areas of collagenolysis. This is a "blue" granuloma because collagenolysis is associated with formation of interstitial mucin. The granulomas are comprised mostly of histiocytes, with few giant cells. Although eosinophils are often seen, plasma cells are absent.

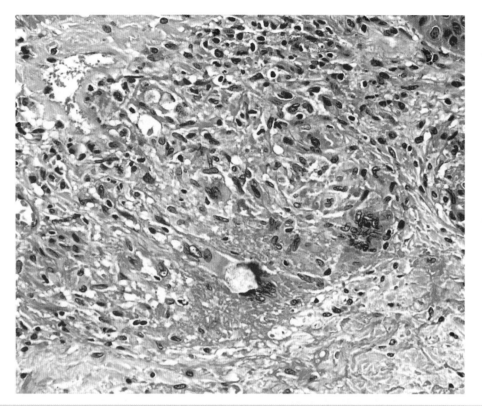

**Fig. 12.16:** Foreign body granuloma
Foreign body granulomas often consist of tightly packed histiocytes and giant cells, and may mimic sarcoidosis. Examination by polarized light microscopy may reveal birefringent material.

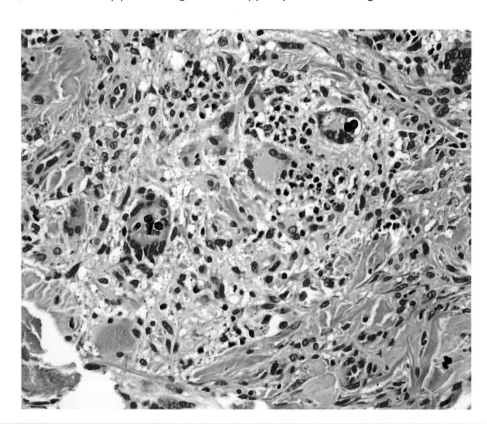

**Fig. 12.17:** Chromoblastomycosis
This is an example of an infectious granuloma. Granulomas with neutrophils suggest infection or a reaction to a ruptured hair follicle. Note the brown ovoid *Medlar bodies* that are specific for chromoblastomycosis.

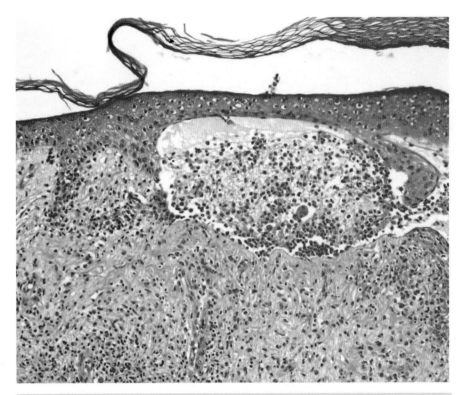

**Fig. 12.18:** Bullous pemphigoid

In this immunobullous disease, the epidermis has lifted off the dermis to form a *subepidermal blister*. The blister cavity often contains eosinophils.

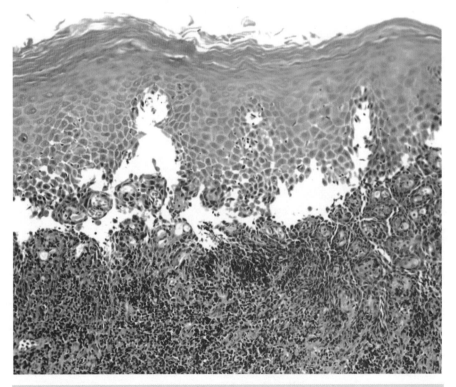

**Fig. 12.19:** Pemphigus vulgaris

The blister forms within the lower layers of the epidermis, with preservation of the papillary pattern at the base of the blister, which is lined by attached basal keratinocytes (a *suprabasilar blister*). Round keratinocytes called *acantholytic cells* are seen in the blister space, which may or may not contain eosinophils.

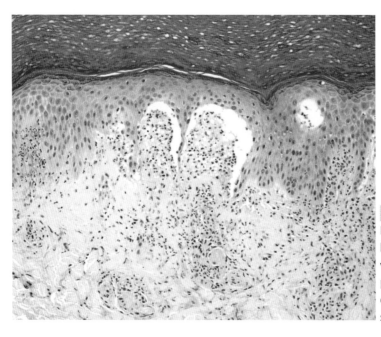

**Fig. 12.20:** Dermatitis herpetiformis In this extremely pruritic immuno-bullous disease, small subepidermal vesicles containing copious neutro-phils are aggregated at the tips of dermal papillae and associated with small subepidermal blisters.

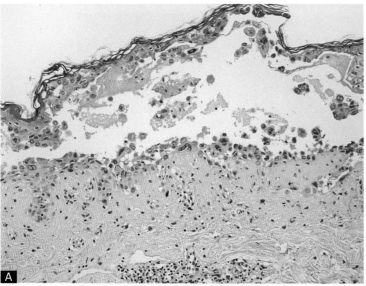

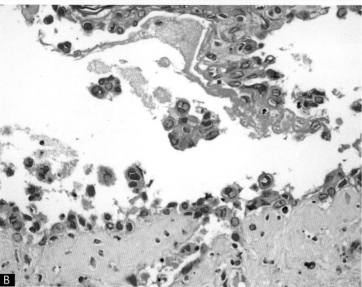

**Figs 12.21A and B:** Herpes simplex **A.** Intraepidermal vesicle contain-ing clusters of ballooned keratino-cytes infected by HSV1. **B.** Multinuc-leated ballooned keratinocytes with "gun-metal gray" nuclei with peri-pheral margination of their chro-matin.

THE SKIN

CHAPTER

**12**

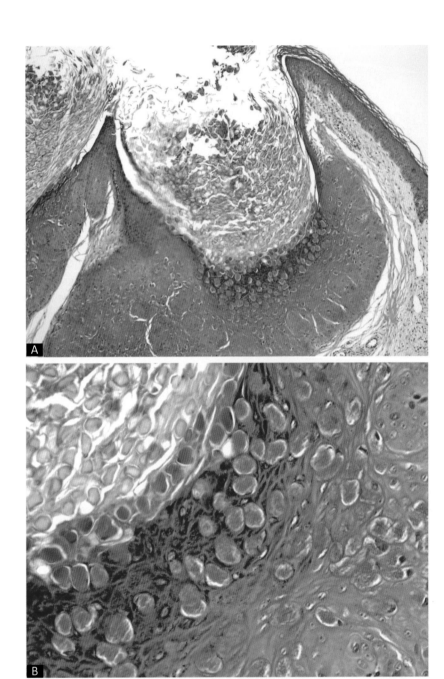

**Figs 12.22A and B:** Molluscum contagiosum
**A.** Infection by this poxvirus produces an umbilicated dell in the epidermis. Molluscum bodies are most numerous in the granular and cornifying layers.
**B.** *Molluscum bodies* are cytoplasmic eosinophilic bodies that are divided into small packets by septa and squeeze the nucleus to one side of the cell.

**12**

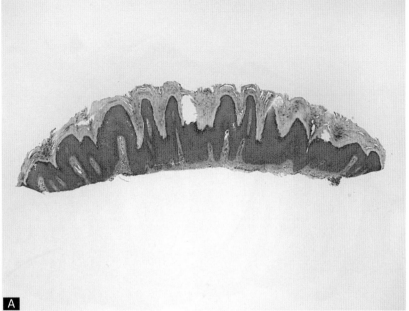

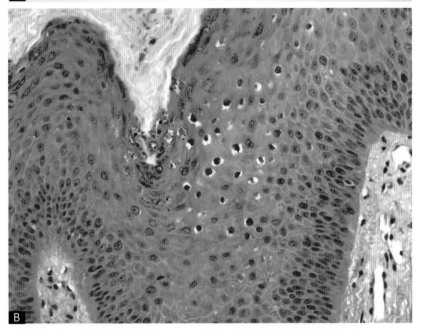

**Figs 12.23A and B:** Common wart

**A.** Infection by human papillomavirus induces rounded to pointed epidermal papillomatosis with a thick blue-staining cornified layer and inward bowing of the rete ridges. **B.** Clues to human papillomavirus infection include *koilocytes* and *hypergranulosis*.

THE SKIN

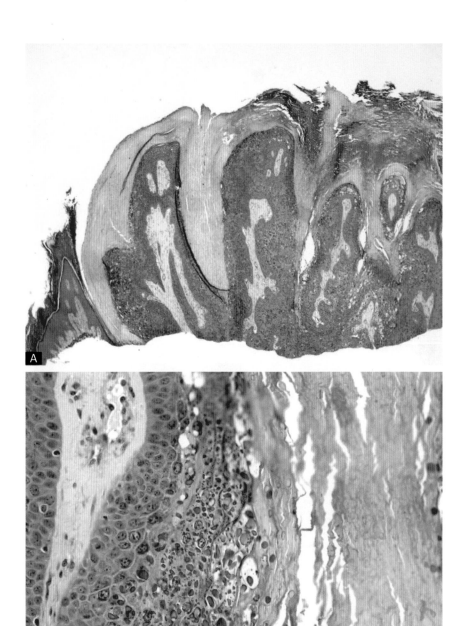

**Figs 12.24A and B:** Palmoplantar wart

**A.** Warts on palmar or plantar skin induce marked papillomatous hyperplasia of the epidermis with a thick blue-staining cornified layer and inward bowing of the rete ridges. **B.** Human papillomavirus cytopathic effect is particularly prominent in palmoplantar warts, where they induce marked hypergranulosis with pink keratohyaline intracytoplasmic bodies and rounded parakeratosis.

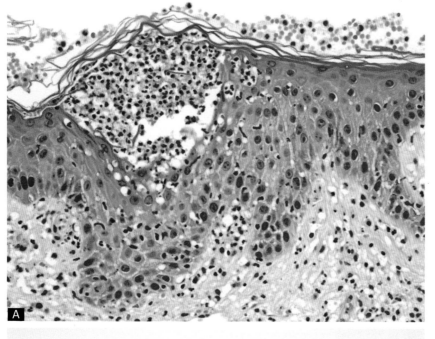

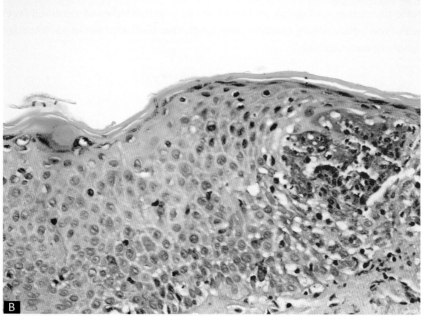

**Figs 12.25A and B:** Tinea corporis

**A.** A subcorneal pustule with neutrophils is often a clue to tinea/dermatophytosis. Careful inspection of the cornified layer to the right will reveal a few punched out spaces corresponding to tangentially sectioned hyphae at the base of the cornified layer. **B.** Periodic acid-Schiff (PAS) staining highlights the fungal hyphae within the cornifying layer.

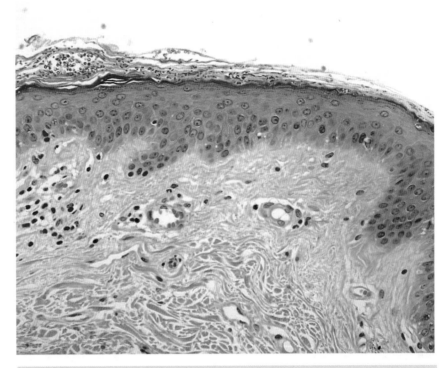

**Fig. 12.26:** Tinea versicolor

Note the numerous hyphae and yeast in the slightly thickened cornified layer with little inflammatory reaction. The fungi have been compared to "*chopped spaghetti and meatballs*".

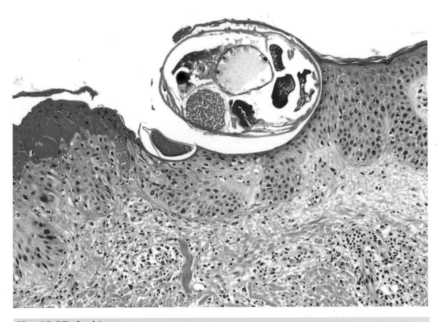

**Fig. 12.27:** Scabies

Scabies mites burrow just below the cornified layer. Be careful not to confuse the much more common and usually innocuous Demodex mite with scabies. Demodex mites are seen within hair follicles of normal skin, particularly of oily skin such as the face. Scabies mites spare the follicles and roam the epidermis, sometimes leaving ova, egg casings and fecal detritus (scybala).

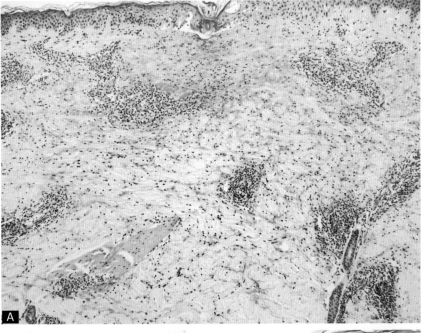

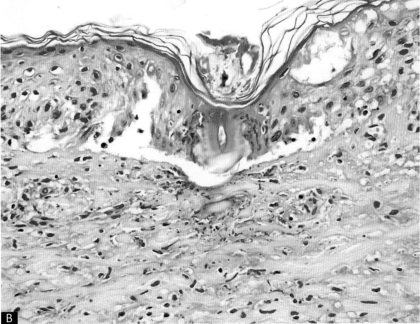

**Figs 12.28A and B:** Chigger bite

**A.** Arthropod bites usually produce an inflammatory infiltrate that extends deep into the dermis and includes either eosinophils or neutrophils. There is often interstitial mucin, edema and fibrin, and bites are often located near adnexa. **B.** The mouthparts of the arthropod were fortuitously captured in the biopsy. Arthropod mouthparts are deeply eosinophilic and sometimes associated with a basophilic cement-like substance that helps them adhere to the skin and creates a physical channel for ingesting dissolved human tissue.

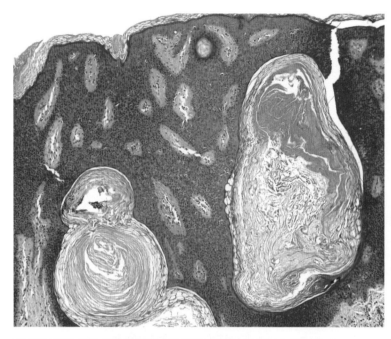

**Fig. 12.29:** Seborrheic keratosis
Seborrheic keratoses are comprised of small basaloid cells that form ramifying struts and infundibular *pseudohorn cysts* containing circular lamellae of orthokeratin.

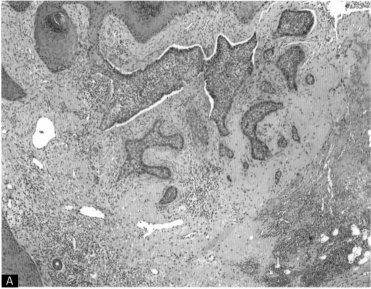

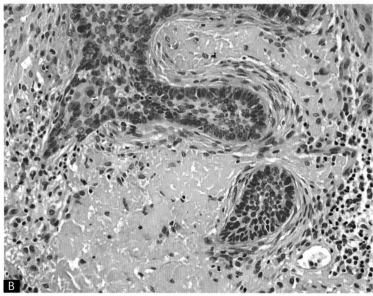

**Figs 12.30A and B:** Basal cell carcinoma
**A.** This is the most common malignant neoplasm in humans. Basal cell carcinomas form rounded or infiltrating aggregations of dark blue cells which connect with the epidermis. *Separation artifact* between tumor nodules and the surrounding stroma is a helpful clue to the diagnosis. **B.** The cells at the edges of the tumor aggregations line up in a *palisade*. Basal cell carcinomas possess a unique azure fibromyxoid stroma peripheral to the tumor aggregates that can facilitate distinction from innocent hair follicles.

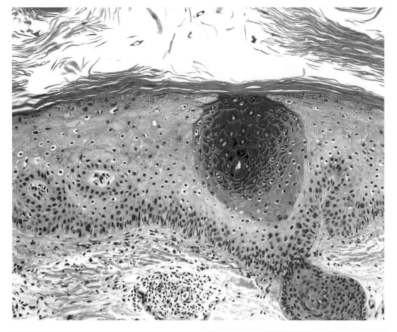

**Fig. 12.31:** Actinic keratosis

The affected epidermis keratinizes abnormally into parakeratin. Since the adnexal stem cells are deeper in the skin, they are more resistant to the effects of solar irradiation and the adnexal epithelium is spared. This leads to a skipping pattern of parakeratosis with intervening zones of blue-colored normal orthokeratin, a helpful clue—the *flag sign*. Note the prominent *solar elastosis*. Always make sure there are signs of sun damage prior to diagnosing actinic keratosis.

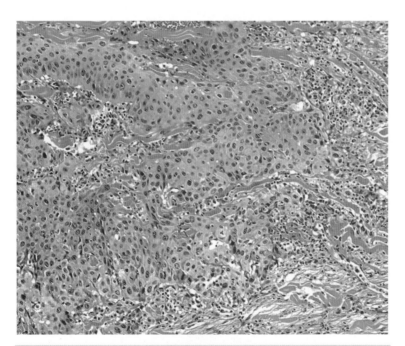

**Fig. 12.32:** Squamous cell carcinoma

The tumor is comprised of cell with large pleomorphic nuclei and arranged in variably shaped aggregates that infiltrate into the dermis.

THE SKIN

CHAPTER
**12**

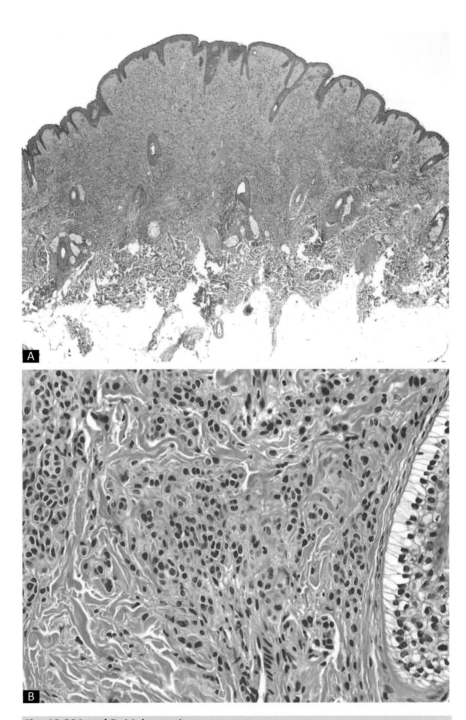

**Figs 12.33A and B:** Melanocytic nevus

**A.** This intradermal melanocytic nevus is comprised of small nests of melanocytes that have small, uniform nuclei and become smaller toward the base. **B.** Melanocytes in nevi differ from lymphocytes by exhibiting a tendency toward clustering into nests, and paler and more irregular nuclei than lymphocytes.

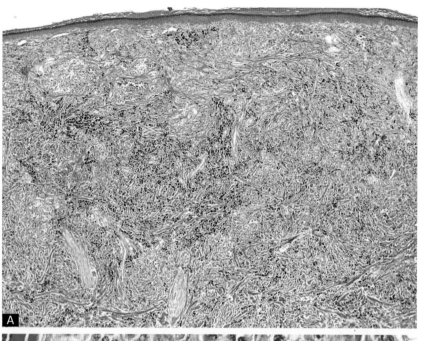

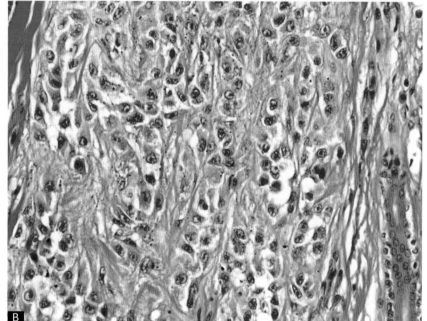

**Figs 12.34A and B:** Melanoma

**A.** This nodular melanoma is comprised of confluent sheets of melanocytes which do not break into smaller groups at the base and have an asymmetric pigment distribution (more pigment on left than the right). **B.** The melanocytes of melanoma have enlarged nuclei with brick-red nucleoli and show preservation of melanin pigment formation in the deep portions of the lesion. Mitoses and foci of necrosis are easily found.

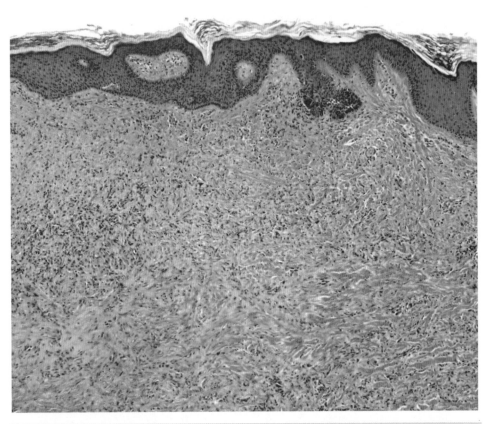

**Fig. 12.35:** Dermatofibroma

In this intradermal tumor, there is a proliferation of fibrocytes with entrapment of eosinophilic collagen bundles at the periphery of the lesion. There may be hyperplasia of hyperpigmented rete ridges overlying the dermatofibroma, leading to misdiagnosis as a lentigo or melanocytic nevus if the dermal changes are not recognized.

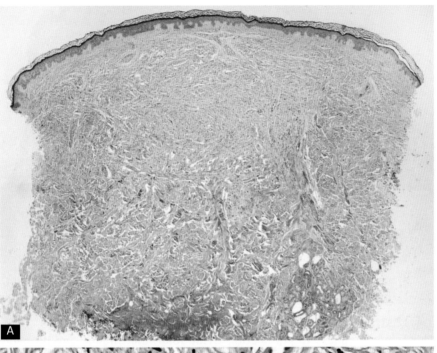

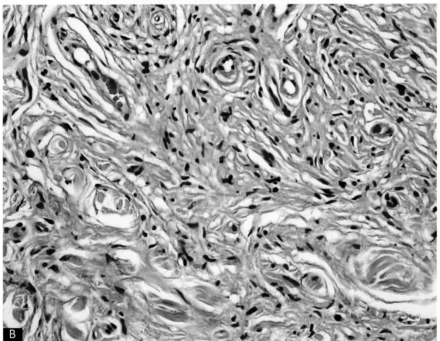

**Figs 12.36A and B:** Neurofibroma

**A.** This dermal proliferation of spindled cells is comprised of Schwann cells, perineural cells, fibrocytes, axons and mast cells. The wavy nuclei, minimal collagenization, and admixed mast cells and mucin help to differentiate it from a dermatofibroma. **B.** Schwann cells with wavy buckled nuclei and tapered eosinophilic cytoplasms comprise the bulk of the tumor.

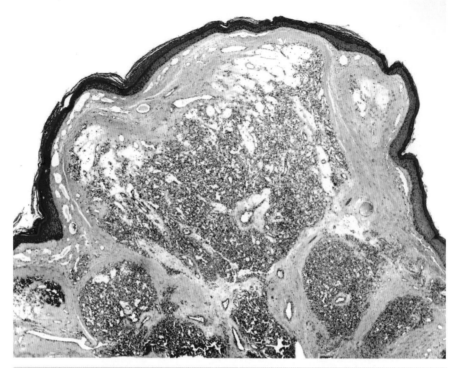

**Fig. 12.37:** Pyogenic granuloma

This tumor is similar to granulation tissue following trauma, and probably represent an abnormal vascular reaction to injury. The lobulated architecture and peripheral collarette of epidermis differentiate it from simple granulation tissue.

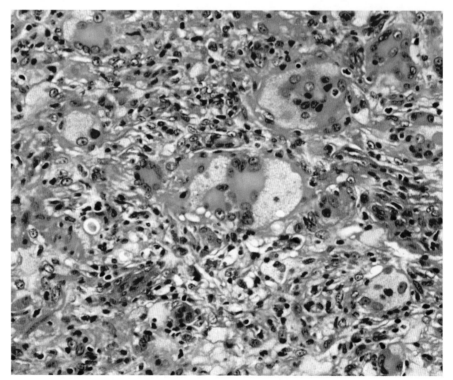

**Fig. 12.38:** Juvenile xanthogranuloma

This tumor consists of a mixed proliferation of histiocytes, lymphocytes and eosinophils. Xanthogranulomas have a yellow hue due to the lipidized histiocytes. *Touton giant cells* with a ring of nuclei and peripherally xanthomatized cytoplasms are characteristic of the lesion.

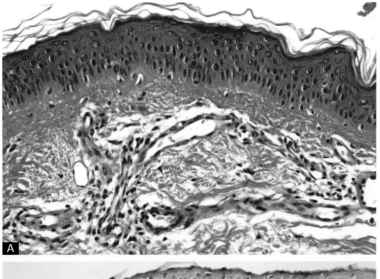

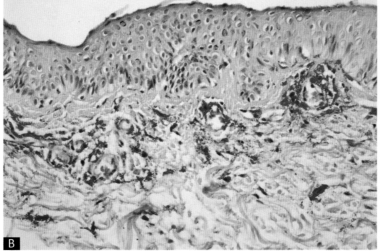

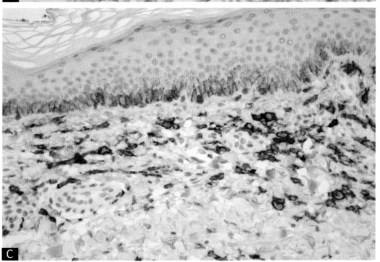

**Figs 12.39A to C:** Mastocytosis

**A.** The mast cells are easily overlooked in this example of adult mastocytosis, *telangiectasia macularis eruptiva perstans*. **B.** The mast cells are highlighted in red with Leder's histochemical preparation. **C.** Mast cells can also be highlighted with CD117 immunohistochemistry.

CHAPTER

**12**

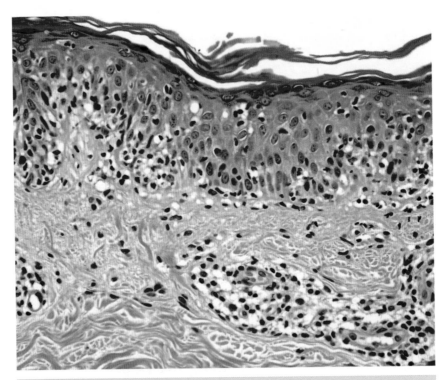

**Fig. 12.40:** Mycosis fungoides

Diagnosis of mycosis fungoides depends heavily upon correlation with the clinical findings, patient history and generous biopsies. This example highlights the disproportionate exocytosis of *epidermotropic T-cells* into the epidermis, where they line up along the dermoepidermal junction. Intraepidermal T-cells in mycosis fungoides are often surrounded by a halo and may be slightly larger, darker and more convoluted than the reactive lymphocytes in the underlying dermis.

# 13 Bones, Joints and Soft Tissues

*Katie L Dennis, Fang Fan*

## Introduction

*The bones, joints and soft tissues constitute the main portion of the solid body mass. They provide the support and the protection to other organs and enable the body to move. In this chapter we will discuss the most important histopathologic changes involving the bones and joints, and also review the most common soft tissue tumors.*

## Bones

Bones are made of the organic matrix (osteoid) and mineral calcium hydroxyapatite, which make them hard and imparts them strength. Bones provide not only the body framework but also support and protect other organs. Bones also provide the microenvironment for hematopoiesis, and are the major store for calcium and phosphates, thus playing a role in mineral homeostasis.

Bones consist of several cell types; the most important are: (a) pluripotent mesenchymal cells; (b) osteoblasts; (c) osteocytes; (d) osteoclasts (Fig. 13.1). Pluripotent mesenchymal stem cells are osteoprogenitor cells which under proper stimulation may differentiate into bone forming cells called *osteoblasts*. Osteoblasts are located on the surface of the bone trabeculae and cortical bone. Osteoblasts synthesize bone matrix proteins and initiate bone mineralization. With time they become surrounded by newly formed osteoid, whereupon they become *osteocytes*. Osteoblasts remaining on the bone surface appear flattened and are also called bone lining cells. *Osteoclasts* are large macrophage-derived multinucleated giant cells with abundant cytoplasm responsible for bone resorption.

The most important bone disorders are:
- Developmental disorders
- Metabolic disorders
- Inflammation
- Neoplasms.

### Developmental Disorders

During bone development osteoblasts initially produce *woven bone* which is then remodeled into mature *lamellar bone*. The majority of bones are developed via *endochondral ossification*, preceded by formation of cartilage, which is then progressively replaced by bone. The bones of the skull vault, the maxilla and the mandible are formed by the direct deposition of bone in mesenchymal tissues in a process known as *intramembranous ossification*. Bone development is controlled by growth hormone, thyroid hormones and sex hormones. Parathyroid hormone (PTH) also acts on osteoblasts and indirectly on osteoclasts.

Developmental abnormalities belong to the group of genetic diseases which typically become symptomatic during early stages of life. Numerous genetic abnormalities may affect bone formation and are the underlying cause of diseases such as achondroplasia, osteogenesis imperfecta, osteopetrosis and several others. Histologic changes in these diseases are mostly nonspecific and nondiagnostic.

*Osteopetrosis* is a group of rare genetic diseases characterized by deficient osteoclast function leading to reduced bone resorption and diffuse bone sclerosis. It is also known as "marble bone disease" because the bones have a stone-like quality; but they are abnormally brittle and fracture easily. Osteopetrosis occurs in an autosomal dominant and an autosomal recessive form, and the disease may clinically present with varying severity. Histologically, the bone lacks a medullary canal and is filled with primary spongiosa. Osteoclasts may be normal, increased or decreased depending on the underlying genetic defect. Deposited bone is not remodeled and tends to be woven instead of forming mature trabeculae in architecture **(Fig. 13.2)**.

### Metabolic Disorders

Metabolic disease may affect the bones of children or adults. In children, metabolic disorders may affect the growth and formation of bones, whereas in the adult these disorders usually change the structure of bones and lead to bone remodeling or deformities, or cause bone fragility leading to increased incidence of fractures.

*Osteoporosis* refers to a condition of reduced bone mass characterized by proportional loss of both the organic matrix (osteoid) and the mineral components of the bone. Depending on the cause, osteoporosis may be classified as *primary* or *secondary*.

*Primary osteoporosis*, which typically includes senile and postmenopausal osteoporosis, is the most common form of this disease. Thoracic and lumbar vertebral fractures are painful and may lead to significant deformity and loss of height. Histologically, the cortex is thinned; the bone trabeculae are thinned and lose their interconnections **(Fig. 13.3)**. The hypotheses about the pathogenesis of primary osteoporosis include age-related changes (reduced function of osteoblasts with aging), reduced physical activity (increased bone loss with reduced physical activity), genetic factors, and body's calcium level and hormonal effect (estrogen deficiency plays a major role in postmenopausal bone loss). *Secondary osteoporosis* may be a consequence of bone mass loss due to endocrine disorders, malnutrition and malabsorption, tumors, drugs and a variety of other diseases.

*Osteomalacia* is caused by a defect in bone matrix mineralization most commonly associated with vitamin D deficiency. Osteomalacia due to vitamin D deficiency in children, called *rickets*, affects the growth of long bones, which become soft and deformed **(Fig. 13.4A)**. In adults, osteomalacia is characterized by softening of bones which consist of predominantly uncalcified osteoid **(Fig. 13.4B)**.

*Paget disease* is a disease of unknown etiology that affects elderly persons. It is characterized by an initial osteolytic stage, followed by a mixed osteoclastic-osteoblastic stage, ending in a third "burnt-out" phase characterized by abnormal sclerosis of the bone. The microscopic hallmark of late-stage Paget's disease is the mosaic pattern of lamellar bone produced by cement lines that anneal haphazardly deposited units of lamellar bone **(Fig. 13.5)**. Most cases are mild clinically and discovered as an incidental radiologic finding, but the disease may also cause bone deformities, and represents a risk factor for late-age malignant bone tumors.

*Hyperparathyroidism* produces characteristic bone lesions. It may be *primary*, which is related to autonomous parathyroid hyperplasia or adenoma and *secondary* when the prolonged states of hypocalcemia, as in chronic renal disease, result in compensatory hypersecretion of PTH. The PTH stimulates osteoblasts to release factors that activate osteoclasts and accordingly hyperparathyroidism is characterized by unopposed osteoclastic bone resorption **(Fig. 13.6)**. Subperiosteal resorption produces thinned cortices. In cancellous bone, groups of osteoclasts tunnel into and dissect centrally along the bone trabeculae, making an appearance of railroad tracks known as *dissecting osteitis*. Generalized *osteitis fibrosa cystica* (von Recklinghausen disease) is the result of severe hyperparathyroidism. The bone loss may cause fracture and hemorrhage that elicit reactive changes forming a mass-like lesion containing macrophages, giant cells, granulation tissue and fibrous tissue, known as *"brown tumor of hyperparathyroidism"*.

## Inflammation

*Osteomyelitis*, or the inflammation of bone and marrow, is most often caused by bacteria. It may be a manifestation of systemic infection or a localized disease. Osteomyelitis is categorized as acute or chronic depending on the stage of the inflammation.

*Acute pyogenic osteomyelitis* is most often caused by *Staphylococcus aureus*, but in neonates it may be related to infection with *Escherichia coli*. In drug addicts it may be caused by *Pseudomonas aeruginosa* and in patients with sickle cell anemia is often caused by *Salmonella sp*. Microscopically it is characterized by exudates of neutrophils, sometimes associated bone necrosis and intraosseous abscess formation (Fig. 13.7).

*Chronic osteomyelitis* usually results from unresolved acute infection or it may be caused by *Mycobacterium tuberculosis* or fungi. Protracted infection usually leads to fibrosis of the medullary spaces, which also contain infiltrates of lymphocytes and plasma cells (Fig. 13.8). The adjacent bone may show remodeling and reactive changes.

## Neoplasms and Related Lesions

Primary bone tumors can be classified into several groups such as: (a) bone forming tumors; (b) cartilage forming tumors; (c) fibrous and fibro-osseous tumors and (d) miscellaneous tumors. These tumors may be benign or malignant. For the final diagnosis of bone tumors the histologic findings should always be correlated with the clinical and imaging data. Bones are often involved by metastatic tumors from primaries in other sites. Multiple myeloma originating in the bone marrow is a common tumor of older adults, and it may cause prominent destructive lesions of the bone.

*Osteomas* are round to oval nodular tumors protruding from the subperiosteal surface of the cortex. They often arise from the facial bone or within the skull. Microscopically they resemble mature bone composed of a composite of woven and lamellar bone (Fig. 13.9). Osteomas are slow growing tumors and only raise clinical concern when they cause obstruction of a sinus cavity or press against the brain or eye. Multiple osteomas are associated with Gardner syndrome.

*Osteoid osteomas* are small (< 2 cm) well-circumscribed bone-forming tumors affecting adolescents and young adults. These tumors are composed of randomly arranged osteoid and bone trabeculae rimmed by osteoblasts (Figs 13.10A and B). The osteoblasts appear morphologically benign. Osteoid osteoma may elicit marked reactive new bone formation around the lesion, making itself the nidus of the tumor. *Osteoblastomas* are morphologically identical to osteoid osteomas but larger in size (> 2 cm) and more frequently involve the spine. In contrast to osteoid osteomas they do not induce a strong bony reaction.

*Osteosarcoma* is the most common primary malignant tumor of the bone. Tumors have their peak incidence in adolescence, most often affecting the metaphysis of long bones. Two-thirds of tumors originate around the knee joint. The histologic hallmark of osteosarcoma are atypical spindle cells resembling osteoblasts. These cells form osteoid which usually undergoes ossification. The neoplastic bone/osteoid is coarse and lace-like and there are usually prominent areas of necrosis (Fig. 13.11). Osteosarcomas frequently destroy the overlying normal cortical bone and tend to extensively involve the marrow cavity.

*Chondromas* are benign tumors of hyaline cartilage. When they arise within the medullary cavity, they are called *enchondromas*. Enchondromas occur as solitary metaphyseal lesions of the short tubular bones of hands and feet. Microscopically, they are well-circumscribed nodules of hyaline cartilage containing cytologically benign chondrocytes (Fig. 13.12). The peripheral region of the tumor may undergo ossification. A syndrome of multiple enchondromas or enchondromatosis is called Ollier disease. When enchondromatosis is present with soft tissue hemangiomas, it is referred to as Maffucci syndrome.

*Chondrosarcomas* are malignant tumors containing neoplastic cartilage. They tend to occur in adults and involve the central portion of the skeleton including pelvis, shoulder and ribs. Histologically they are divided into conventional (most common, 90%), clear cell, dedifferentiated and mesenchymal types. The tumor is grossly bulky and gelatinous, eroding the adjacent cortex and infiltrating through the bone trabeculae and marrow space. Chondrosarcomas are microscopically graded as low, intermediate and high grade based on cellularity, cytologic atypia and mitotic activity (Figs 13.13A and B). High-grade chondrosarcomas demonstrate high cellularity, marked pleomorphism and frequent mitoses. Areas of necrosis are often present.

*Fibrous cortical defects* are very common benign bone lesions. The vast majority occur in the metaphysis of the distal femur and proximal tibia, and have characteristic radiologic features. Most are discovered incidentally and may undergo spontaneous resolution. Few grow large (5–6 cm) and develop into *non-ossifying fibroma*. Both lesions contain proliferating fibroblasts in storiforms and sheets of foamy macrophages, giant cells and hemosiderin deposition (Fig. 13.14).

*Fibrous dysplasia* is a benign tumor composed of fibrous tissue and bone growing in a disordered pattern. The lesions arise during skeletal growth and development, and are considered to be localized developmental arrest. The lesional tissue is gritty and composed of irregularly shaped trabeculae of woven bone surrounded by proliferating fibroblasts (Figs 13.15A and B). The bone trabeculae lack osteoblastic rimming. Fibrous dysplasia is clinically divided into *monostotic fibrous dysplasia* (single bone involvement), *polyostotic fibrous dysplasia* without endocrine dysfunction (multiple bone involvement) and polyostotic fibrous dysplasia associated with café-au-lait skin pigmentations and endocrine abnormalities (*McCune-Albright syndrome*).

*Ewing sarcoma/primitive neuroectodermal tumor (Ewing/PNET)* is a primary malignant small round cell tumor of the bone and soft tissue of children and young adults. Both the bone and the soft tissue tumors share an identical chromosomal translocation t (11;22)(q24;q12). Microscopically, the tumors are composed of hypercellular sheets of small round cells and scant intervening stroma (Fig. 13.16). Tumor cells are slightly larger than lymphocytes and have scant cytoplasm. Mitoses are easily identified and necrosis may be prominent. The extraosseous PNETs tend to show more neural differentiation than the osseous Ewing sarcoma. The diagnosis is usually confirmed by demonstrating the characteristic chromosomal translocation in the tumor cells.

*Giant-cell tumor* of the bone is a benign tumor of adulthood, typically affecting the bones around the knee. It is composed of mononuclear cells admixed with multinucleated osteoclast-like giant cells (Figs 13.17A and B). The nuclei of the giant cells resemble those of mononuclear cells in the background. Necrosis, hemorrhage, hemosiderin deposition, fibroblastic proliferation and reactive new bone formation may be present.

*Metastatic tumors* are the most common malignancy of the bone. In adults, common primary sites include prostate, breast, kidney and lung. In children, common metastatic tumors originate from neuroblastoma, Wilms tumor, Ewing sarcoma and rhabdomyosarcoma. Metastatic tumors may produce osteolytic, osteoblastic or mixed lytic and blastic lesions. Most metastases produce a mixed lytic and blastic reaction; prostatic adenocarcinoma commonly elicits an osteoblastic lesion while tumors from lung, kidney and gastrointestinal tract produce lytic bone lesions (Figs 13.18A and B).

## Joints

Normal joints bridge the ends of the bones. The solid (nonsynovial) joints provide mechanical stability and allow minimal movement; the cavitated (synovial) joints have a joint space that allows for a wide range of movements.

The most important diseases of joints are:
- Osteoarthritis
- Rheumatoid arthritis
- Gout (tophus)
- Pigmented villonodular synovitis.

## Osteoarthritis

*Osteoarthritis*, also called *degenerative joint disease (DJD)*, is a multifactorial disease of old age characterized by progressive erosion of the articular cartilage and deformity of the joints. The eroded and dislodged cartilage and underlying bone may protrude into the joint space forming *loose bodies* (joint mice) **(Figs 13.19A and B)**. The exposed subchondral bone becomes the new joint surface and causes friction with the opposing degenerated articular surface. The subchondral bone plates may undergo sclerosis and the reactive new bone formation may result in osteophytes protruding into the joint capsule and periarticular soft tissue.

## Rheumatoid Arthritis

*Rheumatoid arthritis* is a chronic systemic inflammatory disorder that affects many tissues and organs of the body including joints. The joint involvement is symmetrical and usually starts at small joints followed by larger joints. Histologically, it is characterized by nonsuppurative chronic and proliferative synovitis **(Fig. 13.20)** that may eventually progress to destruction of the articular cartilage. The inflammatory infiltrate is composed of CD4+ T helper cells, B cells, plasma cells and macrophages.

## Gout

*Gout* refers to transient attacks of acute arthritis initiated by deposition of urate crystals within the joint and surrounding tissues. Gout is associated with a state of hyperuricemia due to primary or secondary causes. *Tophi* are the pathognomonic hallmark of gout. They are formed by large aggregations of urate crystals surrounded by an intense inflammatory reaction of foreign body giant cells, macrophages and lymphocytes **(Figs 13.21A and B)**. The urate crystals may be seen in the cytoplasm of the giant cells.

## Pigmented Villonodular Synovitis

Pigmented villonodular synovitis is a diffuse form of tenosynovial giant-cell tumor which is a benign tumor of synovial lining of joints, tendon sheath and bursae. Pigmented villonodular synovitis grossly presents as nodules and papillary projections of soft tissue with a red-brown color. Microscopically it is composed of sheets and nodules of bland mononuclear cells underneath the synovium **(Figs 13.22A and B)**. Multinucleated giant cells may be seen. Hemosiderin-laden macrophages are usually abundant.

# Soft Tissue Tumors

Soft tissues of the body refer to all non-epithelial and extraskeletal connective tissues, including adipose tissue, fibrous tissue, smooth muscle, skeletal muscle, blood vessels and neural tissue. Most soft tissue tumors are benign and occur sporadically. Common sites are lower extremities (40%), trunk and retroperitoneum (30%), upper extremities (20%) and head and neck (10%).

Soft tissue tumors may be benign or malignant. Tumors are usually classified according to the predominant cell type forming them, on the assumption that they have originated from the precursor of that cell type.

The most important soft tissue tumors are:
- Tumors of adipose tissue: lipoma and liposarcoma
- Tumors of fibrous tissue: fibromatoses (desmoid tumor) and fibrosarcoma
- Tumors of fibrohistiocytic origin: malignant fibrohistiocytoma
- Tumors of smooth muscle: leiomyoma and leiomyosarcoma
- Tumors of skeletal muscle: rhabdomyoma and rhabdomyosarcoma
- Tumors of vascular tissue: hemangioma and angiosarcoma
- Tumor of uncertain histogenesis: synovial sarcoma.

## Tumors of Adipose Tissue

*Lipoma* is the most common soft tissue tumor of adulthood. It usually presents as a soft, painless and superficial subcutaneous mass. The excision specimen shows a well-encapsulated mass composed of mature fat (Fig. 13.23).

*Liposarcoma*, in contrast to its benign equivalent, arises most often in the deep soft tissue of extremities and retroperitoneum. It is one of the most common sarcomas of adulthood. It occurs in several microscopic subtypes including: (a) well-differentiated; (b) myxoid and (c) pleomorphic types. *The well-differentiated liposarcoma* morphologically resembles mature adipose tissue and has an indolent clinical course. Lipoblasts, the hallmark of liposarcoma, may be difficult to find. Well-differentiated liposarcoma is characterized by amplification of the *MDM2* gene which can be used as a diagnostic tool to differentiate it from a lipoma in difficult cases. *Myxoid liposarcoma* has an intermediate clinical behavior and is associated with chromosomal abnormality t(12;16)(q13;p11). The characteristic histological features include myxoid background, rich vascular channels ("chicken-wire" vascular pattern) and abundant lipoblasts (Figs 13.24A to C). *Pleomorphic liposarcoma* is composed of poorly differentiated anaplastic cells with scant fat cell differentiation. These tumors have more aggressive clinical behavior and may metastasize. All liposarcomas are treated by wide local excision and have potential to recur locally.

## Tumors of Fibrous Tissue

Common benign tumors of fibrous tissue are divided into superficial fibromatosis and deep-seated fibromatosis. *Superficial fibromatosis* includes palmar (Dupuytren's contracture), plantar and penile (Peyronie's disease) fibromatoses. The lesions are nodular or poorly defined masses. Histology shows abundant dense collagen with fascicles of mature-appearing fibroblasts (Fig. 13.25). Superficial fibromatosis may resolve spontaneously, stabilize or recur after excision. *Deep-seated fibromatoses*, or *desmoid tumors*, occur more frequently in younger patients (teens to thirties). Depending on the location, it is divided into abdominal, intra-abdominal and extra-abdominal desmoids. Intra-abdominal desmoid tumors often occur in patients with familial adenomatous polyposis (Gardner's syndrome). The majority of these tumors have mutations in the beta-catenin gene, a useful feature for diagnosis. Desmoid tumors are grossly gray white infiltrative tumors with firm cut surfaces and ill-defined borders. Microscopically they are similar to superficial fibromatosis and are composed of proliferating fibroblasts and dense collagenous background (Fig. 13.26). Complete excision with clear margins is important in preventing local recurrence. The tumor may also respond to tamoxifen, chemotherapy or radiation therapy.

*Undifferentiated pleomorphic sarcoma*, previously known as malignant fibrous histiocytoma (MFH) is thought to represent a high-grade fibrosarcoma (Figs 13.27A and B). It is composed of spindle shaped cells showing marked pleomorphism, and commonly contains scattered multinucleated giant cells, atypical mitoses and broad areas of necrosis. These tumors may occur in any part of the body and usually have a poor prognosis.

## Tumors of Skeletal Muscle

*Rhabdomyosarcoma* is the most common sarcoma of childhood and adolescence (less than 20 years of age). Most of the tumors occur in the head and neck or genitourinary tract. The characteristic diagnostic tumor cell is called a rhabdomyoblast, which has an eccentric nucleus and abundant eosinophilic cytoplasm with striations (Figs 13.28A and B). Rhabdomyosarcomas have three subtypes: (a) embryonal; (b) alveolar and (c) pleomorphic. The embryonal rhabdomyosarcoma is most common; within this category is the most common variant, so-called "sarcoma botryoides".

## Tumor of Uncertain Histogenesis

The cell origin of *synovial sarcoma* is uncertain. Synovial sarcoma occurs in younger patients (20–40 years), in the deep soft tissue around large joints of extremities. It is a unique biphasic tumor with both epithelial and mesenchymal components (Figs 13.29A and B) and is associated with a specific chromosomal translocation t(X;18). Synovial sarcoma is treated with wide excision and chemotherapy and may metastasize to regional lymph nodes and lung.

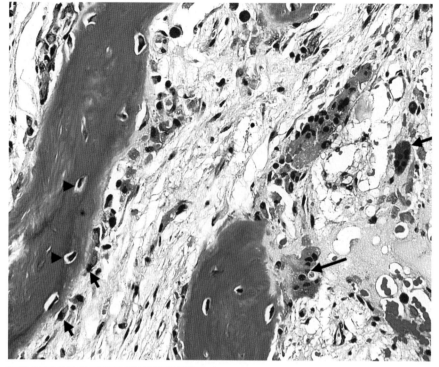

**Fig. 13.1:**
Normal bone histology showing osteoblasts rimming the bone (short arrow), multinucleated osteoclasts (long arrow) and osteocytes (arrowhead).

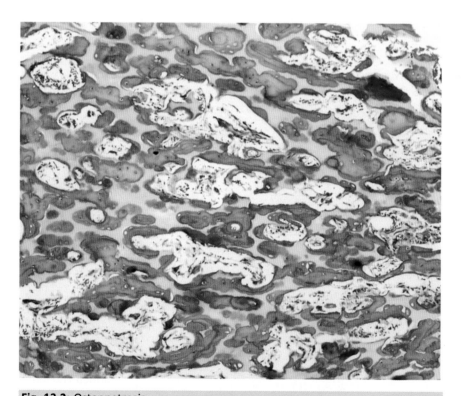

**Fig. 13.2:** Osteopetrosis
The bone lacks medullary cavity. Deposited bone is not remodeled and tends to be woven instead of forming mature trabeculae in architecture.

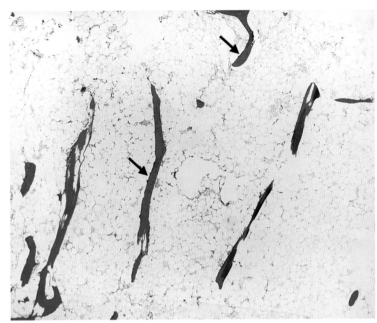

**Fig. 13.3:** Osteoporosis
The bone trabeculae are significantly thinned (arrows) and the bone marrow is replaced completely by adipose tissue.

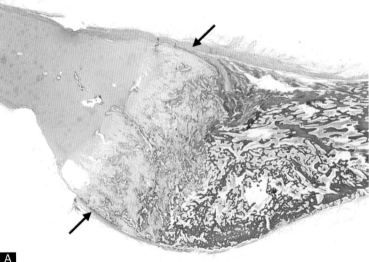

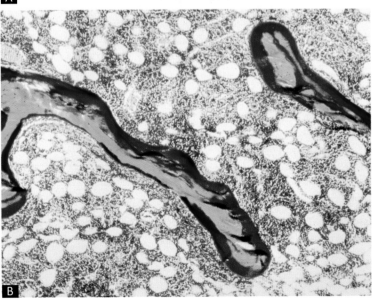

**Figs 13.4A and B:** Osteomalacia (rickets)
**A.** This rib section from a child with rickets shows a widened and deformed chondro-osseous junction (arrows) with an irregular zone of enchondral bone formation. **B.** Ostomalacia in an adult presents with broad seams of osteoid (red) rimming the centrally ossified trabeculae (green).

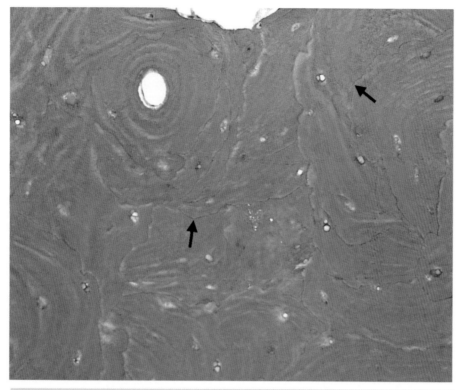

**Fig. 13.5:** Paget disease

Sclerotic bone with characteristic irregular cement lines (arrows) in a mosaic or jigsaw pattern that anneal haphazardly deposited units of lamellar bone.

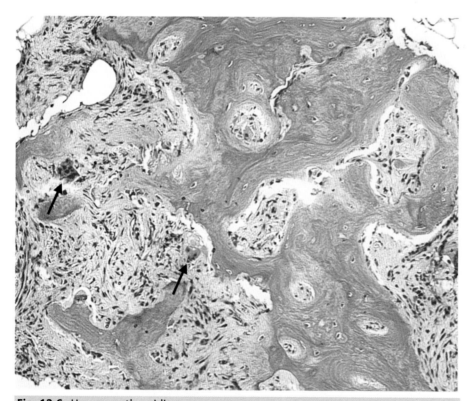

**Fig. 13.6:** Hyperparathyroidism

Hyperparathyroidism results in increased osteoclastic activity (arrows) and consequent bone loss.

BONES, JOINTS AND SOFT TISSUES

CHAPTER
**13**

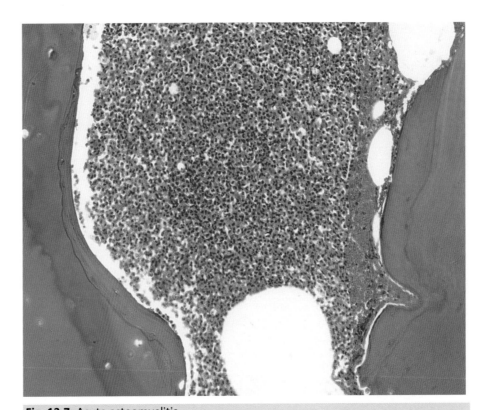

**Fig. 13.7:** Acute osteomyelitis
Collections of neutrophils are seen within the bone marrow cavity.

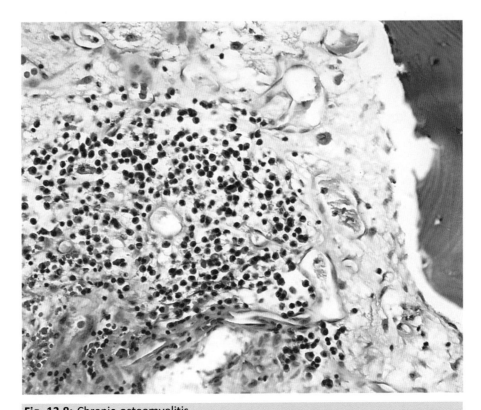

**Fig. 13.8:** Chronic osteomyelitis
The bone marrow space shows collections of plasma cells and lymphocytes scattered in fibrous tissue replacing the normal bone marrow.

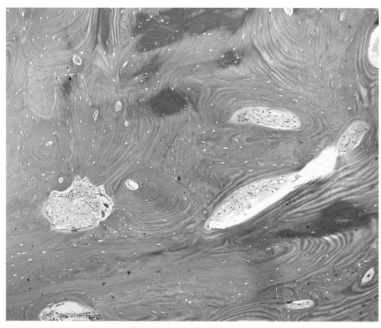

**Fig. 13.9:** Osteoma
It most commonly occurs in the skull or facial bone and is composed of mature bone.

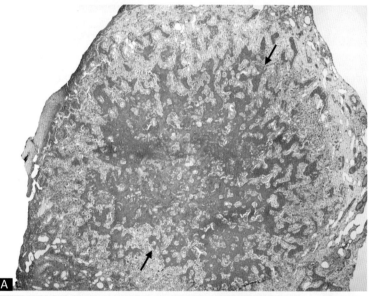

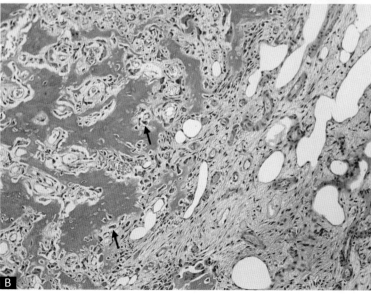

**Figs 13.10A and B:** Osteoid osteoma
**A.** This low power view of an osteoid osteoma nidus (arrows) shows randomly arranged osteoid and bone trabeculae. **B.** At the center of the nidus, the irregular bone trabeculae are rimmed by osteoblasts (arrows) and lie in a background of hypocellular fibrovascular tissue.

CHAPTER
**13**

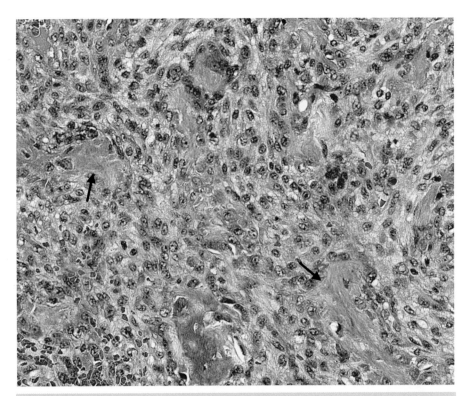

**Fig. 13.11:** Osteosarcoma

The neoplastic cells are densely packed, pleomorphic and form lace-like osteoid (arrows).

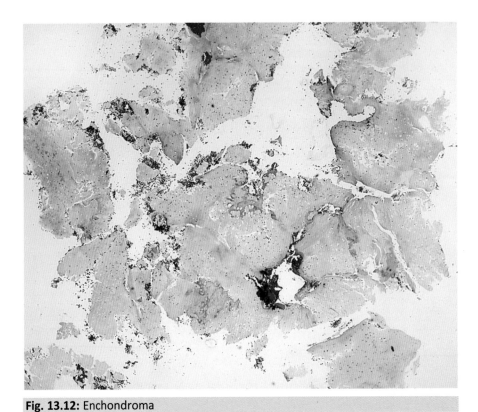

**Fig. 13.12:** Enchondroma

This radiologically well-circumscribed lesion is composed of nodules of hyaline cartilage containing cytologically benign chondrocytes.

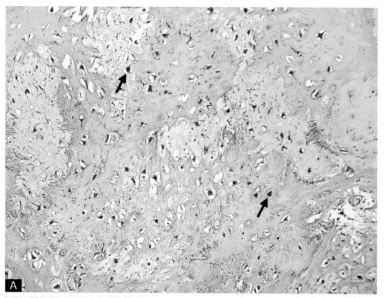

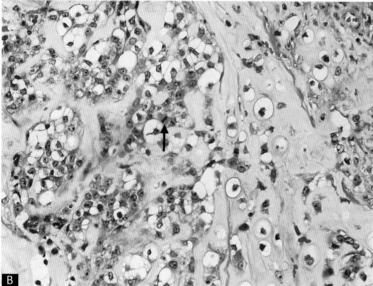

**Figs 13.13A and B:** Chondrosarcoma
**A.** Low to intermediate grade chondrosarcoma shows increased cellularity with chondrocytes containing enlarged and atypical nuclei (arrows). The distinction between low-grade chondrosarcoma and enchondroma relies on radiological, clinical and histological features. **B.** High-grade chondrosarcoma is characterized by high cellularity, marked cytologic atypia and easily identified mitosis (arrow).

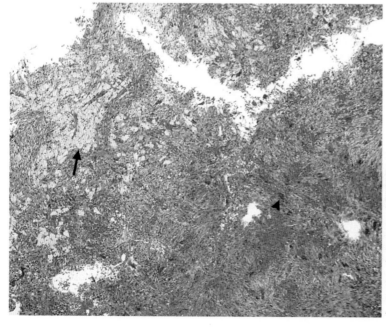

**Fig. 13.14:** Fibrous cortical defect (non-ossifying fibroma)
This very common benign bone lesion contains proliferating fibroblasts in storiforms and sheets of foamy macrophages (arrow). Giant cells (arrowhead) and areas of hemorrhage are also common findings.

CHAPTER
**13**

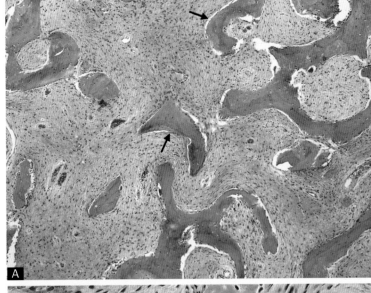

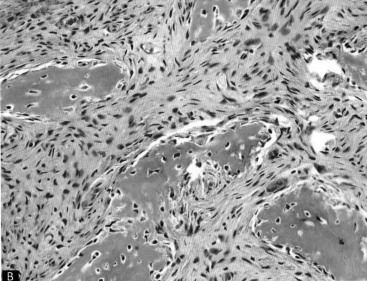

**Figs 13.15A and B:** Fibrous dysplasia
**A.** The lesion is characterized by haphazardly distributed irregular bone trabeculae (arrows) surrounded by proliferating fibroblasts. **B.** In contrast to normal newly formed bone, these bone trabeculae are not rimmed by osteoblasts.

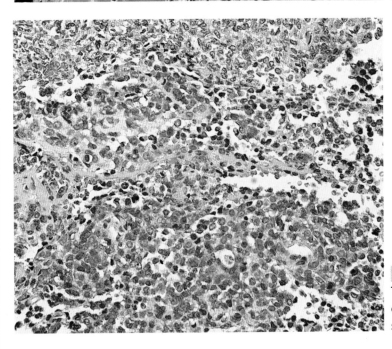

**Fig. 13.16:** Ewing sarcoma
The tumor is composed of sheets of malignant small blue cells with scant cytoplasm.

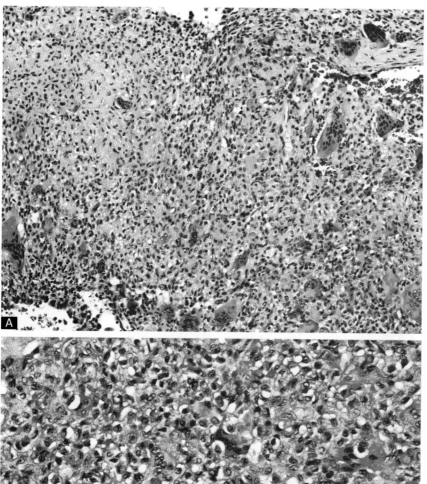

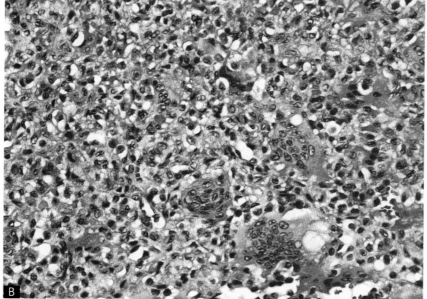

**Figs 13.17A and B:** Giant cell tumor of the bone

**A.** It is a benign tumor composed of mononuclear cells admixed with multinucleated giant cells. **B.** The nuclei of the giant cells resemble the nuclei of the mononuclear cells in the background.

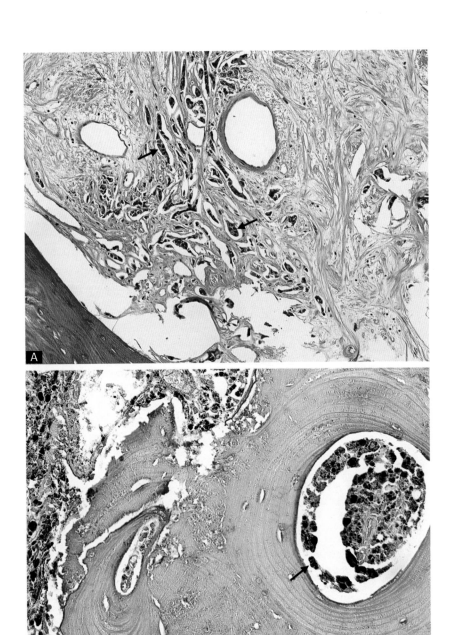

**Figs 13.18A and B:** Metases to the bone

**A.** This lesion represents metastatic breast carcinoma to the bone (arrows).
**B.** Metastatic melanoma in the bone is shown here with malignant cells containing melanin pigment (arrow).

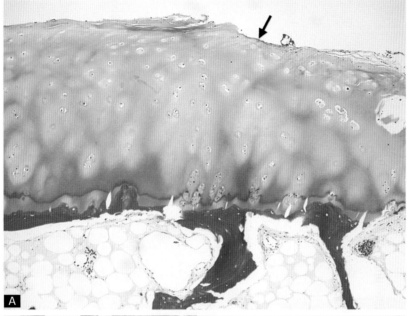

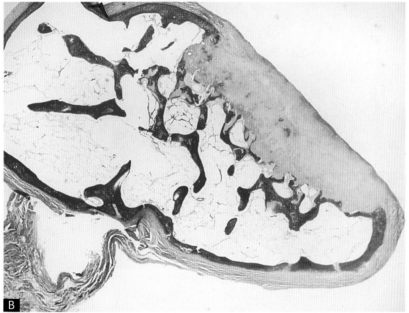

**Figs 13.19A and B:** Degenerative joint disease (osteoarthritis)
**A.** The articular cartilage is eroded (arrow). **B.** The eroded and dislodged cartilage and underlying bone may protrude into the joint space forming *loose bodies* (joint mice).

BONES, JOINTS AND SOFT TISSUES

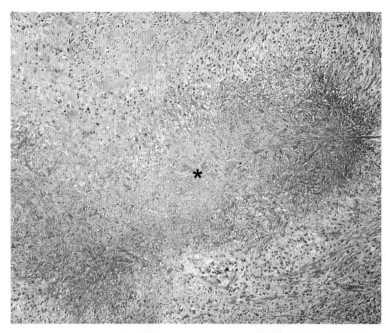

**Fig. 13.20:** Rheumatoid arthritis
A rheumatoid nodule shows a necrotic center (\*) surrounded by palisading histiocytes.

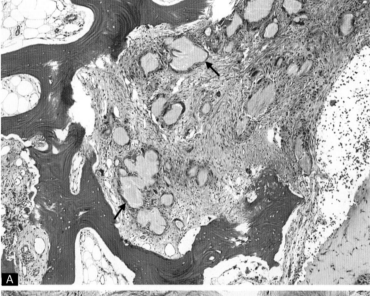

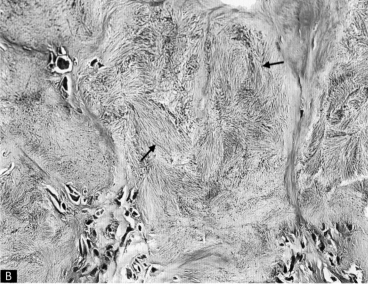

**Figs 13.21A and B:** Gout
**A.** Low-power view shows dense eosinophilic deposits of urates surrounded by foreign body giant cells and histiocytes, so-called tophi (arrows). **B.** Higher magnification shows slender needle-shaped crystals (arrows). These crystals are negatively birefringent.

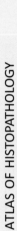

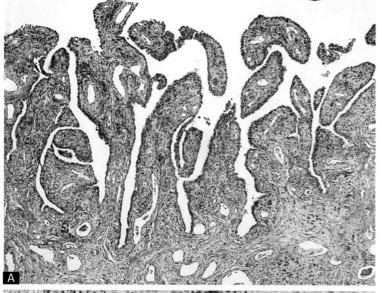

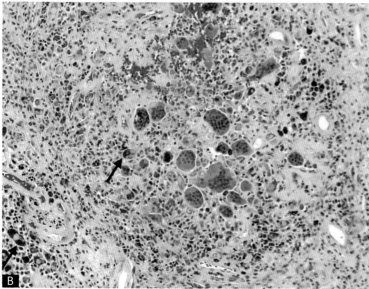

**Figs 13.22A and B:** Pigmented villonodular synovitis
**A.** Low-power view shows surface villous proliferation of synovium.
**B.** Underneath the surface synovium, there are nodular sheets of histiocytes and giant cells with hemosiderin deposition (arrow).

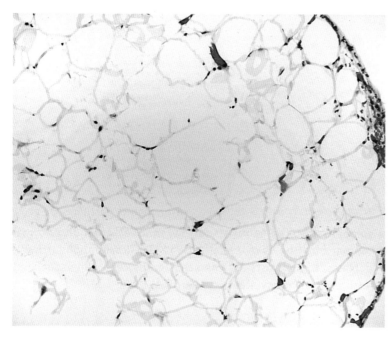

**Fig. 13.23:** Lipoma
It is a well-circumscribed, encapsulated tumor composed of mature adipose tissue.

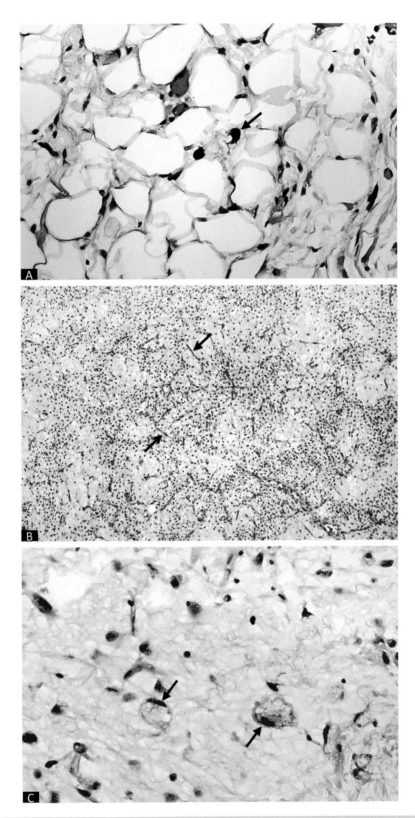

**Figs 13.24A to C:** Liposarcoma

**A.** Well-differentiated liposarcoma contains scattered lipoblasts (arrow) in a background of normal appearing adipose tissue. **B.** Myxoid liposarcoma shows characteristic vascular proliferation (arrows), myxoid background and abundant lipoblasts. **C.** Lipoblasts are characterized by cells with vacuolated lipid-laden cytoplasm pushing on hyperchromatic and atypical nuclei (arrows).

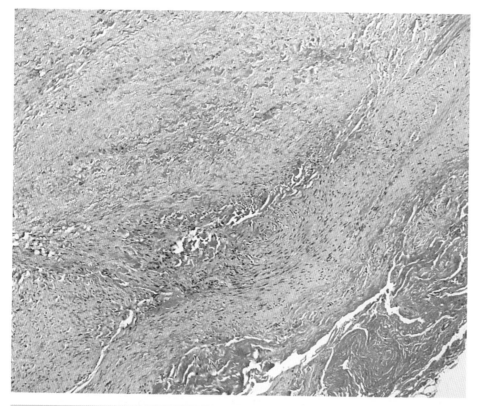

**Fig. 13.25:** Palmar fibromatosis (Dupuytren's contracture)
The lesion is usually ill-defined from surrounding tissue and composed of bland fibroblasts in a dense collagenous background.

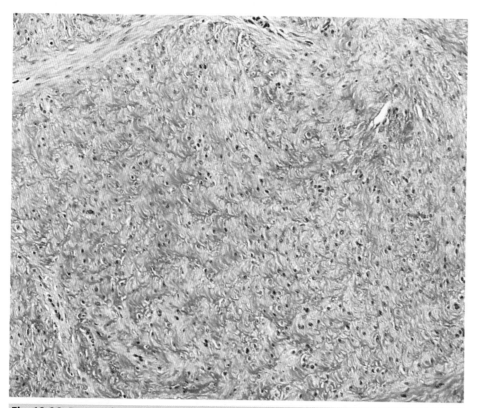

**Fig. 13.26:** Desmoid tumor
This deep-seated fibromatosis has similar features as superficial fibromatosis and is composed of bland fibroblasts with dense collagenous deposition.

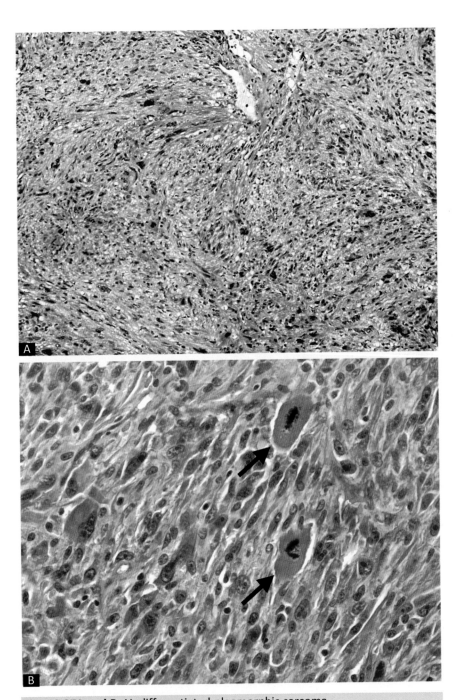

**Figs 13.27A and B:** Undifferentiated pleomorphic sarcoma
**A.** The tumor is composed of malignant spindle cells. **B.** It typically contains cells with frequent and atypical mitoses (arrows).

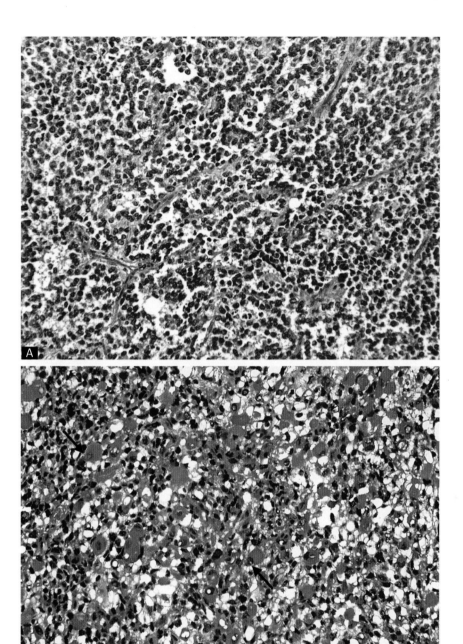

**Figs 13.28A and B:** Rhabdomyosarcoma

**A.** Alveolar rhabdomyosarcoma shows a typical alveolar growth pattern. Tumor cells are small and uniform with scant cytoplasm. **B.** An aggregate of rhabdomyoblasts (strap cells) are shown here (arrows) with eccentric nuclei and abundant eosinophilic cytoplasm.

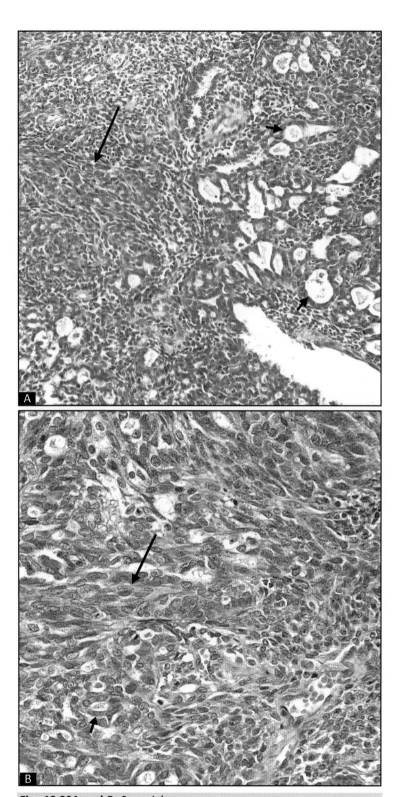

**Figs 13.29A and B:** Synovial sarcoma
**A.** Low-power view shows typical biphasic components: an epithelial component (short arrow) and a spindle cell component (long arrow).
**B.** High-power view demonstrates the juxtaposed epithelial glandular component (short arrow) and spindle cell component (long arrow). Tumor cells from each phase have similar morphology.

# 14 Skeletal Muscles

*Ivan Damjanov*

## Introduction

*Skeletal muscles are composed of striated muscle fibers arranged into fascicles (Figs 14.1A and B). Each fascicle has an external connective tissue envelope called perimysium, that contains nerves and blood vessels. Thin strands of connective tissue extend from the perimysium inside the fascicles forming the connective framework called endomysium. Externally the perimysium extends into the thick connective tissue forming the shell of the anatomically recognizable skeletal muscles called epimysium, which in turn is connected to the tendons and periosteum, linking the muscles with other parts of the skeletal system. The main function of the muscles is to move the extremities, some of its external parts, such as the eyeballs, or the body as a whole.*

*Each muscle fiber is innervated by a single axonal branch of a motor neuron axon. This innervation determines whether the muscle fiber will have the properties of slow-twitch (type I) or fast-twitch (type II) fibers. Most human muscles are composed of both type I and type II fibers intermixed at random. These two muscle types cannot be recognized in routine H&E stained slides. Instead, the muscle must be stained using enzyme histochemical techniques on fresh-frozen tissue cut on a cryostat or by immunohistochemistry on paraffin embedded tissue sections, using antibodies to fast or slow myosin. With these techniques one can readily recognize type I and type II fibers arranged normally in a checkerboard manner (Fig. 14.2).*

The most important diseases of the skeletal muscles that cause distinctive histopathologic changes are as follows:
- Neurogenic muscle diseases
- Genetic muscle diseases
- Inflammatory muscle diseases
- Rhabdomyolysis.

It should be noted that many muscle diseases may present with distinct clinical signs and symptoms, but do not produce any microscopic changes in the diseased muscles. Myasthenia gravis and Lambert-Eaton syndrome, two autoimmune diseases affecting the transmission of neural impulses onto the striated muscles belong to clinical diseases that produce no microscopic changes in the affected muscles. Furthermore, there are numerous genetic muscle diseases that produce initially minimal morphologic changes. Some of these diseases can be recognized in muscle biopsy by electron microscopy, whereas in others the abnormality can be definitely identified only biochemically or by means of molecular biology.

## Neurogenic Muscle Diseases

*Neurogenic muscle atrophy* results from a loss of innervation resulting from: (a) pathologic changes in axonal branches (e.g. in diabetic neuropathy); (b) injury of the axon (e.g. transection of the peripheral nerve); (c) injury of the lower motor neuron in the spinal cord (e.g. poliomyelitis or

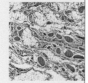

amyotrophic lateral sclerosis); (d) transection of the upper motor neuron axons (e.g. spinal cord injury) or (e) a loss of upper motor neuron (e.g. cerebral cortical infarct). Microscopically, neurogenic muscle atrophy can present in three forms:

- Single muscle fiber atrophy
- Group atrophy
- Panfascicular atrophy.

*Single muscle fiber atrophy* results usually from a loss of the axonal branch innervating that particular muscle fiber (Fig. 14.3). The atrophic fibers, scattered at random among the fibers of normal caliber, appear thin or angulated, but have a normal internal structure. This type of atrophy is most often found in diabetic neuropathy, but is also an early sign of amyotrophic lateral sclerosis. Both type I and type II fibers are affected (Fig. 14.4A). It must be distinguished from *selective type II fiber atrophy*, a common consequence of immobility and is frequently found in elderly persons confined to bed or armchair (Fig. 14.4B). This "disuse" atrophy is also a common consequence of corticosteroid treatment.

*Group atrophy* results from injuries of small nerves and their branches. Typically it is found in amyotrophic lateral sclerosis (lower and upper motor neuron degeneration and loss) or after peripheral nerve injury (Fig. 14.5A). Group atrophy involves both type I and type II muscle fibers (Fig. 14.5B). If the traumatic peripheral nerve injury is repaired, muscle may become reinnervated and may recover its strength. However, since the atrophic fibers will be usually reinnervated by axons stemming from a single motor nerve, these fibers will all be either type I or type II. This type of fiber grouping is characteristic of reinnervation (Fig. 14.5C).

*Panfascicular atrophy* involves all or most of the muscle fibers within a fascicle. Typically atrophy involves an entire motor unit and is a consequence of destruction or loss of a groups of spinal motor neurons (Fig. 14.6). It is a typical feature of poliomyelitis or spinal muscular atrophy such as Werdnig-Hoffman disease.

## Genetic Muscle Diseases

This large group of diseases can be divided into several groups:

- Muscular dystrophies
- Congenital myopathies
- Myopathies caused by inborn errors of metabolism.

*Muscular dystrophies* belong to a group of genetic muscle disease that begin in childhood and are characterized by progressive muscle wasting and irreversible loss of muscle strength and function. The most common diseases of this group are: (a) X-linked muscular dystrophy of the Duchenne or Becker type; (b) myotonic dystrophy and (c) limb girdle muscular dystrophies.

*Duchenne and Becker type of muscular dystrophy* are hereditary X-linked diseases caused by mutations of dystrophin gene located on the X chromosome. Muscle biopsy in these diseases shows signs of muscle fiber injury (degeneration or dystrophy) and loss, accompanied by removal of damaged fibers by macrophages and abortive regeneration (Fig. 14.7A). In later stages of the disease the muscle fibers are replaced with fibrous or fat tissue (Figs 14.7B and C), which may cause enlargement of muscles (pseudohypertrophy). These microscopic findings are not pathognomonic and the final diagnosis is usually made by additional immunohistochemical, or molecular biologic and genetic testing.

*Myotonic dystrophy* is an autosomal dominant disease caused by mutation and an expansion of a CTG triplet repeat of a gene on the short arm of chromosome 19. The muscle pathology is highly variable, but in most patients the biopsy shows splitting of muscle fibers, variation in their size and shape, and an increased number of internal nuclei (Fig. 14.8).

*Congenital myopathies* are a group of diseases characterized by onset in early life and slowly progressive or even non-progressive muscle weakness and hypotonia. Muscle biopsy shows subtle microscopic changes which are usually non-diagnostic. For example, one may see increased variation in the size and shape of muscle fibers, intramysial fibrous tissue or single muscle fiber changes **(Fig. 14.9)**. Clinical pathologic studies make it possible to classify congenital myopathies into several entities, such as central core disease, centronuclear myopathy or nemaline myopathy. In nemaline myopathy one may see typical cytoplasmic rods by electron microscopy **(Fig. 14.10)**.

*Myopathies caused by inborn errors of metabolism* can be classified according to the underlying metabolic disorder that has caused the pathologic changes in the muscle fibers. This group of muscle diseases includes among others mitochondrial myopathies, lipid myopathies, glycogen storage diseases **(Fig. 14.11)**.

### Inflammatory Myopathies

*Myositis* or inflammation of muscle may be limited to a single muscle or it may involve multiple muscle groups, in which case it is called polymyositis. Etiologically and pathogenetically myositis can be classified into several groups:
- Infectious myositis
- Immunologically mediated myositis.

*Infectious myositis* may be caused by viruses, bacteria and other living pathogens. Most often myositis occurs during systemic viral disease or bacterial sepsis, presenting clinically as generalized muscle pain and muscle soreness. The diagnosis is made clinically, and the biopsy is not indicated. Localized *bacterial myositis* may be seen microscopically in the muscle removed during surgical treatment of infected wounds **(Fig. 14.12)**.

*Parasitic myositis* is a feature of infection with *Trichinella spiralis* **(Fig. 14.13)**. Human infection results from eating inadequately cooked infected pork meat. The parasite has a tendency to encyst in the skeletal muscle and cause a local inflammatory reaction. The parasite may remain viable for many years, but when it dies, it is usually replaced by fibrous tissue which may calcify.

*Polymyositis* is the most common immunologically mediated inflammation muscle disease. Clinically it presents with proximal muscle weakness, localized muscle pain, elevation of creatine kinase in serum and typical electromyographic changes. In muscle biopsy one may see infiltrates of lymphocytes and phagocytic macrophages destroying the muscle fibers **(Figs 14.14A and B)**. Destruction of muscle fibers is accompanied by replacement fibrosis and abortive regeneration of muscle fibers.

*Dermatomyositis* is a systemic disease involving the skin and the muscles. Clinically it presents with typical skin rash and muscle weakness. Pathogenetically it is an immune-mediated microangiopathy with deposits of immunoglobulins and complement that can be seen in small blood vessels by immunofluorescence microscopy. Microscopically, in the muscle biopsy one may see typical perivascular infiltrates of T and B lymphocytes and plasma cells **(Fig. 14.15)**.

## Rhabdomyolysis

*Rhabdomyolysis*, also known as *necrotizing myopathy*, denotes muscle injury resulting in nonselective destruction of muscle fibers. Rhabdomyolysis may be caused by toxins, viruses, ischemia, trauma and many other nonspecific forms of muscle injury. Microscopic findings are nonspecific and include muscle fiber destruction, accompanied by infiltrates of macrophages participating in the removal of damaged muscle fibers **(Fig. 14.16)**. The area of injury is ultimately replaced by fibrous tissue or fat cells.

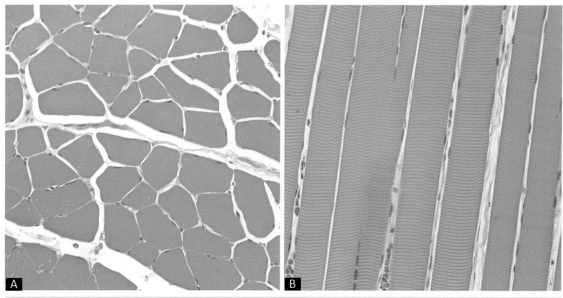

**Figs 14.1A and B:** Normal skeletal muscle

**A.** Cross-section shows mild variation in size and shape of muscle fibers, which are arranged into distinct fascicles. **B.** Longitudinal section shows cross striations and peripherally located subsarcolemmal nuclei. The intercellular fibrous tissue containing capillaries is scant.

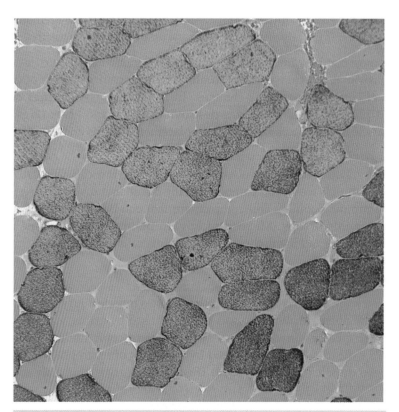

**Fig. 14.2:** Normal skeletal muscle

In this section stained immunohistochemically with antibodies to slow myosin, type I fibers appear brown, and are intermixed at random with type II fibers which appear red.

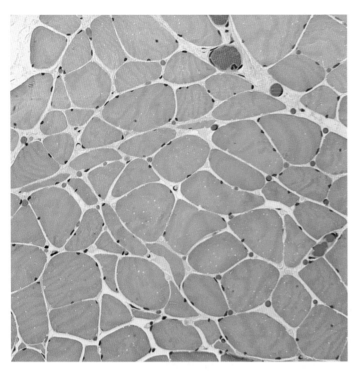

**Fig. 14.3:** Neurogenic atrophy
In this muscle biopsy of a patient suffering from diabetes mellitus there are scattered atrophic muscle fibers.

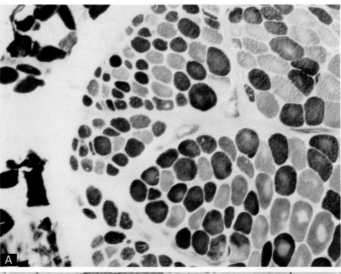

A

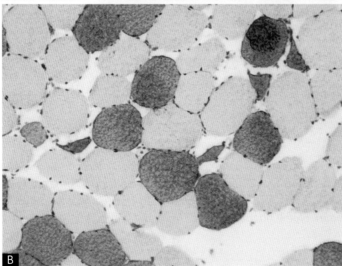

B

**Figs 14.4A and B:** Muscle atrophy
These two biopsy specimens are both stained immunohistochemically to show type I muscle fibers light brown and type II fibers dark brown.
**A.** Nonselective atrophy involving both type I and type II fibers, most prominently in the left side of the figure. **B.** Selective type II atrophy. Note that the lightly stained type I fibers and some darkly stained type II fibers are of normal size, but there are also atrophic type II fibers.

CHAPTER
**14**

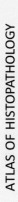

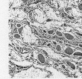

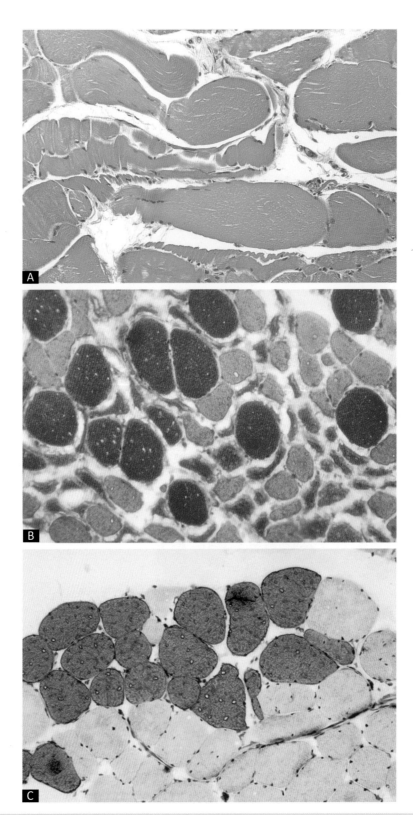

**Figs 14.5A to C:** Group atrophy

**A.** Numerous muscle fibers are atrophic in this biopsy of a patient with amyotrophic lateral sclerosis. **B.** Immunohistochemistry shows that both type I and type II fibers are atrophic, and are intermixed with unaffected fibers which often show signs of compensatory hypertrophy. **C.** In this reinnervated muscle immunohistochemistry shows grouping of dark type II fibers, separate from type I fibers, which are lightly stained.

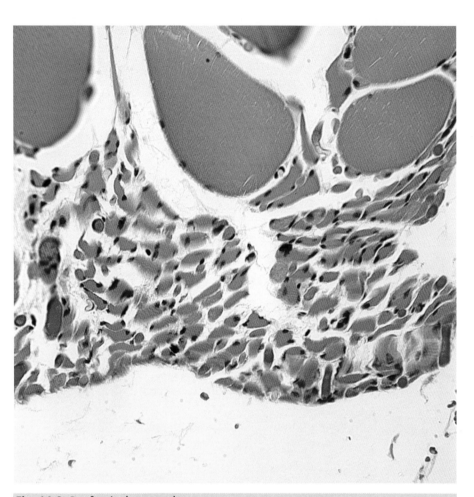

**Fig. 14.6:** Panfascicular atrophy
The entire fascicle is composed of small atrophic fibers, whereas the adjacent fascicle is composed of muscle fibers of normal size.

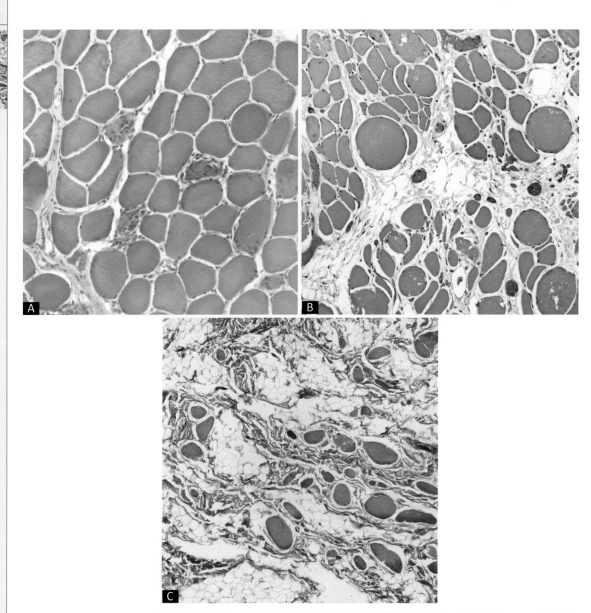

**Figs 14.7A to C:** Muscular dystrophy

**A.** Damaged muscle fibers are being removed by macrophages. **B.** In progressive stages of the disease, the muscle consists small and large fibers and the amount of intramysial fibrous tissue is increased. **C.** In advanced stages of the disease muscle fibers have been replaced by fibrous tissue and fat cells.

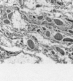

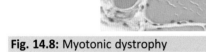

**Fig. 14.8:** Myotonic dystrophy
The biopsy findings include increased variation in size and shape of muscle fibers, splitting of fibers and an increased number of internally located nuclei.

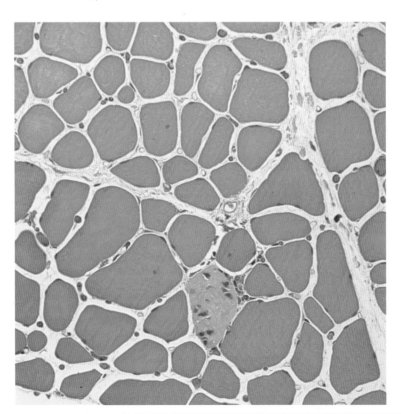

**Fig. 14.9:** Myopathy
The biopsy findings are nonspecific and include single muscle fiber changes, increased variation in size and shape of muscle fibers, some of which appear small and round.

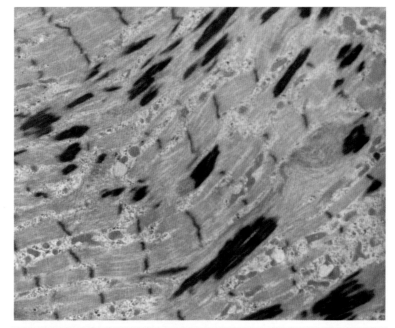

**Fig. 14.10:** Nemaline myopathy

By electron microscopy one may see typical cytoplasmic rods in the affected muscle fibers.

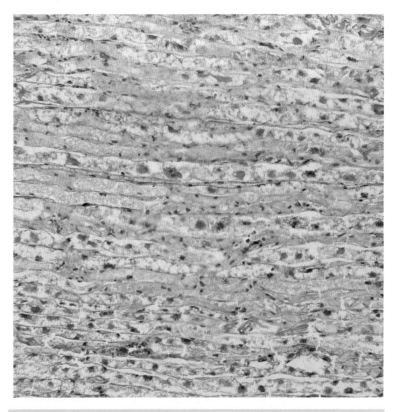

**Fig. 14.11:** Glycogen storage disease

The cytoplasm of muscle cells appears clear rather than eosinophilic, reflecting the abnormal cytoplasmic accumulation of glycogen.

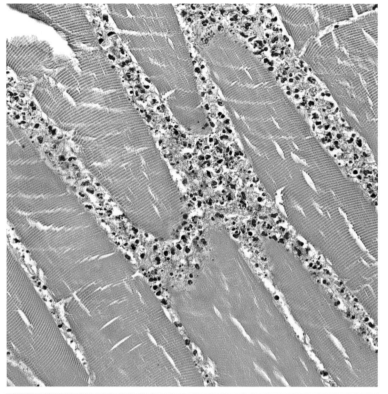

**Fig. 14.12:** Bacterial infection of the muscle
A portion of the muscle has been infiltrated and destroyed by pus, i.e.
dead and dying neutrophils.

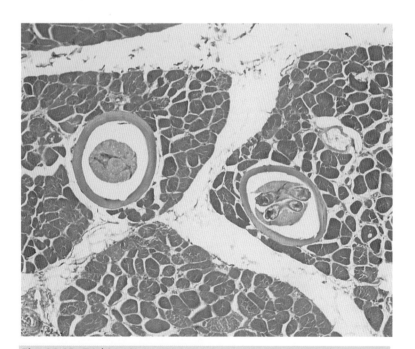

**Fig. 14.13:** Trichinosis
The muscle contains two encysted larvae of *Trichinella spiralis.*

SKELETAL MUSCLES

CHAPTER
**14**

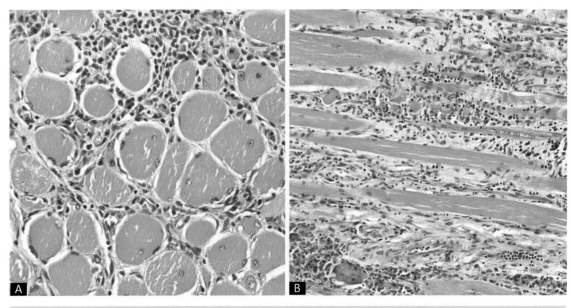

**Figs 14.14A and B:** Polymyositis

**A.** The muscle is infiltrated by lymphocytes which surround individual muscle cells. **B.** The intramysial lymphocytic infiltrates have destroyed focally muscle fibers.

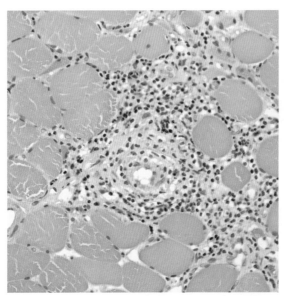

**Fig. 14.15:** Dermatomyositis

The muscle biopsy shows a perivascular infiltrate composed predominantly of lymphocytes and a few plasma cells.

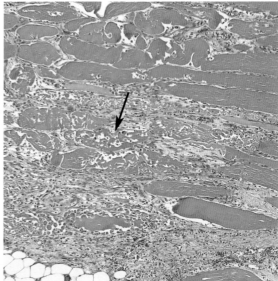

**Fig. 14.16:** Rhabdomyolysis

There are numerous damaged muscle fibers (arrow) and macrophages in process or removing cell debris. In the lower part of the figure one may see fibrous tissue replacing the muscle fibers.

# 15 Central Nervous S

*Paul St. Romain,*

## Introduction

*The nervous system has been traditionally divided into: (a) the central nervous system comprising the brain and the spinal cord; (b) the peripheral nervous system (peripheral ner and (c) the autonomic nervous system (sympathetic and parasympathetic ganglia and nerve. Together, these systems are involved in control of homeostasis, initiation and control of movement, sensory perception, memory, emotion, language, and concrete and abstract reasoning; thus, pathologies leading to neurologic deficits may have diverse manifestations. In this chapter we will discuss only the pathology involving the CNS. We will first deal with the reactions of the CNS cells to injury and then with the most important diseases which can be organized into the following groups:*

- *Cerebrovascular diseases*
- *Infectious diseases*
- *Demyelinating diseases*
- *Degenerative diseases*
- *Neoplasms.*

## Normal Central Nervous System

The CNS is a highly specialized tissue composed primarily of neurons and glial cells. Glial cells are subdivided into astrocytes, oligodendrocytes, microglia and ependymal cells (Figs 15.1A to E). With the exception of microglia, which are derived from the stem cell in the bone marrow (mesoderm), all of these cells are embryologically derived from the neural tube (neuroectoderm). Three layers of tissue, named pia, arachnoid and dura mater, are collectively called meninges and serve to cover and protect the brain and spinal cord. The ventricles of the brain contain choroid plexus, which produces cerebrospinal fluid.

## Cellular Reactions to Injury

Cells of the CNS show unique patterns of injury which merit specific consideration before a discussion of individual diseases listed above. Here we shall illustrate some of the forms of neuronal injury and glial reactions to such injury.

### Neuronal Injury

*Neuronal injury* can take several patterns, which correlate with the nature of injury (Figs 15.2A to E). Here we shall illustrate major forms of neuronal injury including: (a) chromatolysis; (b) hypoxic injury and (c) various inclusions.

- *Chromatolysis* represents a reaction to axonal injury but it may be caused by ischemia and toxic nerve cell injury as well. It represents a loss or dissolution of the basophilic Nissl substance corresponding ultrastructurally to the rough endoplasmic reticulum in the perinuclear cytoplasm (perikaryon).

- *Hypoxic injury* of neurons presents with changes in the nucleus and the cytoplasm, indicative of apoptosis. The nucleus becomes pyknotic and the cytoplasm becomes eosinophilic and shrunken; hence the colloquial term "red neuron" used to describe this injury. The electrical activity of neurons requires large amounts of energy in the form of ATP produced by oxidative phosphorylation, and neurons are thus much more sensitive to hypoxia than other cells of the CNS.
- *Chronic neuronal injury* occurs in most neurodegenerative diseases, such as Alzheimer disease, Pick disease and Parkinson disease. Chronic injury may cause vacuolation of the neuronal cytoplasm (perikaryon) or formation of inclusions and cytoplasmic bodies, such as neurofibrillary tangles in Alzheimer disease, tau protein-rich Pick bodies in Pick disease or α-synuclein-rich Lewy bodies in Parkinson disease. In Lafora body disease, a rare autosomal recessive form of myoclonic epilepsy, neurons contain cytoplasmic polyglycosan bodies, which form due to a mutation of a gene that encodes a protein tyrosine phosphatase called laforin.

Neurons are highly specialized cells whose activity in the form of complex networks forms the biological foundation for the functions of the CNS, and neuronal injury will almost always have functional consequences. Furthermore, neurons are terminally differentiated postmitotic cells that cannot proliferate or divide, and accordingly dead neurons are irrevocably lost and cannot be regenerated.

### Glial Reaction to Injury

*Glial reaction to injury* may involve astrocytes, oligodendrocytes, microglia or ependymal cells. Glial reaction may include quantitative or qualitative changes and thus result in: (a) *gliosis*, an increased number of glia cells and/or (b) *structural changes* resulting in alterations of cell shape, changes in the cytoplasm or the appearance of inclusions **(Figs 15.3A and B)**.

- *Gliosis* may involve any of the four glial cell types, although it is not uncommon that one of the cell types predominates. For example, ischemic necrosis is accompanied by prominent *microglial reaction*, in which these cells phagocytose fragmented myelin and their cytoplasm becomes lipid rich and foamy. *Microglial nodules* are found in response to human immunodeficiency virus infection (HIV). *Astrocytic gliosis* is the most common form of reaction to injury of cortical neurons, and is found in response to trauma, infections, hemorrhage or tumors. Mixed gliosis is often seen in neurodegenerative diseases characterized by a loss of neurons, such as Huntington disease or amyotrophic lateral sclerosis (ALS).
- *Structural changes* involving the glial cells may occur in several forms. For example, astrocytes proliferating in response to injury may undergo a characteristic *gemistocytic transformation*. During this change astrocytes enlarge and acquire abundant eosinophilic cytoplasm. Metabolic injury, typically long-standing hyperammonemia related to liver failure, manifests in astrocytes as vacuolation and intranuclear inclusions of glycogen (*Alzheimer type II astrocytes*).

## Cerebrovascular Disease

The vascular disturbances of the CNS can be broadly classified as: (a) ischemic or (b) hemorrhagic. Stroke and apoplexy are other terms for these cerebral ischemic or hemorrhagic events.

### Cerebral Ischemia

*Cerebral ischemia* may be: (a) focal or (b) global. *Focal ischemia* of the CNS occurs when blood flow is interrupted to an anatomically defined area of the brain. This may be due to occlusion of the lumen of blood vessels due to rupture of an atherosclerotic plaque, embolus or vasculitis. The ischemic area undergoes liquefactive necrosis **(Fig. 15.4)**. Necrotic neurons and glial cells are phagocytosed by microglia cells which transforms into foamy cells (German, "gitterzellen"), and the ischemic area transform into a pseudocyst.

*Global ischemia* of the CNS typically occurs in states of severe hypotension. Purkinje cells of the cerebellum and pyramidal neurons of the cortex and CA1 of the hippocampus are also especially vulnerable to hypoxia and show typical patterns of neuronal ischemic injury **(Figs 15.5A and B)**.

*Intracerebral hemorrhage* may occur due to emboli, rupture of an aneurysm or trauma. Grossly, areas of hemorrhage compress normal brain tissue, which undergoes necrosis due to anoxia (Figs 15.6A and B). With time, the hemorrhage is reabsorbed and a fluid-filled pseudocyst remains surrounded by areas of gliosis with hemosiderin-laden macrophages.

## Infections of the Central Nervous System

Infection may spread to the CNS: (a) hematogenously; (b) by local extension; (c) by direct implantation or (d) by spread from the peripheral nervous system. A variety of pathogens are implicated, including viruses, parasites, bacteria, fungi and prions. Here we will discuss features of: (a) meningitis; (b) encephalitis; (c) subacute sclerosing panencephalitis; (d) AIDS encephalopathy and (e) spongiform encephalopathy.

### Meningitis

*Meningitis* is an inflammation of the arachnoid and pia mater localized to the subarachnoid space (Figs 15.7A to D). Bacterial causes in neonates include *Escherichia coli* and group B streptococci; in children and young adults *Neisseria meningitidis* predominates, while in older adults *Streptococcus pneumonia* and *Listeria monocytogenes* are more common. *Streptococcus pneumoniae* is the most prevalent cause overall and affects all ages. Regardless of the specific bacterial cause, the CSF is frankly purulent with elevated protein, neutrophils, and decreased glucose. Grossly, a fibropurulent exudate covers the surface of the brain. Acute bacterial meningitis is a life-threatening emergency, as increased protein in the CSF leads to a buildup of pressure that can lead to tonsillar herniation and death. By contrast, in *viral meningitis* (aseptic meningitis) the CSF shows increased lymphocytes, normal or slightly elevated protein, and normal glucose. The course of viral meningitis is usually self-limited.

### Encephalitis

*Encephalitis* is parenchymal inflammation of the brain, most often caused by viruses (Figs 15.8A to D). Confusion is a frequent symptom, and meningeal involvement is common (meningo-encephalitis). Insect-borne viruses (arboviruses) are histologically characterized by lymphocytic inflammation surrounding blood vessels (perivascular cuffing) and formation of reactive microglial nodules. Herpes simplex virus encephalitis is the most common viral encephalitis today. The infection preferentially involves the frontotemporal lobes, and is often hemorrhagic and necrotic. Cowdry type A intranuclear inclusions, the hallmark of herpes simplex virus infection in any organ, are present in infected cells. Perivascular cuffing of lymphocytes may also be seen. Poliovirus and rabies virus are rare, but historically significant causes of encephalitis. Poliovirus has a tropism for anterior horn cells in the spinal cord, and infection results in loss of these cells with accompanying paralysis. Rabies virus enters the body through wounds and reaches the CNS via retrograde transport down peripheral nerves. The pathognomonic sign of rabies infection is the presence of eosinophilic inclusions called Negri bodies within neurons. Negri bodies are most commonly found in hippocampal neurons and Purkinje cells.

### Subacute Sclerosing Panencephalitis

*Subacute sclerosing panencephalitis* is a syndrome characterized by cognitive decline, spasticity and seizures years after an infection with measles virus. It is thought to be related to persistent CNS infection by a non-productive measles virus. Measles virions are present as intranuclear inclusions in oligodendrocytes and neurons, and are accompanied by widespread gliosis and demyelination (Figs 15.9A and B).

### AIDS Encephalopathy

*AIDS encephalopathy* is the term given to the complex of CNS changes associated with HIV infection, which result in atrophy and cognitive decline (HIV-associated dementia). It may be related directly to persistent HIV infection of the brain resulting in the formation of microglial cell nodules

(Figs 15.10A and B). The immunosuppressed patients who have AIDS are susceptible to opportunistic infections such as cryptococcal meningitis or toxoplasmic encephalitis.

### Spongiform Encephalopathies

*Spongiform encephalopathies* are rare diseases characterized by rapidly progressive dementia. The etiology lies in the molecular properties of a normal human protein termed prion protein (PrP). This protein can undergo spontaneous conformational change from an alpha-helix-rich secondary structure (PrP$^C$) to a beta-pleated sheet-rich structure (PrP$^{SC}$). PrP$^{SC}$ acts as a catalyst to induce the same change in other PrP$^C$; this beta-sheet-rich form then forms neurotoxic aggregates that are proteinase-K resistant and PAS positive. Vacuolation of the neuropil and of the perikaryon of neurons is another hallmark of these diseases (Figs 15.11A and B).

## Demyelinating Diseases

Loss of myelin in the CNS can be due to autoimmunity (multiple sclerosis), infection (progressive multifocal leukoencephalopathy) and hereditary metabolic derangements (leukodystrophies). The most important example is multiple sclerosis.

### Multiple Sclerosis

*Multiple sclerosis* is a chronic autoimmune demyelinating disorder of unknown etiology, involving both the white and the gray matter of the brain and spinal cord (Figs 15.12A to D). It is thought that in predisposed individuals, an inciting agent results in activation of CD4$^+$ T-cells that trigger humoral and cellular immune responses against self myelin-associated antigens. In early lesions (active plaques), inflammatory cells (predominantly lymphocytes and macrophages) can still be found microscopically, while in late lesions white matter and oligodendrocyte nuclei are absent and gliosis is prominent.

## Neurodegenerative Diseases

Neurodegenerative diseases are characterized by progressive loss of neurons. Most diseases in this category are considered idiopathic and with few exceptions (such as Friedreich ataxia or Huntington disease) they predominantly affect the elderly population. A common feature of this group is degradation-resistant protein aggregates, but the role of these aggregates in the pathogenesis of neuronal death is uncertain. The most important degenerative diseases are: (a) Alzheimer disease; (b) Parkinson disease; (c) amyotrophic lateral sclerosis and (d) subacute combined degeneration of the spinal cord.

### Alzheimer Disease

*Alzheimer disease* is the most common cortical degenerative disease and most common cause of dementia. The pathogenesis of this disease is not fully understood, but most evidence points to the critical events in faulty transmembrane signaling, and formation of amyloid Aβ from amyloid precursor protein (APP) due to the activity of certain proteases. The aggregates of misfolded Aβ protein are deposited in the neuropil in the form of *neuritic plaques*, which are thought to be neurotoxic. Chronic neuronal injury is accompanied by formation of *neurofibrillary tangles* in the neuropil and cytoplasm of neurons; these tangles are composed predominantly of *tau protein*, which is involved in microtubule assembly. These changes cause neuronal loss and brain atrophy, evident on gross examination as widening of sulci and thinning of gyri (Figs 15.13A to D).

### Parkinson Disease

*Parkinson disease* is a neurodegenerative disease that results in loss of the dopaminergic neurons of the substantia nigra, relieving inhibition of several pathways in the basal ganglia that act to dampen movement. Hence, the disease is characterized by rigidity, slowness of movement and difficulty initiating movement. Most often it presents in a primary/idiopathic form. Secondary Parkinsonism as a complication of some infections or drugs is less common. In both forms the brain shows on gross examination depigmentation of the substantia nigra due to death of neuromelanin- and lipofuscin-containing neurons. Microscopically, many neurons have been replaced by gliosis and the remaining neurons contain typical Lewy bodies (Fig. 15.14). These inclusions are composed of α-synuclein and on microscopic examination have a dense core surrounded by a bright pink halo.

### Amyotrophic Lateral Sclerosis

*Amyotrophic lateral sclerosis (ALS)* is an idiopathic degenerative disorder of motor neurons in the brain, brainstem and spinal cord. Sensory neurons are unaffected. The loss of upper motor neurons leads to degeneration of the corticospinal tracts and atrophy of the precentral gyrus, while loss of lower motor neurons leads to gross thinning of the anterior roots (Figs 15.15A and B). Bunina bodies are PAS-positive cytoplasmic inclusions containing ubiquitin that may be found in remaining motor neurons. Loss of motor neurons results in atrophy of skeletal muscles illustrated in Chapter 14—Skeletal Muscles.

### Subacute Combined Degeneration of the Spinal Cord

*Subacute combined degeneration of the spinal cord* is a complication of vitamin $B_{12}$ deficiency. Axons in the posterior columns and in the lateral corticospinal tract undergo degeneration over the course of weeks to months (Fig. 15.16). The function of vitamin $B_{12}$ in the maintenance of these spinal tracts may be related to its role as a cofactor for the conversion of methylmalonic acid to succinyl CoA. Microscopic examination of the affected tracts demonstrates swelling of the myelin layers and vacuolating changes in the early stages, followed by axonal degeneration in the later stage.

## Neoplasms

Tumors in the CNS may be primary or metastatic. Primary tumors can come from glia, immature neural cells, neural sheath cells, meninges, inflammatory cells and blood vessels. In children they most often involve the posterior fossa, while in adults they are more commonly supratentorial. The most important tumors of the CNS are: (a) astrocytic tumors (astrocytoma and glioblastoma); (b) oligodendroglioma; (c) ependymoma; (d) medulloblastoma; (e) meningioma; (f) schwannoma; (g) hemangioblastoma and (h) metastatic tumors.

### Astrocytic Tumors

*Astrocytic tumors* are the most common adult primary brain tumor (80%). Depending on the extent of anaplasia these tumors are graded on a scale from I to IV. Low grade malignant tumors fall into the category of grade II lesions and are called astrocytomas (Figs 15.17A and B). Grade III tumors are more cellular and show more anaplasia and mitotic activity than grade II tumors; hence they are called anaplastic astrocytomas (Fig. 15.18). Grade IV astrocytic tumors are called glioblastoma multiforme. These tumors show increased cellularity, marked nuclear pleomorphism, high mitotic activity, and contain areas of necrosis and hemorrhage (Figs 15.19A to D). Glioblastomas are invariably fatal, whereas the lower grade astrocytomas have a better prognosis.

### Oligodendroglioma

*Oligodendroglioma* is a tumor arising from oligodendrocytes. It generally occurs in the white matter of adults, and is well-circumscribed and slow-growing. Microscopically, the tumor is composed of cells resembling normal oligodendroglial cells (Figs 15.20A and B). These cells have round nuclei and a perinuclear halo. Mitoses are infrequent, and necrosis is uncommon, but calcifications may be prominent. Tumors that exhibit loss of chromosome 1p and 19q have a very favorable prognosis.

*Anaplastic oligodendrogliomas* have more nuclear pleomorphism, mitotic activity and necrosis than typical oligodendrogliomas.

## Ependymoma

*Ependymoma* arises from ependymal cells lining the fourth ventricle of children or the central canal of the spinal cord and filum terminale of adults. Microscopically the tumor is composed of monomorphic cells with round or oval nuclei **(Figs 15.21A and B)**. These cells form perivascular pseudorosettes, in which a blood vessel is encircled by a pinkish nuclear free zone containing thin cellular processes of surrounding tumor cells. Tumor cells may also form tubules or canals, and grow along the surface of papillae that have a central vascular core. The most common adult form is the myxopapillary ependymoma which typically occurs in the filum terminale and is microscopically composed of papillae and myxoid areas.

## Medulloblastoma

*Medulloblastoma* is predominantly a tumor of childhood. It occurs exclusively in the cerebellum and is highly malignant. The microscopic appearance is that of a small blue cell tumor, with sheets of cells that have scant cytoplasm, hyperchromatic nuclei and frequently observed mitoses **(Figs 15.22A and B)**. Occasionally, the tumor cells may form rosettes, or show glial or neuronal differentiation with formation of fibrillar neuropil.

## Meningioma

*Meningioma* is a benign tumor arising from the meningothelial cell of the arachnoid mater **(Figs 15.23A to C)**. The most common microscopic findings are whorled clusters of meningothelial cells with formation of psammoma bodies. Several distinct histologic types are recognized such as meningothelial, fibroblastic, psammomatous, cystic, secretory, etc. Meningiomas are slow-growing tumors, and histologic subtyping is of limited clinical significance for these benign neoplasms. In a small minority of cases meningiomas may show increased mitotic activity (*atypical meningiomas*) or overt malignancy.

## Schwannoma

*Schwannomas* are tumors of cranial and spinal nerves that arise from Schwann cells **(Figs 15.24A to C)**. They are often associated with sporadic or germline mutation of the *NF2* gene. A common location is the cerebellopontine angle harboring tumors attached to the eighth cranial nerve. They are generally well-circumscribed and encapsulated. Microscopically, they show two architectural patterns, termed Antoni A and Antoni B. Antoni A regions are densely cellular regions that may demonstrate nuclear palisading and pink nuclear free areas, termed Verocay bodies. The Antoni B pattern is more myxoid and less cellular than Antoni A.

## Hemangioblastoma

*Hemangioblastoma* is a benign vascular tumor frequently associated with von-Hippel-Lindau disease, an autosomal recessive hereditary disorder characterized by hemangioblastomas and cysts of the cerebellum, retina, pancreas, liver and kidneys, along with renal cell carcinoma and pheochromocytoma. Microscopically, the tumor is composed of irregular thin-walled blood vessels with intervening clear stromal cells **(Figs 15.25A and B)**.

## Metastatic Tumors

*Metastatic tumors* account for a quarter to a half of intracranial tumors. The most common primary sites are lung, breast, skin (melanoma), kidney and gastrointestinal tract. The boundary between tumor and normal parenchyma is usually well-demarcated and the normal brain tissue demonstrates reactive gliosis **(Figs 15.26A and B)**.

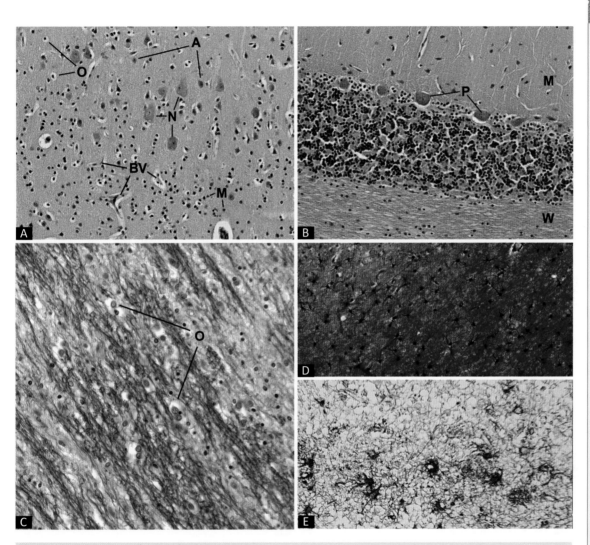

**Figs 15.1A to E:** Normal central nervous system

**A.** Normal cortical white matter contains neurons and glial cell. Neurons (N) stand out as large cells with slightly bluish cytoplasm. Astrocytes (A) have vesicular nuclei. Oligodendrocytes (O) have small round nuclei surrounded with a clear halo (like "fried eggs"). Microglia cells (M) have round or oval small dark nuclei. There are also numerous small blood vessels (BV), some of which are surrounded with a clear space (Virchow-Robin space). **B.** Normal cerebellum consists of several distinct layers: outer molecular layer (M), Purkinje cell layer (P), granular layer and white matter (W). **C.** White matter of the brain consists of myelinated axons and glial cells. Myelin sheaths enveloping the axons stain blue with special stains such as Luxol fast blue. Between the axons one may see oligodendrocytes (O). **D.** Astrocytic processes may be demonstrated with special stains such as gold chloride impregnation or **E.** Immunohistochemically with antibodies to glial fibrillary acidic protein (GFAP).

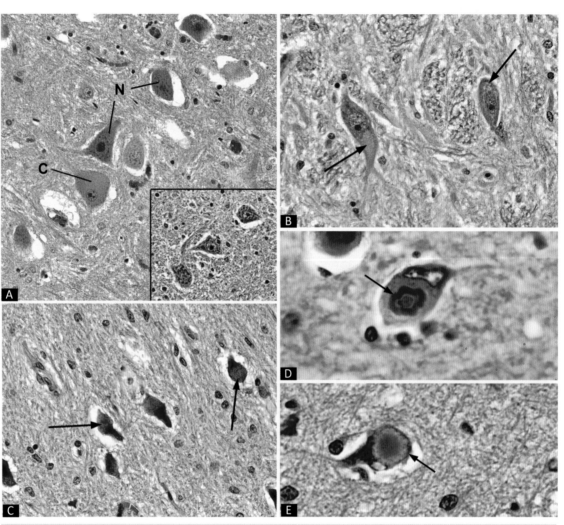

**Figs 15.2 A to D:** Neuronal injury

**A.** The cytoplasm of injured spinal motor neurons (N) appears eosinophilic due to a decreased number of ribosomes on the rough endoplasmic reticulum forming the Nissl substance. Complete disappearance of the Nissl substance from the perikaryon is called chromatolysis (C). Normal motor neurons (photographed at slightly lower magnification) containing perinuclear blue-staining Nissl substance are included in the inset for comparison. **B.** Chronic neuronal injury, as seen in many neurodegenerative diseases, results in vacuolization and swelling of the cytoplasm (arrows). **C.** Some neurodegenerative diseases, such as Pick disease illustrated here, contain cytoplasmic inclusions (arrows). **D and E.** Large intracytoplasmic inclusions (polyglycosan or Lafora bodies) are seen in the perikaryon of neurons in Lafora body disease (arrows).

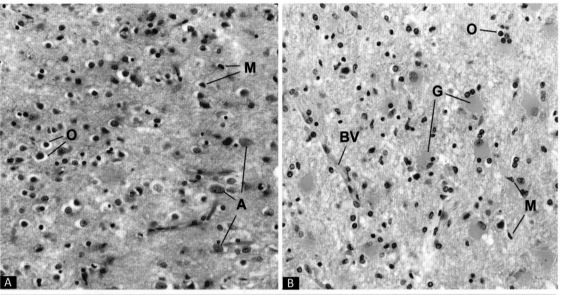

**Figs 15.3A and B:** Glial reaction to injury

**A.** Cortical gliosis in a chronic neurodegenerative disease associated with a loss of neurons. This "glial scar" consists of astrocytes (A), oligodendrocytes (O) and microglial cells (M). **B.** Gliosis with gemistocytic transformation of astrocytes is characterized by the appearance of gemistocytes (G), which have abundant eosinophilic cytoplasm. The area of gliosis also contains oligodendrocytes (O), microglial cells (M) and blood vessels (BV).

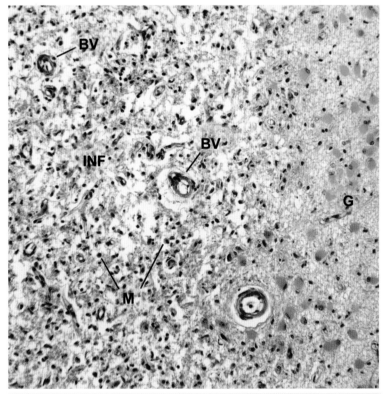

**Fig. 15.4:** Ischemic infarction

The areas of infarction (INF) are infiltrated with microglial cells (M). Due to a loss of neuronal tissue, the blood vessels (BV) that have survived the insult appear more prominent and are spaced closer to one another than normal. The infarct is rimmed with a zone of gliosis (G).

CENTRAL NERVOUS SYSTEM

CHAPTER

**15**

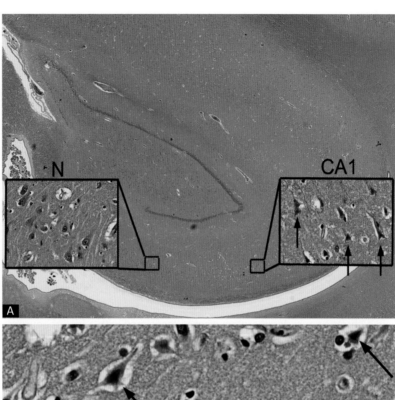

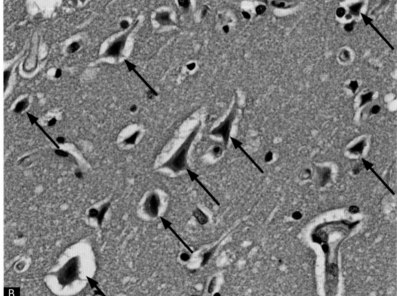

**Figs 15.5A and B:** Global ischemia

**A.** Zonal ischemic necrosis in the CA1 area of the hippocampus can be recognized by the presence of numerous red neurons (arrows). It appears distinctly different from the surrounding normal tissue (N). **B.** Global ischemia causes neuronal injury, evidenced by the appearance of numerous "red neurons".

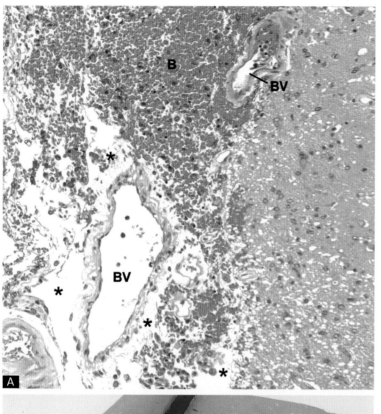

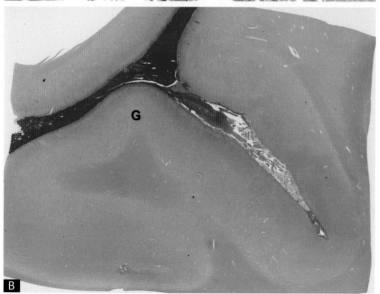

**Figs 15.6A and B:** Cerebral hemorrhage

**A.** In this hemorrhagic infarction the extravasation of blood (B) is accompanied by a loss of brain parenchyma (asterisks) sparing the blood vessels (BV). **B.** Subarachnoid bleeding is characterized by the accumulation of blood in the subarachnoid space on the surface of the cerebral gyri (G).

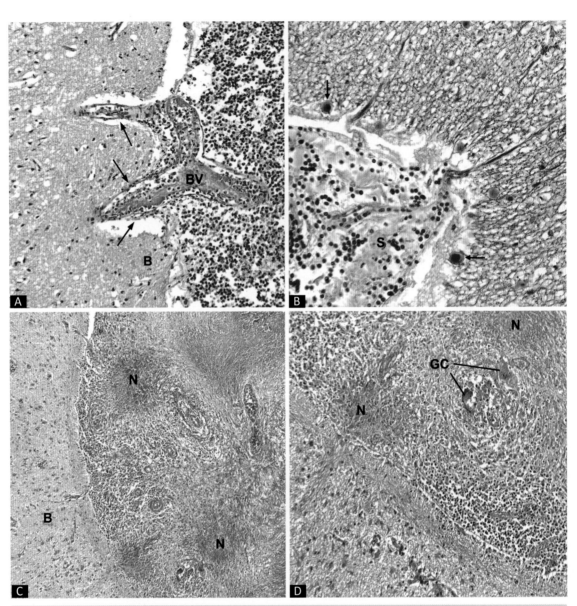

**Figs 15.7A to D:** Meningitis

**A.** Acute purulent meningitis presents with accumulation of neutrophils in the subarachnoid space on the external surface of the brain (B). The infiltrate is most prominent around the meningeal blood vessel (BV) and also extends into the cerebral perivascular spaces (arrows). **B.** Chronic fungal meningitis is characterized by an accumulation of chronic inflammatory cells in the subarachnoid space (S) of this spinal cord. Fungal organisms are not in this figure, but could be demonstrated with special stains such as silver impregnation according to Grocott. The round bodies in the subpial white matter of the spinal cord are called corpora amylacea (arrows). They are of no pathologic significance and are found often in the CNS of older persons. **C.** Tuberculous meningitis is characterized by the formation of necrotizing granulomas (N) in the predominantly mononuclear infiltrate in the subarachnoid space. The inflammation is limited to the subarachnoid space and the brain (B) is not involved. **D.** At higher magnification one can see that the central necrosis (N) of granulomas is surrounded by epithelioid macrophages, lymphocytes, and giant cells (GC).

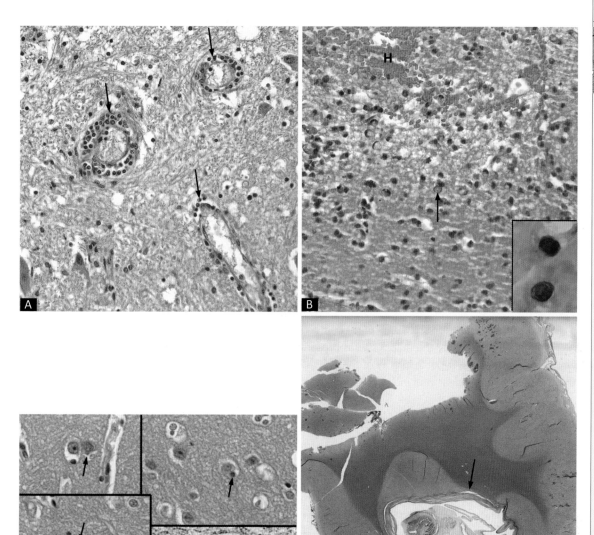

**Figs 15.8A to D:** Encephalitis

**A.** Viral encephalitis presents with infiltrates of lymphocytes in the perivascular spaces (arrows). **B.** Herpes simplex virus (HSV) encephalitis is characterized by hemorrhagic necrosis (H) of the brain and mononculear infiltrates of mononuclear cells, some of which contain intranuclear inclusions (arrow). These inclusions are small and difficult to find, and are best demonstrated by immunohistochemistry using specific antibodies to HSV (inset, higher magnification). **C.** Rabies is characterized by the appearance of eosinophilic Negri bodies in the cytoplasm of neurons (arrows). The right lower quadrant shows the Negri body at higher magnification. **D.** In encephalitis of cysticercosis the brain contains encysted parasites (arrows).

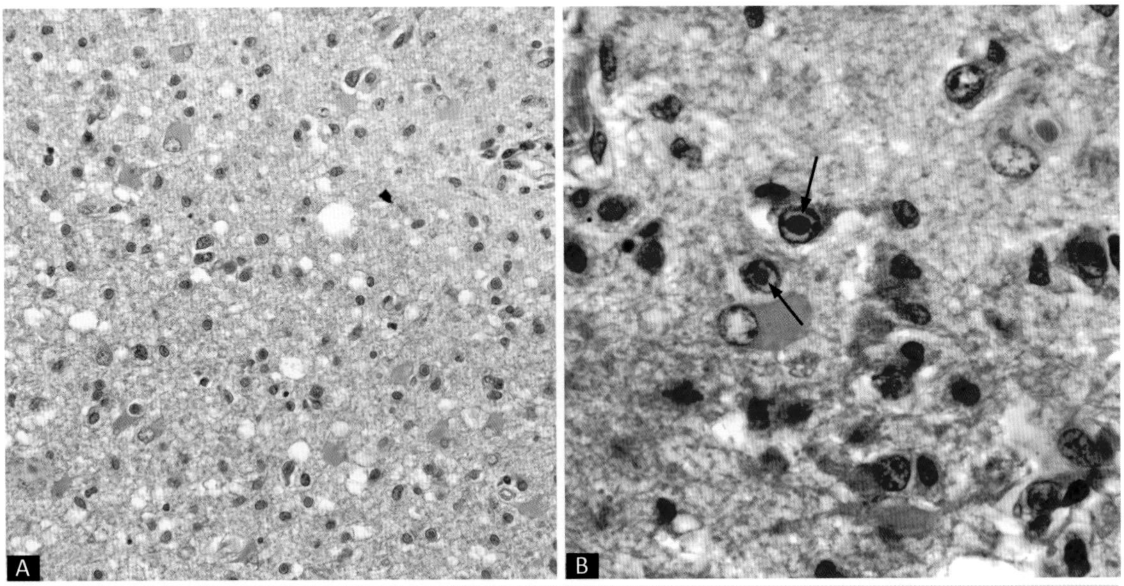

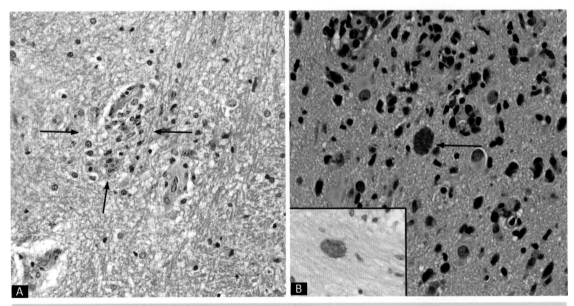

**Figs 15.9A and B:** Subacute sclerosing panencephalitis

**A.** This infection caused by the measles virus presents with neuronal injury and prominent reactive gliosis, which accounts for the hypercellularity of the brain illustrated here. **B.** At higher magnification one may see the bluish-red intranuclear viral inclusions in oligodendrocytes (arrows).

**Figs 15.10A and B:** AIDS encephalopathy

**A.** The infection results in the formation of microglial nodules (arrows). **B.** Toxoplasmosis can be diagnosed by finding the typical toxoplasma cysts (arrow). The diagnosis can be confirmed immunohistochemically with antibodies to toxoplasma (inset).

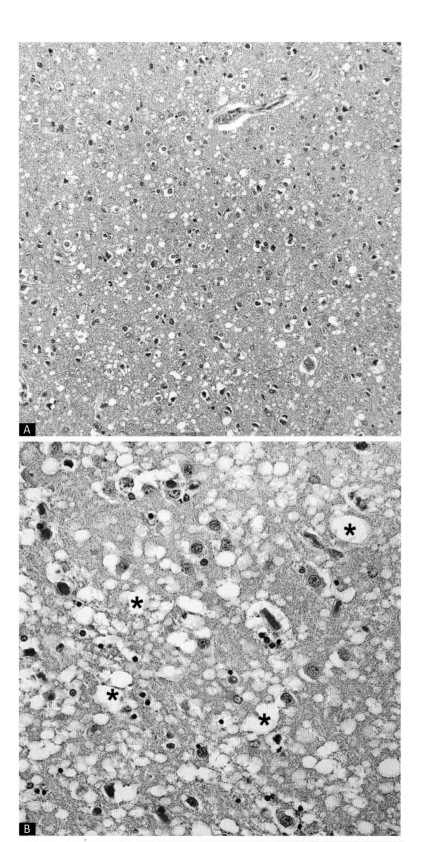

**Figs 15.11A and B:** Spongiform encephalopathy

**A.** Prion diseases produce widespread loss of neurons and vacuolization of the neuropil. **B.** At higher magnification one may appreciate the vacuolization (asterisks) without any noticeable glial or inflammatory reaction.

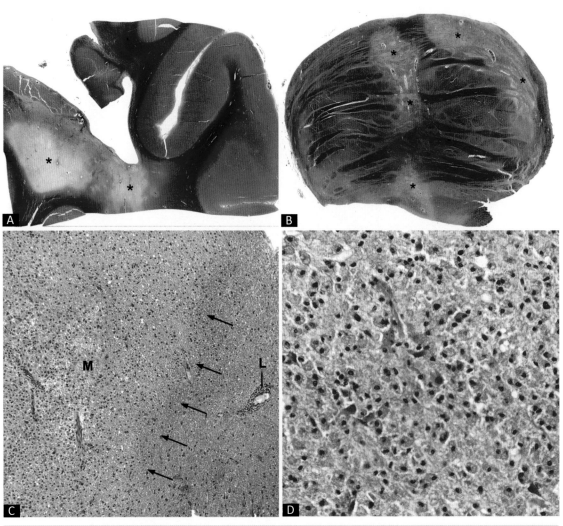

**Figs 15.12A to D:** Multiple sclerosis

**A.** Cerebral cortex at low magnification showing the plaques of demyelination (asterisks) which appear as lightly stained areas. **B.** The plaques of demyelination (asterisks) are irregularly distributed in this brainstem involved by multiple sclerosis. **C.** During active demyelination the plaque (marked by arrows) is infiltrated with numerous macrophages (M), which are most prominent in the central parts of the lesion. The blood vessels in the adjacent brain may be surrounded by lymphocytes (L). **D.** Higher magnification of the central part of an active plaque shows that it is composed of macrophages, which have abundant eosinophilic cytoplasm.

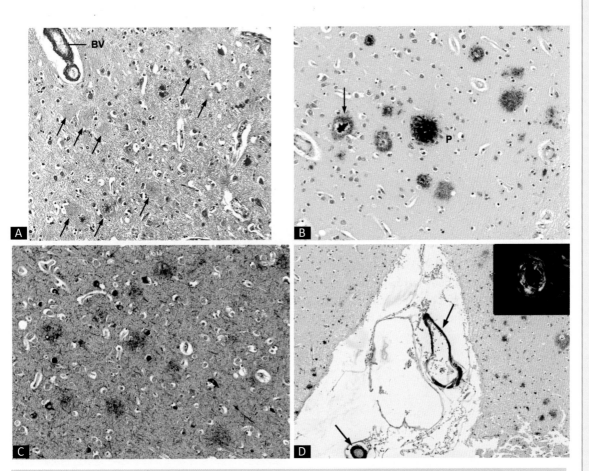

**Figs 15.13A to D:** Alzheimer disease

**A.** In H&E-stained sections of the cerebral cortex one can see the round outlines of numerous neuritic plaques (arrows) in the neuropil. These changes are known as senile plaques since they may be found in limited numbers in aging brains of asymptomatic persons. The wall of a small blood vessel (BV) is infiltrated with amyloid and thus appears homogeneously eosinophilic. **B.** Neuritic plaques stain immunohistochemically with antibodies to amyloid Aβ. In early stages the plaques have a dense core and appear targetoid (arrow), but the older plaques (P) are diffusely permeated with amyloid. **C.** Neuritic plaques stain with antibodies to tau protein. They appear fibrillar because the tau protein forms fibrils in the cytoplasm of grouped neurons. **D.** Amyloid in the blood vessels stains immunohistochemically with the antibodies to Aβ protein (arrows). Inset shows a similar small artery stained with Congo red, showing green birefringence under polarized light.

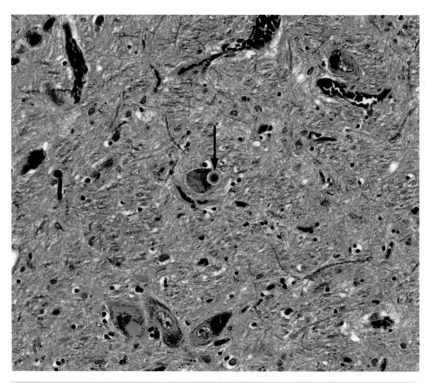

**Fig. 15.14:** Parkinson disease

A Lewy body (arrow) is seen in a pigmented neuron of the substantia nigra as round cytoplasmic inclusion with a dense core. The tissue is stained with Luxol fast blue, which stains the core of the Lewy body blue.

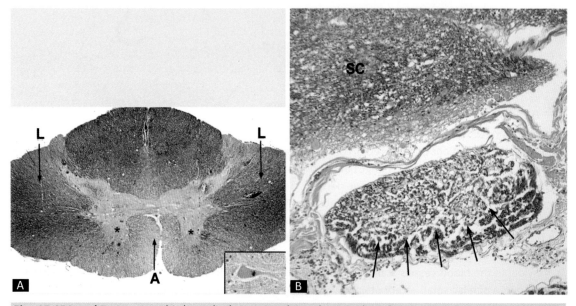

**Figs 15.15A and B:** Amyotrophic lateral sclerosis involving the spinal cord

**A.** Normally myelinated columns of the white matter are stained blue with Luxol fast blue, whereas the demyelinated and atrophic motor columns appear red. In the white matter the areas of demyelination are seen involving the lateral (L) and anterior motor tracts (A). The gray matter, which stains red, shows atrophy of the anterior horns (asterisks). Inset shows a neuron containing a ubiquitin-rich Bunina body, demonstrated immunohistochemically as a brown cytoplasmic body. **B.** The demyelinated portion of an atrophic motor neuron exiting from the spinal cord (SC) appears red and is marked with arrows; the lower rim of the nerve is still preserved and stains blue.

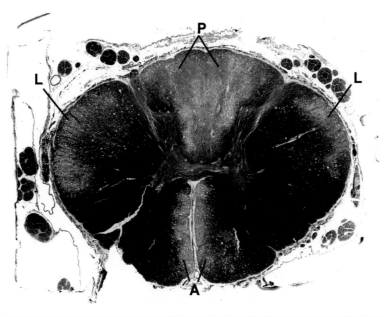

**Fig. 15.16:** Subacute combined degeneration of the spinal cord
In this silver impregnated slide demyelination appears as lighter staining areas in the posterior (P) lateral (L) and anterior (A) columns.

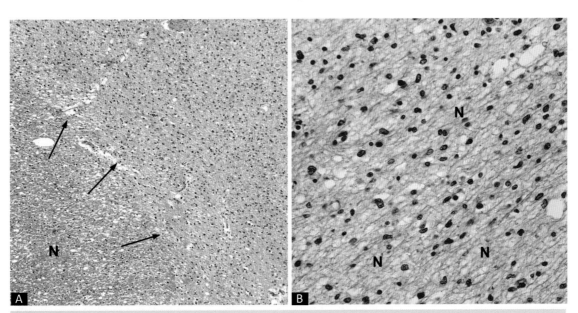

**Figs 15.17A and B:** Astrocytoma, grade II
**A.** The tumor, marked with arrows, is relatively sharply demarcated and appears hypercellular in comparison to normal brain tissue (N). **B.** Higher magnification of this astrocytoma shows that it is composed of fibrillar astrocytes, which form a well developed fibrillar neuropil (N) and show relative uniformity of their nuclei. This indicates that the tumor cells are relatively well differentiated and have a low nucleus to cytoplasm ratio.

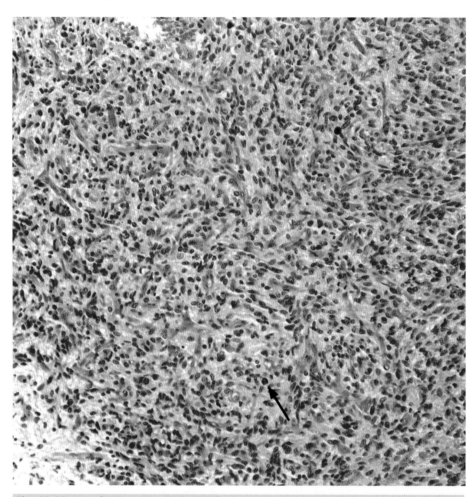

**Fig. 15.18:** Anaplastic astrocytoma grade III

This hypercellular tumor is composed of astrocytes, which show more nuclear polymorphism and have less cytoplasm than normal astrocytes. Mitoses (arrow) may be present, but there is no necrosis.

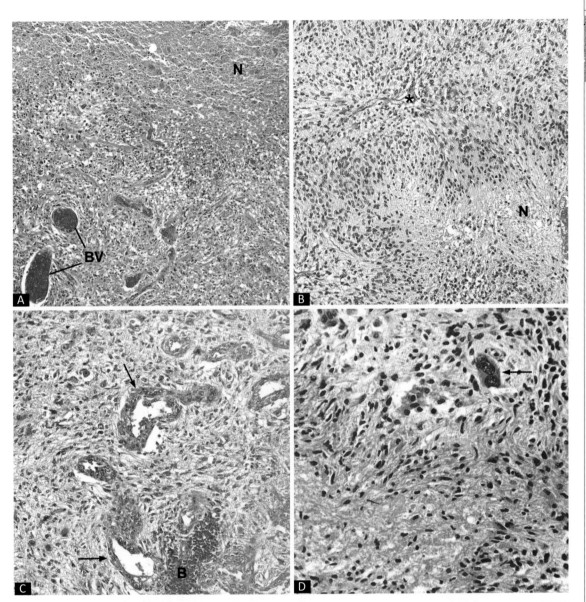

**Figs 15.19A to D:** Glioblastoma

**A.** The tumor shows high cellularity, abundance of blood vessels (BV) and broad areas of necrosis (N). **B.** In another area the tumor shows prominent cellularity around a blood vessel (asterisk) and pseudopallisading around an area of irregular necrosis (N). **C.** The tumor contains numerous small and medium sized blood vessels (arrows), which tend to bleed (B). For their size, these blood vessels have disproportionately thick walls due to the proliferation of endothelial cells. **D.** Nuclei vary in size and shape, and some are markedly enlarged (arrow).

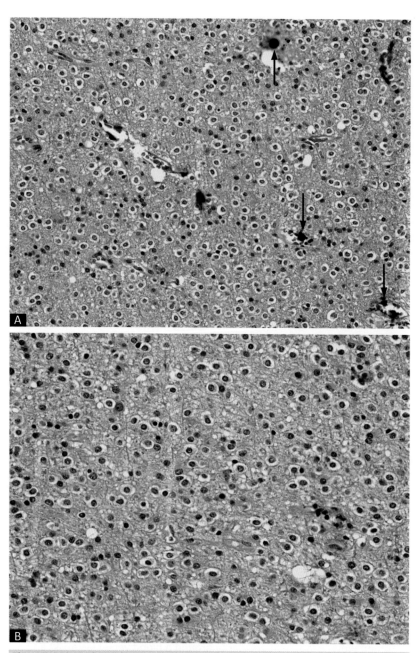

**Figs 15.20A and B:** Oligodendroglioma

**A.** The tumor is composed of relatively uniform cells which have round nuclei and resemble normal oligodendrocytes. There are also foci of calcification (arrows). **B.** Higher magnification view of tumor cells which have relatively uniform round nuclei and clear cytoplasm (fried-egg appearance).

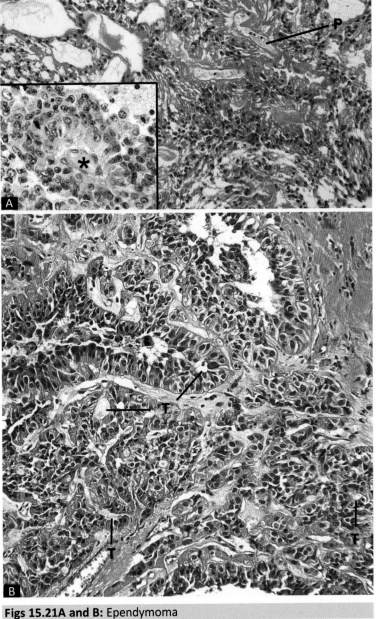

**Figs 15.21A and B:** Ependymoma

**A.** Myxopapillary tumor with wide spaces containing myxoid extracellular material (M) and perivascular pseudorosettes (P). The inset shows a perivascular pseudorosette, with asterisk marking the lumen of the blood vessel. **B.** The tumor forms tubules (T) and canals.

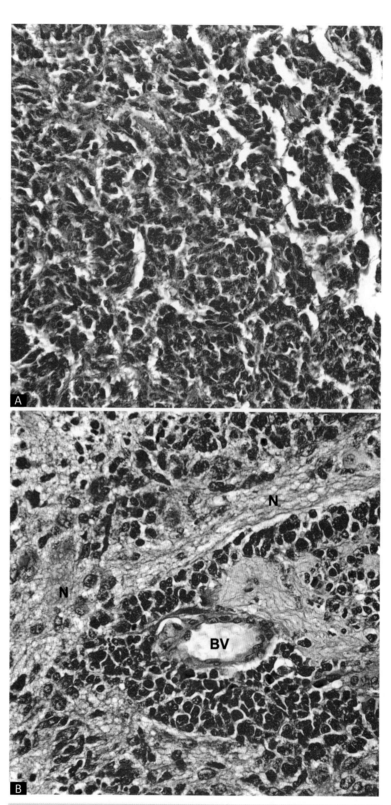

**Figs 15.22A and B:** Medulloblastoma

**A.** The tumor is composed of small blue cells with scant cytoplasm, growing without any distinct pattern. **B.** Groups of dark cells surround a blood vessel (BV). Fibrillar areas nearby show neuropil-like differentiation (N).

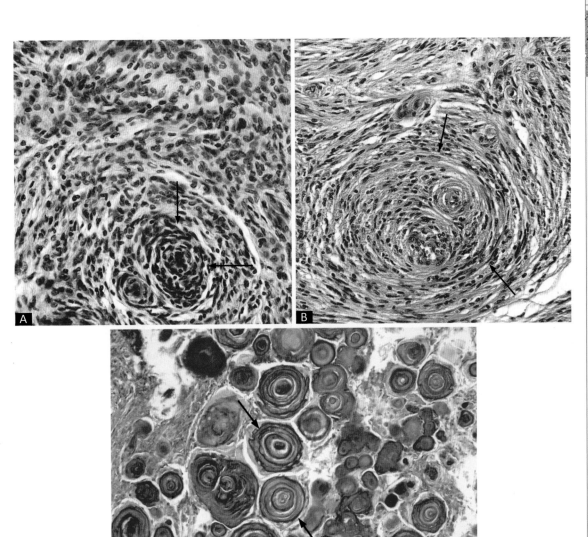

**Figs 15.23A to C:** Meningioma

**A.** Meningothelial cells form whorls (arrows). **B.** Higher magnification of a fibroblastic meningioma that also forms whorls (arrows) shows much more prominent extracellular collagenous matrix. **C.** Psammomatous meningioma consists almost exclusively of numerous concentric calcifications called psammoma bodies (arrows).

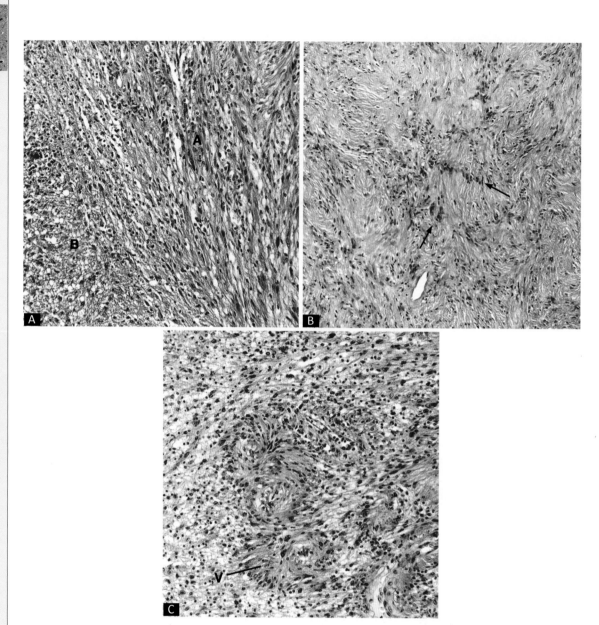

**Figs 15.24A to C:** Schwannoma

**A.** Tumor is composed of spindle cells resembling normal neural sheath cells. In one area the cells are arranged into dense bundles (Antoni A area), whereas in the other they are loosely structured (Antoni B). **B.** Tumor cells show pallisading (arrows). **C.** Pallisading of nuclei arranged in whorls within Antoni A areas are called Verocay bodies (V).

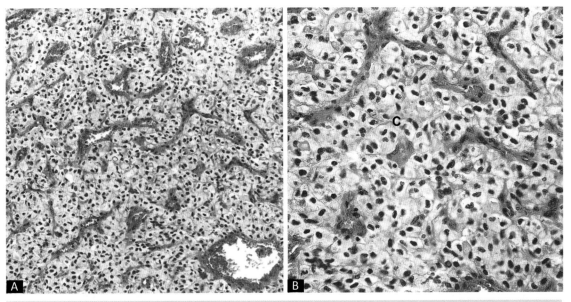

**Figs 15.25A and B:** Hemangioblastoma

**A.** This vascular tumor is composed of numerous blood-filled vessels surrounded by plump spindle-shaped and clear cells. **B.** At higher magnification one may see that the perivascular spaces contain spindle-shaped cells and clear cells (C).

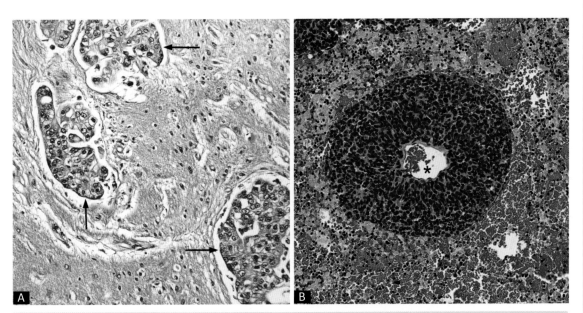

**Figs 15.26A and B:** Metastatic cancer

**A.** Poorly differentiated breast carcinoma forms nests (arrows) in neural tissue. **B.** Small cell carcinoma of the lung arranged around a centrally located small blood vessel (asterisk) has caused hemorrhage which has destroyed and replaced the peritumoral neural tissue.

CENTRAL NERVOUS SYSTEM

CHAPTER

**15**

# *Index*

*(The letter f after page number in the index denotes Figure)*

## A

Acanthocytosis 57
Acinar cell carcinoma 161, 174f
Acne
  rosacea 308f
  vulgaris 298, 308f
Actinic keratosis 301, 323f
Acute
  adrenal insufficiency 277
  and chronic salpingitis 220
  appendicitis 134f
  bacterial epididymitis 204f
  cholecystitis 140, 156f
  endometritis 234f
  gastritis 86
  inflammation 2
  lymphoblastic leukemia/
    lymphoma 60, 71f
  lymphoblastic lymphoma 77f
  mastitis 254
  myeloid leukemia 60, 70f
  osteomyelitis 340f
  pancreatitis 159, 164f
  poststreptococcal
    glomerulonephritis 178,
    183f
  pyelonephritis 180, 193f
  pyogenic osteomyelitis 333
  respiratory distress syndrome
    29, 39f
  salpingitis 241f
  tubular necrosis 180, 193f
  viral hepatitis 138, 143f
Adenosis 254
Adrenal 277
  amyloidosis 293f
  cortical
    adenoma 278, 294f
    carcinoma 278, 295f
    hyperplasia 277
  hemorrhage 293f
  hyperplasia 294f
AIDS encephalopathy 369, 380f
Allergic
  contact dermatitis 304f
  rhinitis 27
Alpha-1-antitrypsin deficiency
  150f
Alveolar proteinosis 39f
Alzheimer disease 370, 383f
Amebic colitis 92, 125f
Amyloidosis 5
Amyotrophic lateral sclerosis
  371

Androgenetic alopecia 298
Anemia 57
Angiofibroma 6, 25f
Angiosarcoma 6, 26f
Anterior pituitary 273
Anthracosis 48f
Aortic dissection 15f
Aplastic anemia 67f
Appendiceal carcinoid 135f
Arterial changes of hypertension
  13f
Arteries 1
Arthropod bites 301
Asbestosis 48f
Aspergillus pneumonia 41f
Astrocytic tumors 371
Astrocytoma, grade II 385f
Atelectasis 37f
Atherosclerosis 2
  of aorta 9f
Atopic dermatitis 298, 305f
Atrial myxoma 5, 22f
Atypical
  ductal hyperplasia 255, 263f
  lobular hyperplasia 255
Autoimmune
  gastritis 87, 107f
  hepatitis 138, 146f

## B

Bacterial
  myocarditis 4
  pneumonia 30
Bacterial infections 300
  of muscle 365f
Barrett esophagus 84, 101f
Basal cell carcinoma 301, 322f
Benign prostatic hyperplasia 201,
  211f
Blighted ovum 223, 250f
Blood vessels 1
Bones, joints and soft tissues 331
Breast 253
Bronchioloalveolar carcinoma 34,
  51f
Bronchopneumonia 40f
Bronchopulmonary infections 29
Bullous pemphigoid 299, 314f
Burkitt lymphoma 79f

## C

Candida esophagitis 84, 100f
Capillaries 1

Carcinoid tumor 89, 91, 96
Carcinosarcoma 220, 241f
Cardiac
  amyloidosis 21f
  glycogenosis 21f
  hypertrophy 3
    caused by hypertension 13f
Cardiomyopathy 5, 20f
Cardiovascular system 1
Cellular reactions to injury 367
Central nervous system 367
Cerebral
  hemorrhage 377f
  ischemia 368
Cerebrovascular disease 368
Cervical
  adenocarcinoma 217
  intraepithelial neoplasia 228f
Chigger bite 321f
Cholesterolosis 141
Chondromas 333
Chondrosarcoma 333, 343f
Choriocarcinoma 208f, 224
Chromoblastomycosis 313f
Chronic
  adrenal insufficiency 277
  bronchitis 33, 49f
  cervicitis 216
  cholecystitis 141, 156f
  cystitis 180
  endometritis 218, 234f
  gastritis 86
    caused by Helicobacter
    pylori 105f
  glomerulonephritis 179, 192f
  inflammation 2
  lymphocytic leukemia 60, 74f
  myeloid leukemia 60, 72f, 73f
  nasal inflammation 35f
  neuronal injury 368
  obstructive pulmonary disease
    33
  osteomyelitis 333, 340f
  pancreatitis 160, 165f
  pyelonephritis 194f
  viral hepatitis 138, 143f
Cirrhosis 139
Clear cell adenocarcinoma 219
  of endometrium 238f
Coal miner pneumoconiosis 32
Colonic
  adenocarcinoma 133f
  adenoma 132f
Common wart 317f

Complete hydatidiform mole 251f
Complex hyperplasia 218
Compression atelectasis 28
Condyloma acuminatum 202, 213, 229f
Congenital
    and inherited conditions 159
    myopathies 356
Conn syndrome 278
Contact dermatitis 298
Contraction band necrosis 2
Coronary
    atheromas 2
    atherosclerosis 10f
    heart disease 2
Crescentic glomerulonephritis 184f
Crohn's disease 126f
Cryptogenic organizing pneumonia 32, 47f
Cryptorchid testes 199, 203f
Cushing syndrome 278
Cystic fibrosis ducts 163f
Cystitis 194f
Cytomegalovirus esophagitis 84, 99f

**D**

Degenerative joint disease (osteoarthritis) 347f
Demyelinating diseases 370
Dermatitis herpetiformis 300, 315
Dermatofibromas 326f, 303
Dermatomyositis 357, 366f
Desmoid tumor 351f
Desquamative interstitial pneumonia 32, 47f
Developmental
    anomalies 83, 86, 90, 92
    disorders 177, 331
Diabetic
    glomerulopathy 179
    nodular glomerulosclerosis 190f
Diffuse large B cell lymphoma 78f
Digestive system 83
Disorders of hair follicle 298
Diverticular disease 93
Diverticulosis and diverticulitis of colon 128f
Drug reaction 299
Ductal adenocarcinoma 169f
    of pancreas 160
Ductal carcinoma *in situ* of breast 255, 264f
Dupuytren's contracture 336, 351f

**E**

Elastic arteries 1
Embryonal carcinoma 200, 206f
Emphysema 33, 49f
Encephalitis 369, 379f
Enchondroma 342f
Endocervical
    adenocarcinoma in situ 217, 230f
    polyp 216, 227f
Endocrine system 273
Endometrial
    epithelial tumors 218
    hyperplasia 218, 235f
    polyp 236f
    stromal nodule 219, 239f
    stromal tumors 219
Endometrioid adenocarcinoma 237f
Endometriosis 221, 244f
Endometritis 218
Eosinophilic
    esophagitis 84, 98f
    gastritis 107f
Ependymoma 372, 389f
Epidermal neoplasms 301
Esophageal adenocarcinoma 102f
Esophagus 83
Ewing sarcoma 344f
    primitive neuroectodermal tumor 334
Exophytic papillomas 28

**F**

Fallopian tube 220
Fat necrosis 260f
Female reproductive system 215
Fibroadenoma 267f
Fibroepithelial lesions 256
Fibrolamellar hepatocellular carcinoma 155
Fibroma 248f
Fibrous cortical defect (non-ossifying fibroma) 334, 343f
Fibrous dysplasia 334, 344f
Focal
    glomerulosclerosis 179
    nodular hyperplasia 140, 152f
    segmental glomerulosclerosis 189f
Follicular
    adenoma 285f
    carcinoma 286f
    cyst 243f
    lymphoma 77f
Foreign
    bodies 299
    body granuloma 313f

**G**

Gallbladder 140
Ganglioneuroma 296f
Gardner syndrome 336
Gastric
    adenocarcinoma 88, 113f
    adenoma 88, 112f
    carcinoid tumor 114f
    lymphoma 116f
Gastrointestinal stromal tumor 89, 91, 115, 121f
Genetic muscle diseases 356
Genodermatoses 297
Germ cell tumors 200, 222
Gestational endometrium 233f
Giant cell
    aortitis 5, 22f
    tumor of bone 345f
Glial reaction to injury 368, 375f
Glioblastoma 387f
Global ischemia 376f
Glomerular diseases 178
Gluten-sensitive enteropathy 90, 118f
Glycogen storage disease 364f
Glycogenoses 5
Goiter 274
Gout 335, 348f
Graft versus host disease 94, 128f
Granuloma
    annulare 299, 312f
    of histoplasmosis 42f
Granulomatous
    de Quervain thyroiditis 274, 282f
    dermatitis 299
Granulosa cell tumor 223, 248f
Graves disease 275, 283f
Group atrophy of muscle fibers 356, 360f
Gynecomastia 272f

**H**

Hairy cell leukemia 75f
Hard atheromas 2
Hashimoto thyroiditis 275, 283f
Hemangioblastoma 372, 393f
Hemangioma 6
Hematolymphoid neoplasms 303
Hematopoietic and lymphoid system 57
Hemolytic anemia 59

Hepatic abscess 148f
Hepatobiliary system 137
Hepatoblastoma 153f
Hepatocellular
    adenoma 140
    carcinoma 140, 154f
Hereditary
    hemochromatosis 139, 150f
    spherocytosis 58
Herpes esophagitis 84
Herpetic esophagitis 99f
High grade dysplasia 101f
Hodgkin lymphoma 61, 81f
Honeycomb lung 46f
Human papillomavirus 216
Hyalinization of arterioles 14f
Hydatidiform mole 223
Hyperparathyroidism 339f
Hyperplasia 276
Hyperplastic polyp 88, 94, 130f
    of stomach 110f
Hypersensitivity
    pneumonitis 31, 44f
    vasculitis 6, 24f
Hypertension 3
Hypoxic injury 368

**I**

Ichthyosis vulgaris 297, 304f
Idiopathic pulmonary fibrosis 32,
    46f
IgA nephropathy 178, 185f
Immature teratoma 247f
Immunologic lung diseases 31
Infections of
    central nervous system 369
    heart 4
Infectious
    diseases 180
    endocarditis 18f
    esophagitis 84
    folliculitis 298, 309f
    granulomas 299
    myositis 357
    rhinitis 27
Inflammatory
    bowel disease 93, 126f
    dermatoses 297
    diseases 137, 159
    fibroid polyp 88
    fibroid polyp of stomach 112f
    myopathies 357
Interface dermatitis 298
Interstitial
    lung diseases 31
    pneumonia caused by viruses
        41f
Intracerebral hemorrhage 369
Intraductal
    papillary mucinous neoplasm

161, 172f
    papilloma 256, 268f
    proliferative lesions 254
Intratubular germ cell neoplasia
    205f
Invasive
    breast carcinoma 256
    ductal carcinomas 269f
    endocervical adenocarcinoma
        217, 231f
    lobular carcinoma 257, 270f
    mucinous carcinoma 271f
    squamous cell carcinoma 217
        of cervix 229f
    tubular carcinoma 270f
Iron
    deficiency anemia 63f
    related gastropathy 108f
Ischemic
    colitis 92, 123f
    infarction 375f

**J**

Joints 334
Juvenile
    polyp 94, 129f
    xanthogranuloma 303, 328f

**K**

Kaposi sarcoma 6, 26f
Keratinizing carcinomas 28
Kogoj collections 306f
Krukenberg tumor 249f

**L**

Large cell undifferentiated
    carcinoma 34, 51f
Leiomyoma 220, 240f
Leiomyosarcoma 240f
Lentigo maligna 302
Leukocytoclastic vasculitis 299,
    309f
Leydig cell tumors 201, 209f
Lichen
    planus 298, 307f
    sclerosus 215, 226f
Lipoma 349f
Liposarcoma 350f
Liver 137
Lobar pneumonia 40f
Lobular neoplasia 255, 266f
Low grade
    appendiceal mucinous
        neoplasm 96, 136f
    ductal carcinoma in situ 255
    dysplasia 101f
    endometrial stromal sarcoma
        219, 239f
Lungs 28

Lupus
    erythematosus 298, 307f
    nephritis 178, 186f
Lymphoma 61, 89, 91
Lymphoplasmacytic sclerosing
        pancreatitis 160, 167f

**M**

Macrocytic anemia 57, 58
Male breast
    carcinomas 257
    lesions 257
    tissue 272f
Male genital system 199
Malignant hypertension 14f
Mammary duct ectasia 254, 260f
Marble bone disease 332
Massive hepatic necrosis 138
Mastocytosis 329f
Mature teratoma 247f
Mean corpuscular
    hemoglobin 57
    volume 57
Medullary carcinoma 257, 271f,
    288
Medulloblastoma 372, 390f
Megaloblastic anemia 64f
Melanocytic
    neoplasms 301
    nevus 324f
Melanoma 325f
Membranous nephropathy 179,
    187f
Ménétrier disease 88
    of stomach 109f
Meningioma 372, 391f
Meningitis 369, 378f
Mesothelioma 54f
Metabolic disorders 139, 332
Metases to bone 346f
Metastatic
    cancer 393f
    tumors 223, 234, 372
Microangiopathic
    diseases 59
    hemolytic anemia 69f
Microcystic
    anemia 57
    hypochromic anemia 58
    serous cystadenoma 161, 170f
Microglandular hyperplasia 216,
    227f
Microinvasive squamous cell
    carcinoma 217
Microscopic (collagenous) colitis
    127f
Minimal change disease 179,
    188f
Molluscum contagiosum 300,
    316f

Morbilliform drug reaction 311f
Mucinous
    carcinoma 257
    cystic neoplasm 161, 171f
    tumors 222, 246f
Multicystic renal dysplasia 177,
    182f
Multiple
    myeloma 80f
    sclerosis 370, 382f
Muscle atrophy 359f
Muscular dystrophies 356, 362f
Mycosis fungoides 303, 330f
Myelofibrosis 68f
Myelophthisic anemia 69f
Myocardial
    infarct 2
    infarction-temporal changes
    12f
Myocarditis 19f
Myopathy 363f
Myotonic dystrophy 356, 363f

## N

Nasopharyngeal
    carcinomas 28, 36f
Nemaline myopathy 364f
Neonatal respiratory distress
    syndrome 38f
Neoplasms 96, 139, 141, 160, 180,
    273, 275, 371
    and related lesions 333
Nephroangiosclerosis 192f
Neuroblastoma 278, 296f
Neurodegenerative diseases 370
Neurofibroma 303, 327f
Neurogenic
    atrophy 359f
    muscle diseases 355
Neuronal injury 367, 374f
Nodular
    goiter 274, 282f
    melanomas 302
    sclerosis Hodgkin lymphoma 61
Nonkeratinizing carcinomas 28
Non-neoplastic
    cysts 221
    epithelial vulvar disorders 215
    lesions of cervix 216
Nonproliferative fibrocystic
    change 254
Nonseminomatous germ cell
    tumor 200
Normal
    adrenal 292f
    appendix 134f
    blood smear and bone marrow
    62f
    blood vessels 8f
    breast 253

central nervous system 367,
    373f
chorionic villi of a term
    placenta 250f
colonic mucosa 122f
endometrium 232f
esophagus 97f
hematopoietic and lymphoid
    system 57
histology 1, 177
liver 142f
lung 37f
myocardium 7f
nasal respiratory mucosa 35f
ovary 243f
pancreas 163f
parathyroid 290f
pituitary 279f
prostate 210f
skeletal muscle 358f
skin 304f
small intestine 117f
stomach 104f
testis 203f
thyroid 281f
urinary system 181f

## O

Oligodendroglioma 371, 388f
Osteoarthritis 335
Osteoblasts 331
Osteoclasts 331
Osteoid osteoma 333, 341f
Osteoma 333, 341f
Osteomalacia 332
    rickets 338f
Osteopetrosis 332, 337f
Osteoporosis 338f
Osteosarcoma 333, 342f
Ovary 221

## P

Paget disease 332, 339f
    of nipple 255, 265f
Palmar fibromatosis 351f
Palmoplantar wart 318f
Pancreas 159
Pancreatic
    intraepithelial neoplasia 160, 168
    neuroendocrine tumor 161, 175f
    pseudocyst 160, 166f
Panfascicular atrophy 356, 361f
Papillary
    carcinoma 287f
    lesions 256
Parasitic myositis 357
Parathyroid 276
    adenoma 291f
    hyperplasia 290f

Parkinson disease 370, 384f
Partial hydatidiform mole 251f
Pemphigus vulgaris 300, 314f
Penis 201
Peptic ulcer disease 87, 106f
Pericarditis 20f
Periductal mastitis 254
Peripheral T-cell lymphoma 76f
Perivascular dermatitis 299
Peyronie's disease 336
Pheochromocytoma 278, 295f
Phyllodes tumor 256, 267f
Pigmented
    purpuric dermatitis 299
    villonodular synovitis 335,
    349f
Pituitary 273
    adenoma 280f
Pneumoconioses 32
Pneumocystis jiroveci 30
Polyarteritis nodosa 5, 24f
Polycystic kidney disease 177,
    182f
Polymyositis 357, 366f
Polyps and neoplasms 88, 91, 94
Posterior pituitary 273
Pregnancy
    related changes 223
    lactational changes 259f
Preneoplastic conditions and
    neoplasms 84
Primary
    biliary cirrhosis 138, 147f
    osteoporosis 332
    sclerosing cholangitis 139,
    148f
Prostate 201
Prostatic intraepithelial neoplasia
    211f
Pseudomembranous colitis 92,
    124f
Psoriasiform dermatitis 298
Psoriasis 306f
Pulmonary
    alveolar proteinosis 29
    edema 29
        and congestion 38f
    neoplasms 33
    tuberculosis 30
Pyogenic granulomas 328f, 303

## R

Rapidly progressive
    glomerulonephritis 178
Reactive and inflammatory
    lesions 254
Reflux esophagitis 84, 98f
Renal
    cell carcinoma 180, 196f
    oncocytoma 195f

Reperfusion of myocardial
    infarction 11f
Respiratory system 27
Rhabdomyolysis 357, 366f
Rhabdomyosarcoma 353f
Rheumatic
    endocarditis 3, 16f
    heart disease 3
    myocarditis 4, 17f
    pericarditis 4, 17f
Rheumatoid arthritis 335, 348f
Riedel thyroiditis 275, 284f
Ringworm 300

S

Sarcoidosis 31, 44f
Scabies 320f
Schwannoma 372, 392f
Sclerosing adenosis 262f
Seborrheic keratosis 322f
Seminoma 206f
Serous
    adenocarcinoma 219, 222, 245f
        of endometrium 238f
    borderline tumor 245f
    cystadenoma 222, 244f
Serrated adenoma 94, 131f
Sertoli
    cell tumors 201, 209f
    only syndrome 204f
Sessile serrated polyp 94, 131f
Sex cord
    cell tumors 200
    stromal tumors 222
Sickle cell anemia 57, 58, 66f
Simple hyperplasia 218
Single muscle fiber atrophy 356
Sinonasal
    inflammations 27
    papilloma 28, 36f
Skeletal muscles 355
Skin 297
    tags 303

Small
    cell carcinoma 34, 52f
    intestinal carcinoid tumor 120f
    intestinal lymphoma 122f
    intestine 90
Smooth muscle tumors 219
Soft tissue tumors 335
Solid pseudopapillary neoplasm
    161, 173f
Spherocytosis 57, 65f
Spongiform encephalopathies
    370, 381f
Spongiotic dermatitis 297
Squamous
    carcinoma 85
    cell carcinoma 33, 202, 301
        of penis 213f
    cell hyperplasia 215, 226f
Stomach 85
Subacute
    combined degeneration of
        spinal cord 371, 385
    sclerosing panencephalitis
        369, 380f
Subareolar abscess 254
Superficial spreading melanoma
    302
Surface epithelial-stromal tumors
    221
Synovial sarcoma 336, 354

T

Takayasu disease 5
Temporal arteritis 5, 23f
Teratocarcinoma 207f
Testis 199
Thalassemia 58, 67f
Thyroiditis 274
Tinea 300
    corporis 319f
    versicolor 300, 320f
Trichinella spiralis 357
Trichinosis 365f

Trypanosoma cruzi 4
Tubal pregnancy 221, 242f
Tuberculosis 43f
Tubular carcinoma 257

U

Undifferentiated
    carcinomas 28
    pleomorphic sarcoma 352f
Upper respiratory system 27
Urinary system 177
Urothelial
    carcinoma of bladder 198f
    carcinomas 180
Urticaria 299, 310f
Usual ductal hyperplasia 254,
    262f
Uterine corpus 217

V

Vascular kidney diseases 180
Vasculitis 5
Veins 1
Verrucae/warts 300
Vesiculobullous/blistering
    dermatitis 299
Viral
    infections 300
    myocarditis 4
    orchitis 205f
    pneumonia 30
Vulva, vagina and cervix 215
Vulvar Paget disease 217, 231f

W

Wegener granulomatosis 31, 45f
Whipple disease 91, 119f
Wilms' tumor 180, 197f

Y

Yolk sac tumor 200, 208f